Synthetic Biology - New Interdisciplinary Science

Edited by Madan L. Nagpal, Oana-Maria Boldura, Cornel Baltă and Shymaa Enany

Published in London, United Kingdom

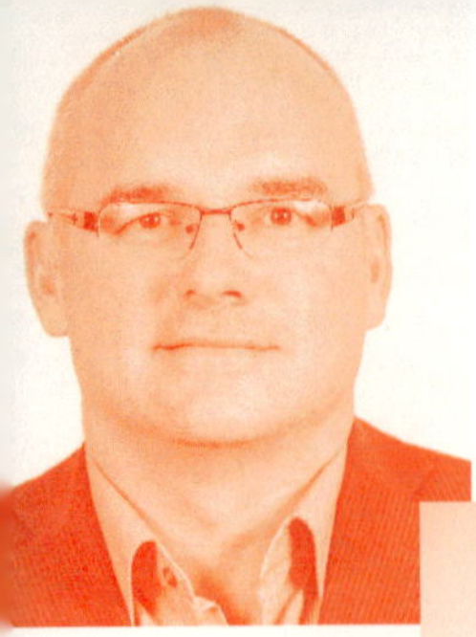
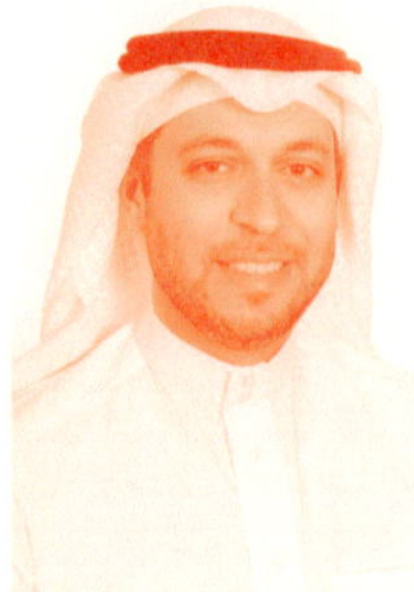
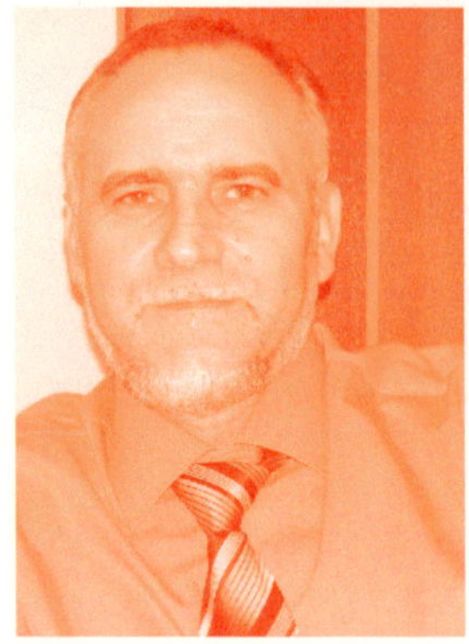
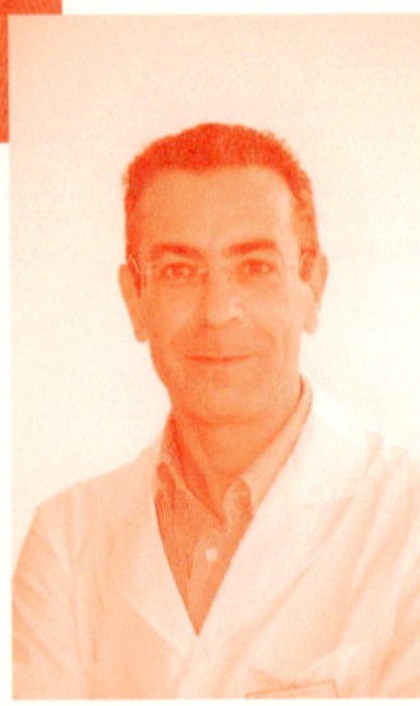
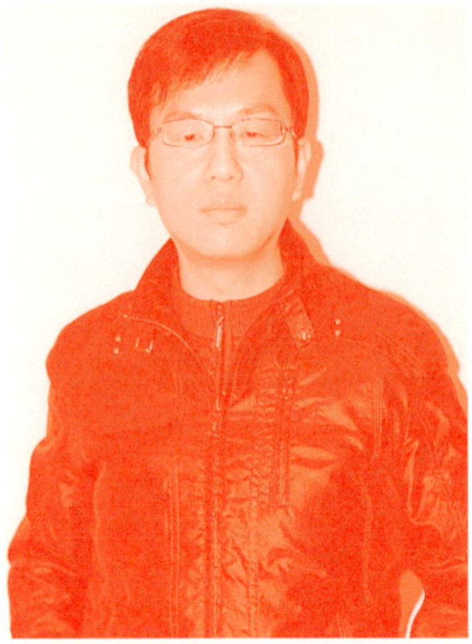
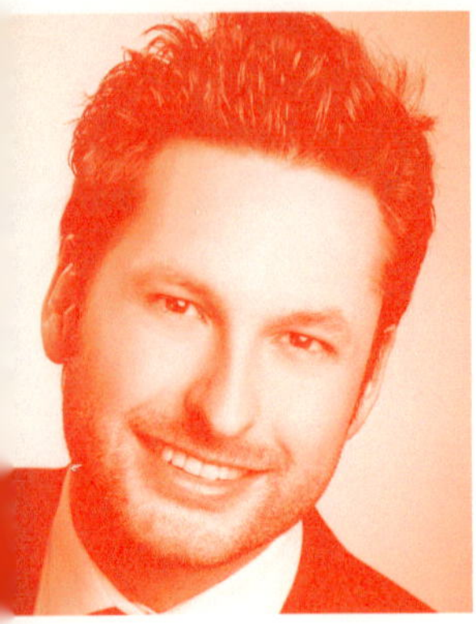
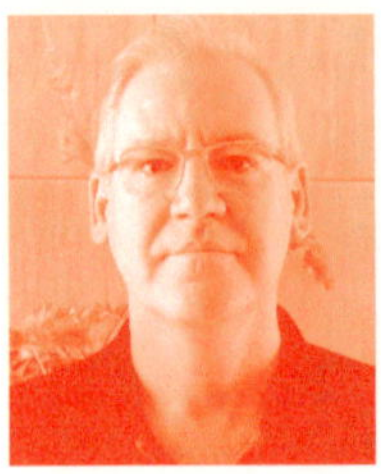

IntechOpen

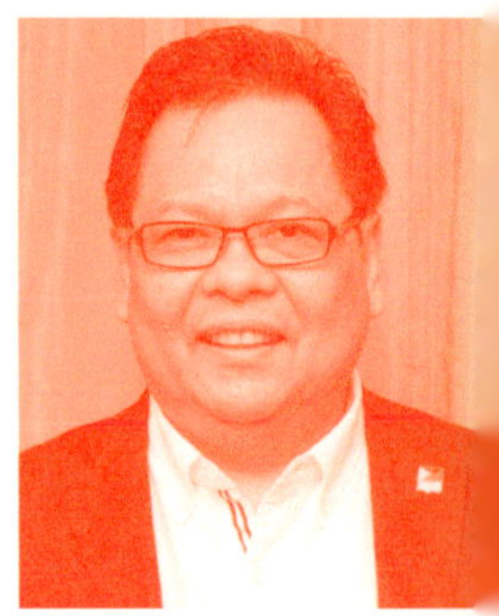
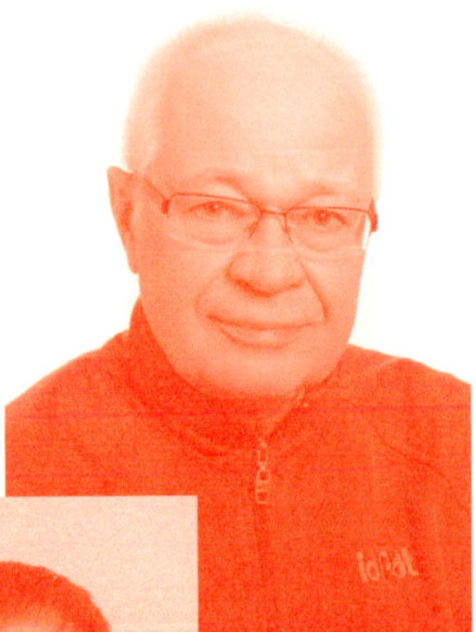
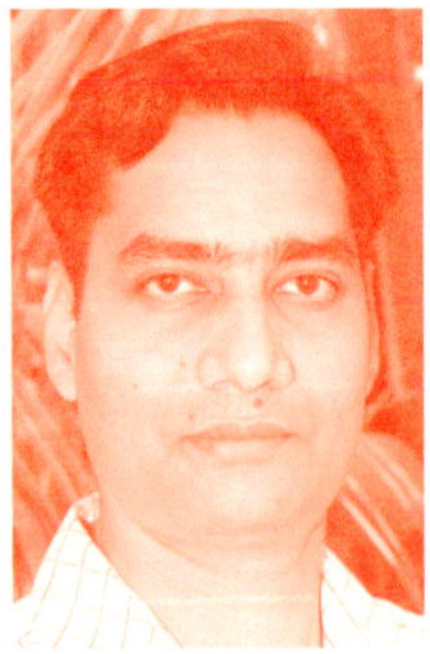
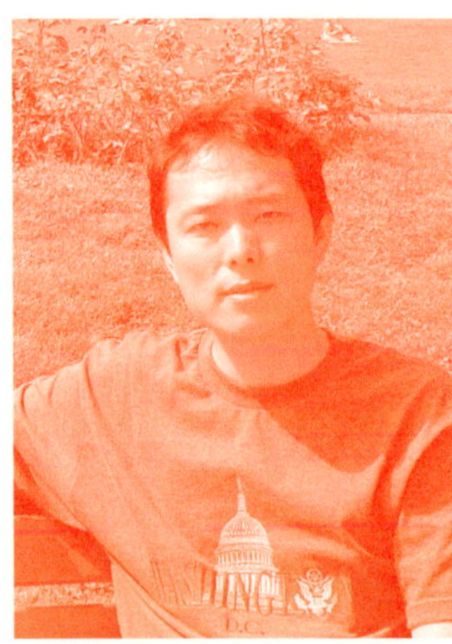
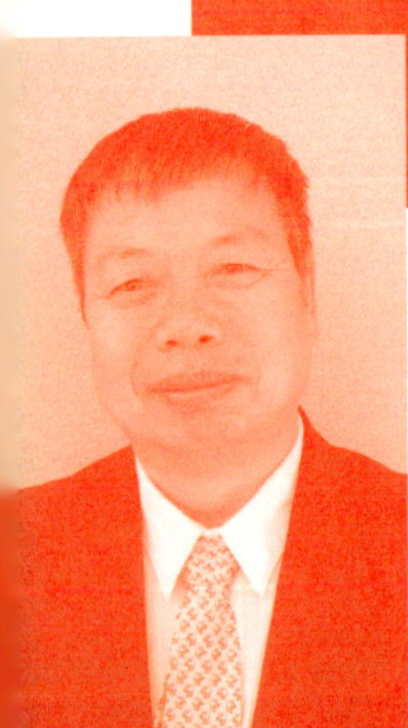
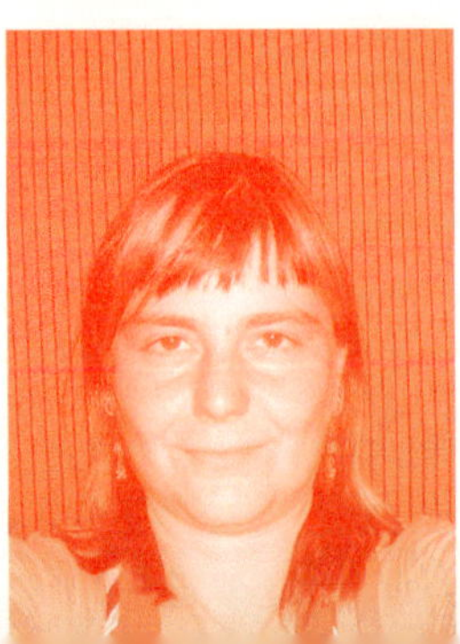

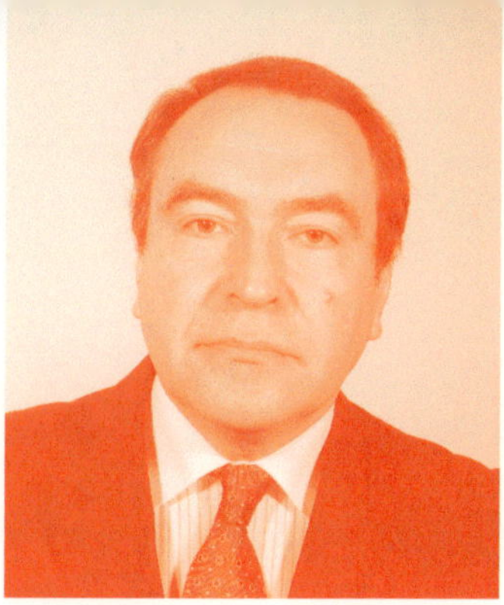
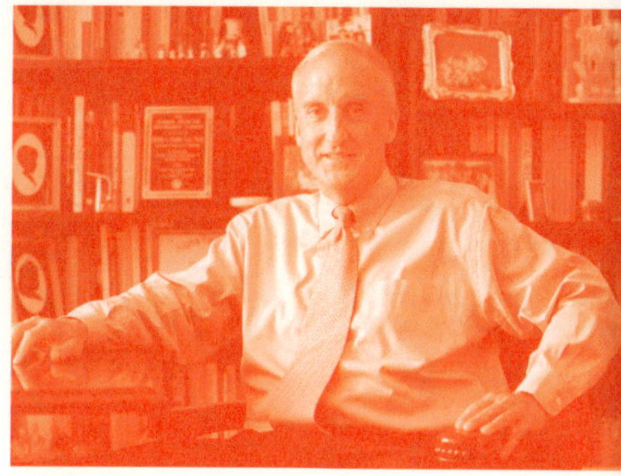
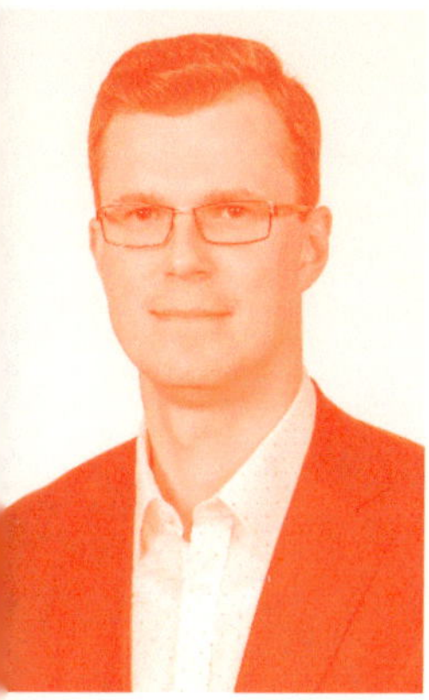
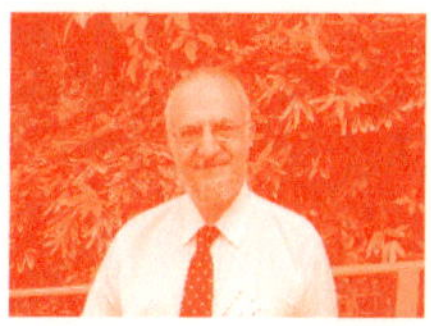
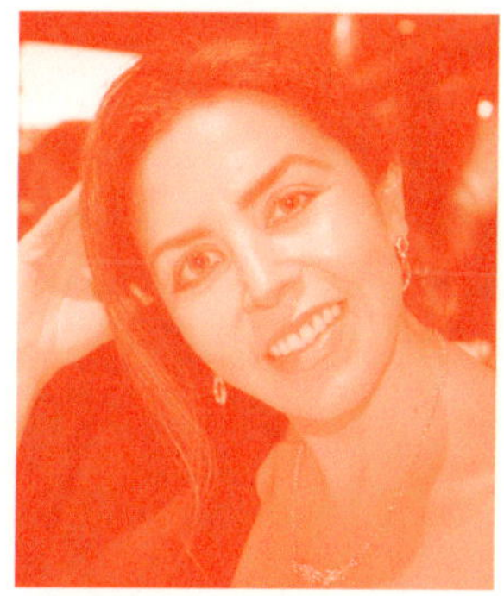

Supporting open minds since 2005

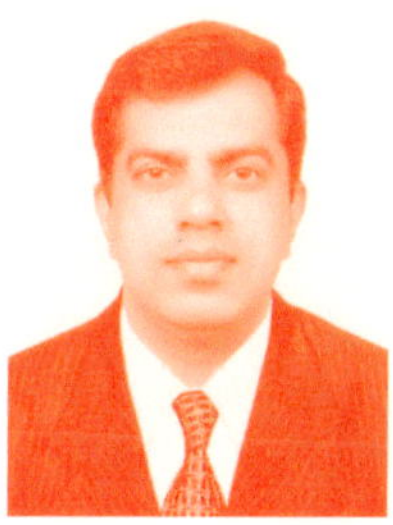
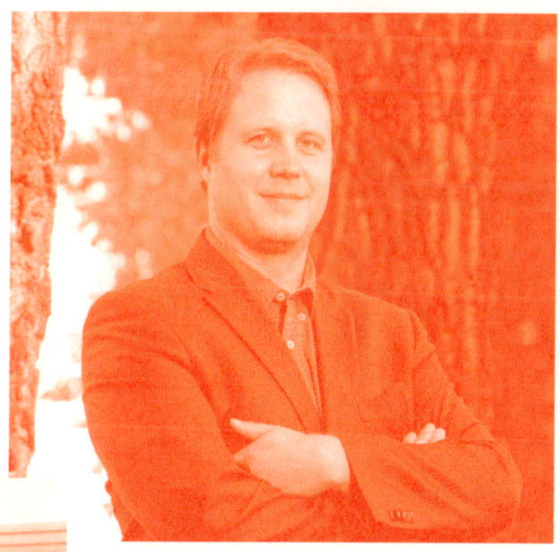
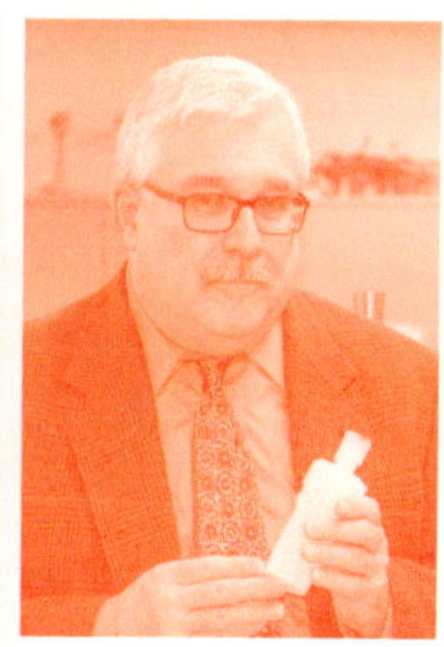
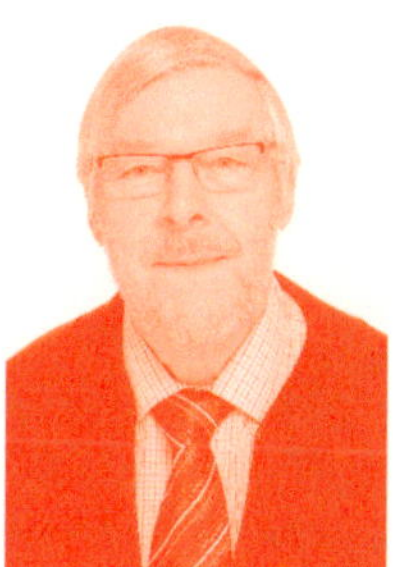
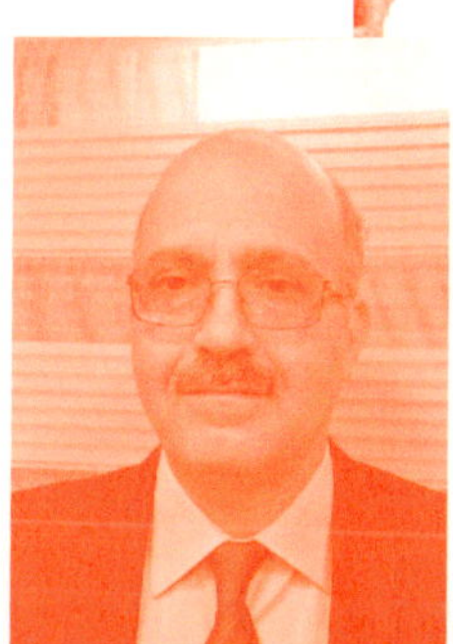
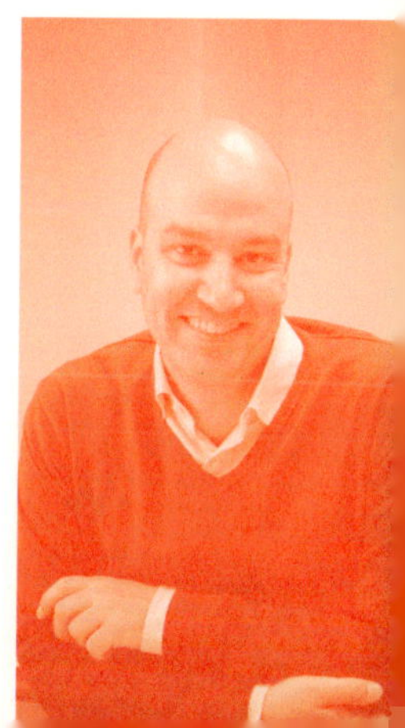
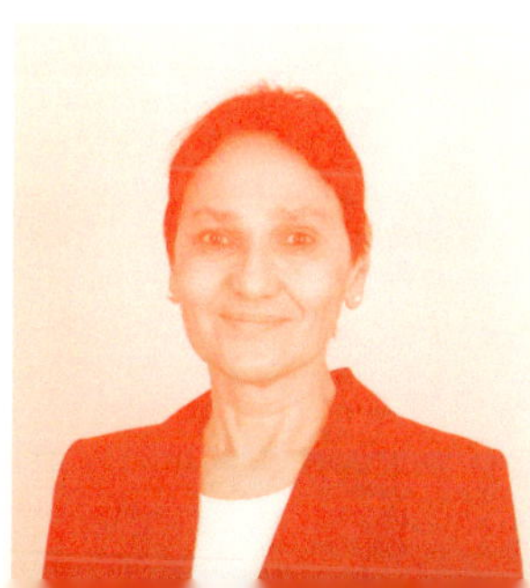

Synthetic Biology - New Interdisciplinary Science
http://dx.doi.org/10.5772/intechopen.77541
Edited by Madan L. Nagpal, Oana-Maria Boldura, Cornel Baltă and Shymaa Enany

Contributors
Rajendra Bera, Danielle Zauli, Bianca Mendes Maciel, Amanda Teixeira Sampaio Lopes, Marjanca Starčič Erjavec, Kadri Karim, Tapas Chakraborty, Sipra Mohapatra, Dipak Pandey, Chimwar Wanglar, R. Holland Cheng, Shizuo Kamita, Mo Baikoghli, Luis De La Maza, Muhd Danish-Daniel, Mohd Ezhar Mohd Noor, Yik Sung Yeong, Tan Min Pau, Gires Usup, Zakiah Jubri, Afiah Nasuha Aznan, Xiangyuan Wan, Suowei Wu, Madan L. Nagpal

First published in London, United Kingdom, 2020 by IntechOpen
IntechOpen is the global imprint of INTECHOPEN LIMITED, registered in England and Wales, registration number: 11086078, 7th floor, 10 Lower Thames Street, London, EC3R 6AF, United Kingdom
Printed in Croatia

British Library Cataloguing-in-Publication Data
A catalogue record for this book is available from the British Library

Additional hard and PDF copies can be obtained from orders@intechopen.com

Synthetic Biology - New Interdisciplinary Science
Edited by Madan L. Nagpal, Oana-Maria Boldura, Cornel Baltă and Shymaa Enany
p. cm.
Print ISBN 978-1-78984-089-6
Online ISBN 978-1-78984-090-2
eBook (PDF) ISBN 978-1-78985-329-2

For EU product safety concerns:
IN TECH d.o.o., Prolaz Marije Krucifikse Kozulić 3, 51000 Rijeka, Croatia, info@intechopen.com or visit our website at intechopen.com.

Meet the editors

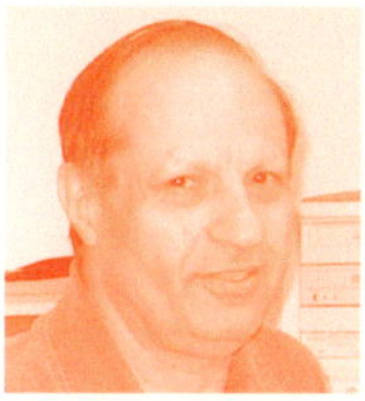

Madan L. Nagpal, PhD, FLS, has been Research Associate Professor at the Department of Microbiology and Immunology, University of South Carolina, Columbia, SC, and Research Chemist at the Dorn Veterans Medical Center, Columbia, SC, USA for 10 plus years. He has published 40 research articles, one book chapter, and edited one book. He was awarded a Research and Productive Scholarship by the University of South Carolina in 1990. He was funded by grants as a co-investigator by the National Institutes of Health and VA Merit Review. His contributions include gene regulation in steroid hormone biosynthesis and the characterization of *Bacillus* species. He is a member of the American Society of Cell Biology, American Association of Advancement of Science, American Association for Laboratory Animal Science, International Who's Who Professionals, and Marquis Who's Who in America.

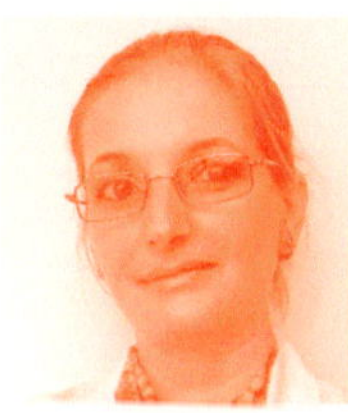

Assist. Prof. Dr. Eng. Oana-Maria Boldura is licensed in genetic engineering with specialization in Molecular Biology (2005). She is a Master of Science in Genetic Manipulation (2007) and Pharmacy (2014), and has a PhD in Biotechnology (2010). From 2015 she has been an assistant professor at the Banat University of Agricultural Sciences and Veterinary Medicine, "King Michael I of Romania" Timisoara, Faculty of Veterinary Medicine, Department of Chemistry, Biochemistry and Molecular Biology, and a researcher in the "Horia Cernescu" Research Unit. Her main scientific competences are in the fields of molecular biology, biotechnology, genomics, and biosecurity with technical aptitudes in the manipulation and experimentation of nucleic acid and proteins (purification, sequencing, gene expression studies, SDS-PAGE analysis of proteins fractions, "lab-on-chip" electrophoresis, and immunological testing). Her areas of interest are molecular forensic methods and apoptotic process pathways.

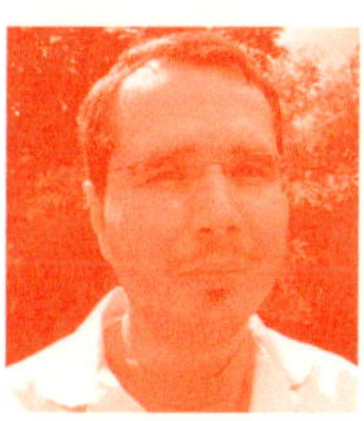

Dr. Cornel Baltă, MD, DVM, is licensed in veterinary medicine. He has a PhD in Veterinary Medicine (2011), qualified as a medical doctor (2018), and is a researcher at the Institute of Life Sciences, "Vasile Goldis" Western University Arad, Romania. His main scientific competences are in the fields of laboratory animals, molecular biology, physiology, histology, and clinical laboratory with competences and technical aptitudes in nucleic acid examination by electrophoresis techniques, PCR and qPCR, and qualitative and quantitative determination of proteins by Western blot and microelectrophoresis. His areas of interest are the study of molecular mechanisms involved in the evolution of liver and gastrointestinal diseases and the study of molecular mechanisms involved in bone regeneration and remodeling using different types of polymers as scaffolds.

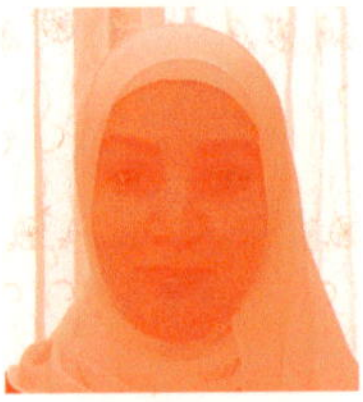

Dr. Shymaa Enany is an associate professor of microbiology and immunology at the Suez Canal University, Egypt. She received her PhD from the School of Medical and Dental Sciences, Niigata University, Japan, and completed her postdoctoral work in collaboration with many laboratories in San Diego, California, USA, and in Niigata, Japan. She is an editorial board member and reviewer in many journals and scientific associations and has many publications in eminent journals as well as books. She has excellent experience in bacterial genomics and proteomics.

Contents

Preface

Synthetic biology can broadly be defined as an applied science for the synthesis of biological components of organisms. It is a novel interdisciplinary science with contributions from genetics, biology, chemistry, physics, engineering, computer science, mathematics, and other disciplines. Its application leads to the creation or modification of genetic materials in living organisms. Thus, synthetic biology has a very wide and complex scope: it is interdisciplinary and can be applied to microbiology, biochemistry, and molecular biology. Synthetic biology gives us a new hope because it is a novel interdisciplinary science. We can foresee the creation of the new world of vegetation, animals, and humans with the interdisciplinary system of biological sciences. By understanding various parts and bringing them together, we can build coherent theories in this complex world of different disciplines and make science more useful and practical.

The first synthetic gene was somatostatin reported in 1977 in *Science*. It was demonstrated that a gene, designed from an amino acid sequence, can be synthesized. Later, improvements in technologies, such as high-performance liquid chromatography for the analysis and purification of DNA fragments, genetic engineering, chemical synthesis, and advances in other branches of biology, led to the production of synthetic organs and manmade biological systems. For example, a synthetic heart has been fabricated from a novel supramolecular elastomer that enables endogenous cells to enter and produce a matrix. Genetically modified yeast produces penicillin and transgenic maize confers resistance to corn rootworms. Gene therapy, which aims to restore correct gene expression in cells that have a defective form, is being developed to prevent diseases such as cancer, muscular dystrophy, diabetes, and many more. Gene therapy is becoming a promising technology for treating hereditary and acquired disorders.

Genetic engineering technologies, such as cloning, custom-designed promoters, and linking genes of one species to another, are being used to produce new characteristics in organisms and thus change the genetic make-up of future generations. The construction of recombinant DNA (i.e., joining DNA of different genes) and its insertion into the host organism creates genetically modified organisms. Genetically modified foods have been developed that are resistant to pests, diseases, and herbicides. Genetic engineering is widely used to produce vaccines, monoclonal antibodies, and animals that can be used as models for diseases or as organ donors (such as pigs) for humans.

The creation of new modern tools in biological disciplines is helping to explore genes and the world of genomes. Recently, the discovery of the technique RNA interference has helped to determine the functions of genes identified by sequencing the genome. Microbes are being designed to break down plastic and clean up pollution. The clustered regularly interspaced short palindromic repeats technology for gene editing is used in the treatment of diabetes and therapeutics of immune diseases. This technology is now applied across various genomes in its role of immunity to genetic diseases.

This book incorporates articles of diverse disciplines. The introductory chapter presents the subject matter in general and the other chapters focus on various important aspects, such as procedures, achievements, and the future ideas and challenges of synthetic biology. These articles are contributed by leading experts in their fields and make this book very special, very useful, and full of knowledge. The field of synthetic biology is growing exponentially and opening up new avenues in multidisciplinary approaches by bringing together theoretical and applied aspects of science.

We convey our appreciations to all the contributing authors and the IntechOpen team, particularly Josip Knapic and Lucija Tomicic-Dromgool, the Commissioning Editor. We believe this book demonstrates the great achievements made by the power of genetic engineering and synthetic biology and that it will be tremendously useful in teaching new perspectives on this fascinating area of science.

Madan L. Nagpal
University of South Carolina,
USA

Oana-Maria Boldura
Banat's University of Agricultural Sciences and Veterinary Medicine,
Romania

Cornel Balta
"Vasile Goldis" Western University of Arad,
Romania

Shymaa Enany
Suez Canal University,
Egypt

Section 1

Genetic Engineering

Chapter 1

Introductory Chapter: The Role of Genetic Engineering Technology in the Manipulation of Genetics of Organisms and Synthetic Biology

Madan L. Nagpal

1. Introduction

Synthetic biology is a new interdisciplinary science that involves synthesis of biological components, systems, and organisms using genetic engineering technology. The manipulation of DNA or the introduction of DNA of one organism into another organism leads to synthetic biology.

The manipulation of the genomes of the organisms is revolutionizing the genetics of the organisms. The cloning of the genes is an important genetic engineering technology and is required for studying the biological properties of the genes, the DNA fragments, and the organization of the genomes. Other techniques that are part of the genetic engineering technology are isolation of DNA, restriction digestion of the DNA, ligation, sequence analyses, and expression.

What
Genetic engineering technology
Does
Turns
Biology to medicine
Genes off and on
Controls gene expressions
Produces transgenic organisms
Synthetic organisms
Organisms with new genes
Modified genes
Man-made genes and genomes
Man-made organisms
Imagine
Man-made men and women
With superintelligence
Superstrength
Super-synthetic biology
Engineered synthetic biology

The genes have specific chromosomal loci and are determined by linkage analysis and deletion mapping. The eukaryotic genes are too large and have introns and exons. The gene is transcribed into mRNA which is further translated into proteins, and the proteins perform various functions in the body.

Genes define the molecular biology of the normal as well as the abnormal states of an organism. Mutations in genes can cause serious changes in the organism. During cell division, DNA is copied, and sometimes, the copy differs in some of the deoxynucleotides, and this is called mutation. Most of the mutations occur naturally and they could lead to evolution. Mutations are also caused by many other ways, such as exposure to chemicals or radiations, and the cell of the organism ends up with DNA slightly different than the original DNA. The DNA damaging agents induce a set of responses, termed as "SOS" in *Escherichia coli*, which involve the transcriptional activation of various genes required for DNA repair. In the yeast *Saccharomyces cerevisiae*, a large number of DNA repair genes have been identified.

The yeast, *Saccharomyces cerevisiae*, is used as a model organism for studying fundamental aspects of eukaryotic cell biology [1]. For understanding the molecular mechanism of DNA repair in eukaryotes, yeast was chosen as a model system to study the role of radiation-repair (*rad*) genes during the cell division cycle [2]. Plasmids containing various RAD-lacZ gene fusions were integrated into the chromosome of haploid yeast cells, and the integrated strains were examined for the expression of beta-galactosidase after treatments with ultraviolet radiation (UV) or 4-nitroquinoline-1-oxide (NQO). It was found that the functions controlled by RAD genes are essential for normal meiosis and DNA replication and recombination [3]. Thus, geneticists can easily manipulate yeast gene expression and study the resulting phenotypic effects. RAD51 gene of yeast is a homolog of RecA gene of *E. coli*. RecA catalyzes repair and recombination and induces SOS response in *E. coli*. SOS system was first described by Miroslav Radman after the distress signal "SOS" in the Morse alphabet (three dots, three dashes, three dots) (https://www.sciencedirect.com/topics/neuroscience/sos-response).

Transfection experiments are carried out in studying the role of viruses in causing diseases. Viruses cause a variety of infectious diseases, and various infections have been linked to atherosclerosis and coronary heart disease [4]. By preparing cDNA and subtraction cDNA libraries from explant and transformed cells, the mechanism of transformation and the role of viruses were studied in causing atherosclerosis [5, 6]. Viruses can precipitate various conditions, including coronary heart diseases and chronic kidney diseases. Understanding the mechanisms could lead to the new areas of investigation and overall cellular pathophysiology.

Gene expression is regulated from DNA to RNA transcription and further to the posttranscriptional modifications of the protein. The expression and regulation of insulin-like growth factor-binding proteins (IGFBPs) -1, -2, -3, and -4 mRNAs in purified rat Leydig cells and their biological effects were studied. The actions of insulin-like growth factors (IGFs) are modified by IGFBPs. IGFBPs may potentiate or inhibit the effects of IGFs on cell growth and protein synthesis. Leydig cells are found in the testis, and the major physiological role of Leydig cells is to produce androgens required for spermatogenesis and development of male characteristics. The testis is a dynamic tissue, containing many cell types that produce a variety of compounds that affect Leydig cell function. The pituitary dependency of IGFBP mRNA expression in Leydig cells was studied by isolating and culturing rat Leydig cells from normal male Sprague Dawley rats (50-day-old) and from 50-day-old rats 5 days after hypophysectomy. The results revealed that on hypophysectomy, IGF-I, IGFBP-2, IGFBP-3, and IGFBP-4 mRNA expressions were reduced in Leydig cells, suggesting that their expressions were pituitary dependent. It was also shown that multiple species of IGFBPs are expressed in Leydig cells and that IGFBPs modify the effect of IGF-I on Leydig cell function [7]. Another good example of gene regulation and expression is the process of erythropoiesis. The erythroid cells exhibit patterns of gene expression that direct a precise ensemble of proteins required for cellular structure and function. Erythroblasts decrease in size, cells produce large amounts of hemoglobin, and membranes undergo reorganization and enucleation. Erythropoiesis yields a highly specialized cell type, the mature erythrocyte to meet the organismal needs of increased oxygen-carrying capacity [8].

The cloning of a gene and studying its expression are an important part of biotechnology. It leads to understanding of the functions of the gene in the living organisms and by modifying the cloned gene, could produce novel compounds and new functions in the cells or the living organisms.

A gene was cloned that was differentially expressed in normal adult rat Leydig cells and whose expression was inhibited by *human chorionic gonadotropin* (hCG) but was induced by interferon-gamma (IFN-γ). DNA sequence analysis identified this gene as rat IFN-γ-inducible protein 10 (IP-10), a member of the CXC chemokine superfamily of proinflammatory cytokines. It was found that high levels of IP-10 messenger RNA (mRNA) were constitutively expressed in freshly isolated and primary cultured Leydig cells and may have paracrine and autocrine effects on testicular function [9]. The effects of overexpression of cytokine-responsive gene-2 (CRG-2) (systematic name CXCL10, also known as interferon-γ-inducible protein 10 (IP-10)) on MA-10 mouse were studied in Leydig tumor cell steroidogenesis and proliferation. Chemokines have been implicated in tumor growth, angiogenesis, metastasis, and the host immune response to malignant cells. CXCL10 is a potent chemokine expressed predominantly by macrophages and Leydig cells in the testis. CXCL10 belongs to a large family of chemotactic cytokines, now termed "chemokines," that are expressed in diverse cell types wherein they regulate innate and adaptive immune responses [10]. Chemokines are chemotactic factors and growth regulators, which exert their effects through seven transmembrane domain or G protein-coupled receptors [11, 12]. CXCL10 binds to CXCR3 receptor (a G protein-coupled receptor) and acts via Giα protein. The purpose of this study was to determine the effects of overexpression of CXCL10 by transfection experiments in MA-10 cells on cell growth, CXCR3 expression, progesterone biosynthesis, and steroidogenic acute regulatory protein (StAR D1, a key regulatory factor in steroidogenesis) gene expression. The complete CXCL10 cDNA was cloned in a mammalian expression vector with the CMV promoter, pcDNA3.1D/V5-His-TOPO, and its expression was confirmed with rat CXCL10 antibody and V5 antibody. Results showed large amounts of CXCL10 protein secreted in the medium in the CXCL10 transfectants by Western blotting. The production of CXCL10 mRNA ranged from 30- to 50-fold more (n = 6) in the transfected cells than the control cells, as determined by semiquantitative and real-time RT-PCR. 8-Br-cAMP downregulated CXCL10 mRNA expression and stimulated CXCR3 mRNA expression. Transfection of MA-10 cells with CXCL10 decreased cAMP-induced progesterone synthesis from 38.5 ± 1.7 ng/ml (1.5×10^5 cells/ml) in control cells to 23.2 ± 1.5 ng in transfected cells ($p < 0.01$). 8-Br-cAMP (0.2 mM)-induced StAR D1 mRNA was decreased 30–40% by transfection with CXCL10. Interestingly, overexpression of CXCL10 induced the expression of its receptor CXCR3 gene, as determined by RT-PCR and fluorescence-activated cell sorter (FACS) analysis. Transfection of CXCL10 also significantly decreased [^{3}H]thymidine incorporation into DNA. These data suggested that CXCL10 inhibited StAR D1 expression, decreased progesterone synthesis, and inhibited cell proliferation. CXCL10 has the potential to be used in gene therapy for prostate cancer due to its antiangiogenic effect and its inhibitory effect on steroidogenesis [13]. CXCL10 may be potentially useful in the treatment of prostate cancer. The experiments were designed to study the effects of overexpression of CXCL10 in human prostate LNCaP cells on CXCR3 gene expression and inhibition of cell proliferation. LNCaP cells were transiently transfected with CXCL10 cDNA in pIRES2-EGFP vector. CXCL10, CXCR3, prostate-specific antigen (PSA), and *glyceraldehyde 3-phosphate dehydrogenase* (G3PDH) mRNA levels were determined by semiquantitative conventional and quantitative real-time RT-PCR, and protein expression was determined by fluorescence-activated cell sorting (FACS). The expression of CXCL10 was markedly enhanced in the transfected cells at mRNA and protein levels in the cells. Overexpression of CXCL10 inhibited cell proliferation of the transfected cells by 30–40% in serum-limited medium (1% FCS in RPMI1640 medium) and decreased PSA production. CXCR3 expression was significantly induced by the overexpression of CXCL10 as determined by RT-PCR and FACS. These results indicated that CXCL10 inhibited LNCaP cell proliferation and decreased PSA production by upregulation of CXCR3 receptor. In conclusion, overexpression of CXCL10 may be potentially useful in the gene therapy of prostate cancer [14].

The identification of unknown organisms is carried out on genetic bases, whereas the molecular and chemical characteristics provide the complementary information. The DNA barcoding is one of the technologies for species classification and identification of unknown organisms. DNA barcoding involves tissue sample collection, DNA isolation, amplification of the isolated DNA, sequencing, and analyses of the results in order to identify the organism. The goal of DNA barcoding is to identify biological specimens using a short specific region of DNA. For example, a short fragment (658 bp) of mitochondrial gene cytochrome c oxidase I (COI) DNA from a single individual when amplified by polymerase chain reaction (PCR) was 100% successful in correctly identifying 200 closely allied species of Lepidoptera specimens [15]. Stoeckle and Thaler [16] pointed out that DNA barcode differences within animal species are usually much less than the differences among species, making it generally straightforward to match unknowns to a reference library. The barcodes could provide new insights and innovations into the evolution and diversification of life.

PCR is a technology to amplify a specific piece of DNA or gene and is used for analyses of genetic diseases, genetic fingerprinting, monitoring microbiological quality of food, detection and diagnosis of infectious diseases, and for many other uses. PCR is used to create copies of DNA for introduction into host organisms such as *Escherichia coli* in genetic engineering and to amplify stretches of genetic material for Sanger sequencing. PCR is used in archaeology, to identify human or animal remains, including insects trapped in amber, and to track human migration patterns; degraded DNA samples may be able to be reconstructed during the early cycles of PCR. PCR can be used to differentiate between similar organisms or work out relationships between different species (https://www.xxpresspcr.com). PCR technique was developed by Kary Mullis and his group in the 1980s, and in 1993, Kary Mullis and Michael Smith were awarded Nobel Prize in Chemistry for their work. The PCR technique involves the synthesis of a new strand of DNA complementary to the template strand using DNA polymerase and a set of primers. Since then a lot of progress has been made in this technique. Real-time PCR has been developed that monitors the progression of the amplification in real time by using fluorescent signaling as the amplification occurs [17].

Using PCR technology, ribosomal RNA (rRNA) 16S–23S interspace region sequence variability in bacterial species was studied [18]. Two distinct genetic clusters within the species *Bacillus subtilis* and *Bacillus atrophaeus* were selected, and it was concluded that *B. atrophaeus* is distinct genetically from *B. subtilis* subgroups represented by W23 and 168, respectively. This was the first study to make sequence comparisons at the genome, strain, and species level for rRNA interspace region. Considerations of this issue will be important in using ribosomal space region (RSR) methodology to differentiate other closely related bacterial species.

Fox et al. [19] identified *Brucella* spp. by RSR PCR molecular technology and chemical characteristics as complementary information in the differentiation of closely related organisms. PCR products were unique to brucellae, allowing them to be readily distinguished from other gram-negative bacteria (including *Bartonella*

DOI: http://dx.doi.org/10.5772/intechopen.90549

spp. and *Agrobacterium* spp.). Carbohydrate profiles differentiated *B. canis* from the other three *Brucella* species due to their absence of the rare amino sugar quinovosamine. PCR of the rRNA region was useful in identification of the genus *Brucella*, while carbohydrate profiling was capable of differentiating *B. canis* from the other *Brucella* species. Species differentiation can also be achieved by determination of approximate size of PCR products of intergenic spacer region (ISR) of 16S–23S rRNA based upon their relative electrophoretic mobility on agarose gels [20].

One of the major properties of genes is their expression pattern. Notably, genes are often classified as tissue specific or housekeeping [21]. Tissue-specific gene expression experiments in adult male rat (55- to 65-day-old) tissues revealed that glucose transporter 8 (GLUT8) was expressed predominantly in the testis, in smaller amounts in the heart and kidney, and in negligible amounts in the liver and spleen. GLUT8 mRNA was found to be highly expressed in crude interstitial cells, Leydig cells, and testicular and epididymal germ cells. In prepubertal rat (20-day-old) tissues, GLUT8 expression was comparatively much lower than in the adult rat tissues. By comparative reverse transcriptase PCR (RT-PCR), human chorionic gonadotropin (hCG) caused dose- and time-dependent increases of GLUT8 mRNA levels. hCG and IGF-I had synergistic effects on GLUT8 mRNA and protein expression. GLUT1 and GLUT3 were also found to be expressed in Leydig cells. However, neither GLUT1 nor GLUT3 was affected by treatments with hCG, IGF-I, or hCG and IGF-I combined. The addition of murine interleukin-1α (mIL-1α; 10 ng/ml), murine tumor necrosis factor-α (mTNF-α; 10 ng/ml), and murine interferon-γ (mIFN-γ; 500 U/ml) separately or in combination decreased hCG-induced GLUT8 mRNA levels significantly. In conclusion, GLUT8 mRNA in Leydig cells was positively regulated by hCG and IGF-I and downregulated by cytokines, mIL-1α, mTNF-α, and mIFN-γ. These results indicated that hCG, growth factors, and cytokines affect Leydig cell steroidogenesis by modulating GLUT8 expression [22]. Another example of tissue-specific gene expression is that in liver tumorigenesis, it has been shown that pyrroline-5-carboxylate reductase (PYCR1) gene is upregulated and the inhibition of PYCR1 may be a novel therapeutic strategy to target liver tumor cells [23].

This book provides deeper understanding of the recent progresses in biotechnology and genetic engineering contributing to synthetic biology and biological processes. The readers will appreciate the significance of the diverse nature of the articles and the eminence of the authors covered in this book. I hope this book gives you enough information on very specific topics and inspires you to further explore and re-invent the subjects in synthetic biology—a new interdisciplinary science.

Author details

Madan L. Nagpal
University of South Carolina, Columbia, SC, USA

*Address all correspondence to: madannag123@yahoo.com

References

[1] Duina AA, Miller ME, Keeney JB. Budding yeast for budding geneticists: A primer on the *Saccharomyces cerevisiae* model system. Genetics. 2014;**197**:33-48

[2] Nagpal ML, Higgins DR, Prakash S. Expression of the *RAD1* and *RAD3* genes of *Saccharomyces cerevisiae* is not affected by DNA damage or during the cell division cycle. Molecular & General Genetics. 1985;**199**:59-63

[3] Friedberg EC. Deoxyribonucleic acid repair in the yeast *Saccharomyces cerevisiae*. Microbiological Reviews. 1988;**52**(1):70-102

[4] Pothineni NVK, Subramany S, Kurjakose K, Shirazi LF, Romeo F, Shah PK, et al. Infections, atherosclerosis, and coronary heart disease. European Heart Journal. 2017;**38**(43):3195-3201. DOI: 10.1093/eurheartj/ehx362

[5] Nachtigal M, Legrand A, Nagpal ML, Nachtigal SA, Greenspan P. Transformation of rabbit vascular smooth muscle cells by transfection with the early region of SV40 DNA. The American Journal of Pathology. 1990;**136**(2):297-306

[6] Nachtigal M, Legrand A, Greenspan P, Nachtigal SA, Nagpal ML. Immortalization of rabbit vascular smooth muscle cells after transfection with a fragment of the *Bgl*II region of herpes simplex virus type 2 DNA. Intervirology. 1990;**33**:166-174

[7] Lin T, Wang D, Nagpal ML, Shimasaki S, Ling N. Expression and regulation of insulin-like growth factor-binding protein-1, -2, -3 and -4 mRNAs in purified rat Leydig cells and their biological effects. Endocrinology. 1993;**132**:1898-1904

[8] Schulz VP, Yan H, Lezon-Geyda K, An X, Hale J, Hillyer CD, et al. A unique epigenomic landscape defines human erythropoiesis. Cell Reports. 2019;**28**:2996-3009. Available from: http://creativecommons.org/licenses/by-nc-nd/4.0/

[9] Hu J, You S, Li W, Wang D, Nagpal ML, Mi Y, et al. Expression and regulation of interferon-γ-inducible protein 10 gene in rat Leydig cells. Endocrinology. 1998;**139**:3637-3645

[10] Murphy PM, Baggiolini M, Charo IF, Hebert CA, Horuk R, Matsushima K, et al. International Union of Pharmacology, XXII. Nomenclature for chemokine receptors. Pharmacological Reviews. 2000;**52**:145-176

[11] Farber LM. Mig and IP-10 CXC: Chemokines that target lymphocytes. Journal of Leukocyte Biology. 1997;**61**:246-257

[12] Tamaru M, Tominaga Y, Yatsunami K, Narumi S. Cloning of the murine interferon-inducible protein 10 (IP-10) receptor and its specific expression in lymphoid organs. Biochemical and Biophysical Research Communications. 1998;**25**:41-48

[13] Nagpal ML, Chen Y, Lin T. Effects of overexpression of CXCL10 (cytokine-responsive gene-2) on MA-10 mouse Leydig tumor cell steroidogenesis and proliferation. The Journal of Endocrinology. 2004;**183**:585-594

[14] Nagpal ML, Davis J, Lin T. Overexpression of CXCL10 in human prostate LNCaP cells activates its receptor (CXCR3) expression and inhibits cell proliferation. Biochimica et Biophysica Acta. 2006;**1762**:811-818

[15] Hebert PDN, Ratnasingham S, deWaard JR. Barcoding animal life: Cytochrome c oxidase subunit 1 divergences among closely related species. Proceedings of

the Royal Society of London B. 2003;**270**(Suppl):S96-S99

[16] Stoeckle MY, Thaler DS. DNA barcoding works in practice but not in (neutral) theory. PLoS ONE. 2014;**9**(7):e100755. DOI: 10.1371/journal.pone.0100755

[17] Mackay IM. Real time PCR in the microbiology laboratory. Clinical Microbiology and Infection. 2004;**10**(3):190-212

[18] Nagpal ML, Fox KF, Fox A. Utility of 16S-23S rRNA spacer region methodology: How similar are interspace regions within a genome and between strains for closely related organisms? Journal of Microbiological Methods. 1998;**33**:211-219

[19] Fox KF, Fox A, Nagpal M, Steinberg P, Heroux K. Identification of *Brucella* by ribosomal-spacer-region PCR and differentiation of *Brucella canis* from other *Brucella* spp. pathogenic for humans by carbohydrate profiles. Journal of Clinical Microbiology. 1998;**36**(11):3217-3222

[20] Johnson YA, Nagpal M, Krahmer MT, Fox FF, Fox A. Precise molecular weight determination of PCR products of the rRNA intergenic spacer region using electrospray quadrupole mass spectrometry for differentiation of *B. subtilis* and *B. atrophaeus*, closely related species of bacilli. Journal of Microbiological Methods. 2000;**40**:241-254

[21] Kryuchkova-Mostacci N, Robinson-Rechavi M. A benchmark of gene expression tissue-specificity metrics. Briefing. Bioinformatics. 2017;**18**(2):205-214. DOI: 10.1093/bib/bbw008

[22] Chen Y, Nagpal ML, Lin T. Expression and regulation of glucose transporter 8 in rat Leydig cells. The Journal of Endocrinology. 2003;**179**:63-72

[23] Ding Z, Ericksen RE, Escande-Beillard N, Lee QY, Loh A, Denil S, et al. Metabolic pathway analyses identify proline biosynthesis pathway as a promoter of liver tumorigenesis. Journal of Hepatology. 2019. DOI: 10.1016/j.jhep.2019.10.026. [Epub Ahead of print], PMID: 31726117

Chapter 2

Synthetic Biology, Artificial Intelligence, and Quantum Computing

Rajendra K. Bera

Abstract

We envisage a world where genetic engineering, artificial intelligence (AI), and quantum computing (QC) will coalesce to bring about a forced speciation of the *Homo sapiens*. A forced speciation will drastically reduce the emergence time for a new species to a few years compared to Nature's hundreds of millennia. In this chapter, we explain the basic concepts that would allow a forced speciation of the *Homo sapiens* to occur and its consequences on life on Earth thereafter. Accelerating speciation mediated by *Homo sapiens* via domestication, gene splicing, and gene drive mechanisms is now scientifically well understood. Synthetic biology can advance speciation far more rapidly using a combination of clustered regularly interspaced short palindromic repeats (CRISPR) technology, advanced computing technologies, and knowledge creation using AI. The day is perhaps not far off when *Homo sapiens* itself will initiate its own speciation once it advances synthetic biology to a level where it can safely modify the brain to temper emotion and enhance rational thinking as a means of competing against AI-embedded machines guided by quantum algorithms.

Keywords: synthetic biology, artificial intelligence, quantum computing, information theory, genetic engineering

1. Introduction

The great journey of building rational scientific knowledge includes observing, making conjectures, and severely verifying them for flaws, limitations, and errors. When conjectures falter, scientists revisit, revise, abandon, start afresh, search for alternatives, etc. They seek unity in diversity or generalize to include diversity, with the knowledge that "truth" is not knowable. In this journey, they seek to be rational, parsimonious[1] in making conjectures, and methodical, open, transparent, and consistent when sharing them. Conjectures are deemed scientifically valid only if there is potential scope of finding an error [1]. "Though [a mistake] stresses our fallibility it does not resign itself to scepticism, for it also stresses the fact that knowledge can grow, and that science can progress—just because we can learn from our mistakes" [1]. The process is criticism controlled.

[1] Following William Occam (1287–1347) who recommended a principle of parsimony (les parsimoniae), famously known as Occam's razor, "plurality is not to be posited without necessity".

In the last few decades, technology has provided some remarkable tools to accelerate, not merely speed up, this process, and these tools have tremendous potential of becoming even more versatile. In the context of synthetic biology, the tools include the triad: clustered regularly interspaced short palindromic repeats (CRISPR) gene editing technology in genetic engineering, artificial intelligence (AI), and quantum computing (QC). There is also a torrential gathering of data since the Human Genome Project [2] published a draft sequence and initial analysis of the human genome in February 2001 [3]. The new sources include data flowing from the Human Cell Atlas project, which plans to identify and locate every type of cell we possess [4], and various brain projects initiated in the US, Europe, Japan, and Korea, and privately funded Allen Institute for Brain Science. China and Taiwan are also getting in the fray [5]. To make sense of the growing mountains of data in terms of finding "the molecular logic of the living state" in a timely manner rather than drowning in it will require data curation and analysis tools and resources that presently only CRISPR, AI, and QC can provide. This appears fortuitous since we anticipate a catastrophic speciation of the *Homo sapiens* to occur soon because of a rapidly changing environment that will likely lead to its decimation unless synthetic biology comes to the rescue.

This chapter is therefore written for the millennials on whose shoulders will fall the responsibility of navigating through a socioeconomic epochal change that is already under way—the emerging postindustrial era—and a possibly unanticipated speciation of the *Homo sapiens*. The aim is to show that the time is ripe for synthetic biology, AI, and QC to join hands and form a purposeful, integrated discipline to further explore the secrets of life, create new life, and find harmonious ways by which the *Homo sapiens* can speciate in a controlled manner.

2. Time for human speciation is near

Biology is a game of creation, survival by adaptation, and annihilation; it is a game that is "red in tooth and claw". Survival of the fittest (also called natural selection) means survival of those best able to adapt to the environment they are in. This is not about individual survival but of cohesive groups belonging to a species capable of exchanging genes or interbreeding. Natural selection is an ultraslow process in which sudden, dramatic changes in the environment generally mean sudden decimation of species living in it. *Homo sapiens* already find themselves in this unenviable but self-created situation that includes climate change (that also brings deadly heat, spreads diseases, overwhelms hospitals[2]), epidemics, automation initiated unemployment, large-scale immigration due to ism-related (e.g., political, religion related dogmatism) strife, concentration of information and wealth in the hands of fewer and fewer people, depletion of natural resources faster than its replenishment by Nature, the rising irrelevance of rote education, the escalating cost and deterioration of health care, a rising global population that embeds a disproportionately rising population from the less developed countries (see **Figure 1**), the rapidly rising population of the aged whose needs must be paid for by a shrinking, less fecund, younger working population (itself worried about an insecure and financially bleak future), etc. Each by itself is a major stress creator; collectively, they are approaching a crescendo portending an environmental catastrophe that leads to speciation or extinction, and destruction of the biosphere's existing order.

With the benefit of hindsight, we can discern the heralding signs of speciation that went unnoticed. In the rapidly growing global population (presently at 7.7

[2] Its consequences on human health was recently highlighted in [6].

Population of the Earth (in billion markers)

Year	Population	Year	Population
1804	1 billion	1999	6 billion
1927	2 billion	2012	7 billion
1960	3 billion	2024	8 billion
1974	4 billion	2048	9 billion
1987	5 billion		

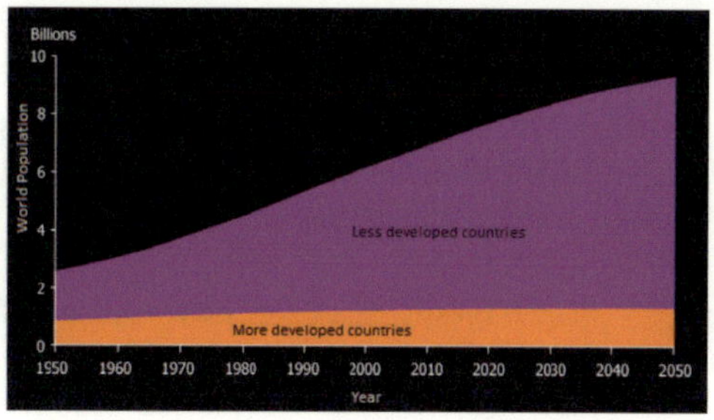

Figure 1.
(Left) World population growth. (Right) World population growth, 1950–2050. Source: World Population Prospects: The 2010 Revision, United Nations, 2011, http://www.un.org/en/development/desa/population/publications/pdf/trends/WPP2010/WPP2010_Volume-I_Comprehensive-Tables.pdf Note the rapidly increasing population size in the less developed countries.

billion plus), the collective population of the more developed countries (characterized by high living standards and education, and low birth rate) since the last several decades has stabilized to about 1.3 billion (including immigrants), while that of the less developed countries (with opposite characteristics) is steadily rising. Concurrently, globally wealth has concentrated into fewer and fewer hands. In January 2018, Oxfam reported that "82% of all wealth created in the last year went to the top 1%, and nothing went to the bottom 50%", that the wealthiest 42 people now had as much wealth as the poorest half, and two-thirds of billionaires wealth come from inheritance, monopoly, and cronyism [7, 8]. The environment for the poorest (hence unfittest) is already brutal.

When natural speciation starts, its largest and earliest victims will come from the less developed countries before it hits the developed ones. In this respect, Africa appears to be highly vulnerable; it "has become the source of some of the greatest threats to the global economic order. Rather than capitalizing on opportunities, international engagement is increasingly focused on mitigating risks" [9]. When speciation begins, these risk mitigation efforts will be in vain because it is the global socioeconomic structure itself that will be disintegrating. The *Homo sapiens'* incommensurate brain power will then make it vulnerable to extinction. The historical legacy of the *Homo sapiens* will not be its fossil record, but its amazing science, technology, engineering, and mathematics (STEM) record for successor species, if any, to peruse.

Speciation is about adapting to the environment. *Homo sapiens* is the only known species to have developed substantial capacity to change the environment to its needs. Thus, it reduced the pressure for speciation since the agricultural era by adopting a socioeconomic structure built around division of labor and a tolerable taxation dogma of "from each according to his ability, to each according to his need" to temper Nature that is "red in tooth and claw". That dogma is increasingly unsustainable because of an escalating need to subsidize the less well off. The affluent 1.3 billion can no longer subsidize the life span of the rest of the unemployable world. But there is the tantalizing possibility that since synthetic biology is ultrafast in editing DNA (deoxyribonucleic acid) and with advancing AI and QC, it will be even faster and better as compared to natural mutation and it may enable the *Homo sapiens* to initiate its own speciation in a programmed manner and survive extinction. What we cannot predict and may even fail to control once initiated are the unintended consequences that will certainly follow. If Ray Kurzweil's prediction about the future capabilities of AI machines ("By 2029, computers will have human-level intelligence" [10]), turn out to be reasonably true, and genetic engineering continues at its present rate of development aided by advances in QC and in understanding RNA (ribonucleic acid)-mediated cellular activity using AI, artificially induced speciation of *Homo sapiens* by the end of this century may become possible before natural selection steps in anger.

Kurzweil also forecasts that the future will provide opportunities of unparalleled human-machine synthesis:

> *2029 is the consistent date I have predicted for when an AI will pass a valid Turing test and therefore achieve human levels of intelligence. I have set the date 2045 for the 'Singularity' which is when we will multiply our effective intelligence a billion-fold by merging with the intelligence we have created. [11]*

Kurzweil's forecasts are based on his "law of accelerating returns" that enunciates that fundamental measures of information technology follow predictable and exponential trajectories seemingly unaffected by dramatic socioeconomic events such as war or peace, and prosperity or recession, paralleling Moore's law in computer technology—the number of transistors on integrated circuit chips doubles approximately almost every 2 years. Indeed, it turns out that once a technology becomes *de facto* information technology, it comes under the grip of the law of accelerating returns because computer simulation of any technology is all about mathematics and computation. The exponential change is the inevitable effect of our ability to conceptualize in larger and larger conceptual blocks by aggregating and augmenting smaller conceptual blocks discovered earlier. This simple mechanism enables the human mind to deal with and find solutions to more complex problems by using the same number of but more versatile concepts rather than an unmanageably larger number of simpler concepts. The method is no different than what mathematicians do. We were first exposed to this method when we studied Euclidean geometry in school. Mathematicians start with simple, primitive concepts they call axioms and build more and more complex theorems as they go along. It works if the axiomatic system is consistent because once a theorem is proven, its validity can be taken for granted even by those who know nothing about mathematics, for example, by machines. This is how machines acquire "intelligence."

During the industrial era just behind us, most people reached their peak capacity to educate and skill themselves in activities (including earning a living) that required mechanizable "intelligent" rote education. That AI machines, in principle, can far surpass humans in such activities had become evident when Alan Turing showed how arithmetical calculations can be mechanized [12] and Gödel had earlier shown that any axiomatic system can be arithmetized [13]. This meant that any form of rational knowledge could be axiomatized and rote education programmed into computers. While creating new knowledge would still require human creativity, once that knowledge had matured and was formalized into an axiomatic system, it would be mechanizable and expandable. It would then be a matter of time that humans would increasingly face competition from machines and eventually be overwhelmed by them. Kurzweil's prediction that this would happen during 2029–2045 is bolstered by recent advances in AI. Ongoing advances in deep learning by machines indicate that through self-learning they can become highly creative and creators of original technology (the patent system will go for a toss) and scientific discoveries without human intervention may well become the norm [14]. Of some 150 predictions since the 1990s, Kurzweil claims an 86% accuracy rate [11, 15, 16]. Since synthetic biology has now come under the grip of mathematics, its exponential development is certain. Synthetic biology is now a part of information technology.

It is only in the last few years that the enormous significance of the exponential growth property of the law of accelerating returns has sunk in the minds of people. As one can see from **Figure 2** (left), till one reaches the vicinity of the knee of the

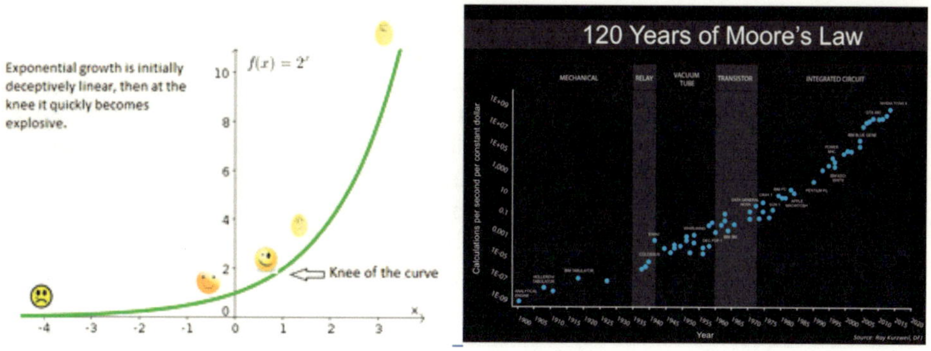

Figure 2.
Exponential growth. Source: (top left) Author. Nature of exponential growth. (Top right) Steve Jurvetson. An updated version of Moore's Law (based on Kurzweil's graph). Wikimedia Commons. https://commons.wikimedia.org/wiki/File:Moore%27s_Law_over_120_Years.png

curve, the curve looks deceptively linear with a mild slope. This allows human minds to extrapolate into the future from gathered knowledge and experience. At the knee, the curve bends upward so rapidly that the human mind cannot respond fast enough to absorb, assess, contemplate, and react rationally. Knee-jerk reaction is about the best humans are capable of in such a situation. *Homo sapiens* now find themselves in an environment which they neither understand nor have the intellectual ability to rationally cope with. This is germane for triggering a speciation event.

Once AI breaches a certain threshold, one should expect a runaway technological growth resulting in a phase transition in human civilization, including perhaps the speciation of the *Homo sapiens*. A likely component of the phase transition may well be that AI enters self-improvement cycles (feedback loops) that eventually cause it to evolve into a powerful level of superintelligence that would qualitatively surpass intelligence levels of all *Homo sapiens*. The accelerating progress of STEM in concert has also brought about commensurate changes in our lifestyle, expectations from life, and erosion of superstition and belief in religion. In the last few decades, the exponential nature of these changes has become noticeable and taxing enough even for the socioeconomic upper strata *Homo sapiens* to cope with. When, to mitigate their anxiety about AI, people claim that AI cannot do this or that which humans can, they often forget to ask if those tasks are worth doing.

Exponential growth in AI has advanced the possibility that artificially induced speciation of *Homo sapiens* may occur by the end of this century. Recent findings show that *Homo sapiens* evolved about 300,000 years ago [17, 18].[3] In recent times, their socioeconomic environment too has changed dramatically. Billions face the prospect of AI machines depriving them of sustainable livelihood and a dignified existence in society. Under such dramatic conditions of environmental change, Nature will force speciation toward life forms with an evolved brain far superior to that of the *Homo sapiens*. The very process may start too late and move too slowly and lead to the extinction of the *Homo sapiens*. Artificially induced speciation may therefore be the only means that may allow the *Homo sapiens* to transition to a new species in a controlled manner. On the flip side, one or more renegade group of *Homo sapiens* may strategize to surreptitiously create a colony of new species with the aim of dominating the Earth and decimating the *Homo sapiens* as an unnecessary burden on Earth.

[3] Prior to these papers, *Homo sapiens* were said to have been around for about 200,000 years.

3. DNA is an information molecule

The language of information now pervades molecular biology—genes are linear sequences of bases (like letters of an alphabet) that carry information (like words) to produce proteins (like sentences). For the process of going from DNA sequences to proteins, we use words like "transcription" and "translation," and of passing genetic "information" from one generation to another. It is rather uncanny that molecular biology can be understood by ignoring chemistry and treating the DNA as a computer program (with enough input data included) in stored memory residing in a computer (the cellular machinery). It is this aspect that bioinformatics exploits. It is analogous to viewing Euclidean geometry not in terms of drawings but in terms of algebra.

In a sense, in the DNA sequences in our cells, written using an alphabet of only four letters, lies hidden the story of who we are and where we come from. For all we know, it might even tell us where we might be going. Albert Lehninger wrote:

> *... living organisms are composed of lifeless molecules ... that conform to all the laws of chemistry but interact with each other in accordance with another set of principles—the molecular logic of the living state. [19]*

It is this "molecular logic of the living state" that is yet to be completely understood, and therein may lie our ability to understand emotion, cognition, and intelligence. So, in a deep sense, the DNA is the master molecule of life. A marvelous thing about cells is that they are so designed that for many purposes one can totally ignore their chemistry and think just about their logic. The fact that one can get away with this is one of the most elegant aspects of molecular biology. The algorithmic side of molecular biology is bioinformatics, the study of information flows in living matter. Bioinformatics is about the development and application of algorithms and methods to turn biological data into knowledge of biological systems. Of fundamental interest is the organization and control of genes in the DNA sequence, the identification of transcriptional units in the DNA, the prediction of protein structure from sequence, and the analysis of molecular function. If there is mathematical logic in living things, then one naturally seeks to determine the formal mathematical system that governs life, that is, how information in the DNA is stored and used by the rest of the cell's machinery to do the myriad of things that it does.

We already know that a DNA molecule—a genotype—is converted into a physical organism—a phenotype—by a very complex process, involving the manufacture of proteins, the replication of the DNA, the replication of cells, the gradual differentiation of cell types, and so on. This epigenetic process is guided by a set of enormously complex cycles of chemical reactions and feedback loops. By the time the full organism appears, there is no discernible similarity between the physical characteristics of the organism and its genotype. Yet molecular biologists attribute the physical structure of the organism to the information encoded in its DNA, and to that alone. This is because there is overwhelming experimental evidence that only DNA transmits hereditary properties. The genotype and the phenotype are isomorphic. However, this isomorphism is so complex that so far it has not been possible to divide the phenotype and genotype into parts, which can be mapped onto each other directly, unlike as, say, in the case of a music record and a record player where portions of a record's track can be easily mapped to specific musical notes [20]. One hopes that AI and QC together will enable us to find this complex mapping. It is all about information processing.

By information we mean the precise determination of sequence, either of bases in the nucleic acid or of amino acid residues in the protein. We gain knowledge of biological systems when we can interpret information in some "meaningful" way without it being easily refuted. That is, we make conjectures and put them through rigorous tests of refutations. Molecular biologists are becoming increasingly sure that "life is a partnership between genes and mathematics" [21]. Indeed, we increasingly tend to believe as Max Tegmark does about the Universe itself:

> *Our reality isn't just described by mathematics – it is mathematics ... Not just aspects of it, but all of it, including you. [In other words,] our external physical reality is a mathematical structure. [22]*

One can well imagine the enormous strides synthetic biology will make when researchers get a deeper understanding of the Book of Life, with AI software becoming their research assistant, and quantum computers executing all the computing required by the AI software.

4. The technology triad

The time has come for synthetic biology, AI, and QC to join hands and form a purposeful, integrated discipline to further explore the secrets of life, create new life, and find harmonious ways by which *Homo sapiens* can speciate. The main responsibility will fall on the shoulders of the millennials. The technology triad (CRISPR, AI, and QC) share some important properties, the ability to create, share, process, and communicate information in digital form. This means they can be supported and integrated with the full power of mathematics and physics. As Richard Feynman notes:

> *Mathematics is a language plus reasoning; it is like a language plus logic. Mathematics is a tool for reasoning. ... [I]t is impossible to explain honestly the beauties of the laws of nature in a way that people can feel, without their having some deep understanding of mathematics. [23]*

Mathematics is the *lingua franca* of the physicists because a formal mathematical statement to be of any value is either true or false; it cannot be true to some and false to others. This is the reason why knowledge based on any axiomatic system, that is, a consistent system in which every valid statement or query has a "yes" or "no" answer, can be arithmetized (i.e., translated into arithmetical statements), encoded in a binary string, and processed in a digital computer. Mathematics is the language that binds men and machine together in a rational dialog. In short, axiomatic systems permit men and machines to mutually communicate without ambiguity or confusion. This is the foundation on which artificial intelligence (AI) rests. It is why Pierre Simon Marquis de Laplace did not even acknowledge God as the creator of the Universe in his mathematical magnum opus on celestial mechanics [24]. He famously told Napoleon Bonaparte, "I had no need of that hypothesis" [25].

Creating and advancing rational knowledge, *inter alia*, requires an ability to communicate thoughts concisely, precisely, and accurately apart from refining knowledge by trial and error, that is, by making our conjectures fitter and fitter for survival. Benjamin Lee Whorf (1897–1941) said, "Language shapes the way we think, and determines what we can think about." And Ludwig Wittgenstein (1889–1951) said, "The limits of my language mean the limits of my world." Mathematics provides fewer limitations than any other language known to *Homo sapiens*. The power of mathematics lies in its ability to extract unity from diversity by abstraction, that is, by eliminating unnecessary context; it helps in discovering group properties (abstract or otherwise) common to all members of the group, for example, the DNA of a species.

Both AI and QC are inseparable from mathematics; they are powerful means of processing and interpreting information (e.g., in the DNA) as well as aiding in inventing novel DNA for specific purposes. Both support and are supported by 3D printing that began by making plastic widgets, but now make guns, houses, prosthetic limbs, vehicle parts, etc. from inanimate matter. The day is not far off when it will advance to printing living, breathing, bio-organs, such as hearts [26] and kidneys, using nanotechnology, computer-aided engineering, and inanimate biodegradable or biocompatible materials and chemicals to build stem cells. Replicating and growing cells, say, in petri dishes is well established, and such cells are already in use as bioink in bioprinters. 3D printing offers the possibility of printing an entire organ, along with a system of arteries, capillaries, and veins that can support it [27, 28]. A major issue in developing this technology is to make it immune-system friendly, since the body may reject organs or cells thus produced, something that can occur even when tissue from one area of the body is put into another.

4.1 CRISPR technology connects synthetic biology with information technology

CRISPR technology has enabled a simple and affordable method of manipulating and editing DNA that has radically changed the ambitions of synthetic biologists. The technology promises to revolutionize how *Homo sapiens* may deal with the world's biggest problems, for example, finding cures for cancer, blindness, and Alzheimer's disease, improving food and eliminating food shortages, fulfilling organ transplant needs, and producing fuel and manufacturing chemicals. Biotechnologists are racing to develop the most efficient, precise, versatile, affordable, and commercially viable genome-editing tools possible. This will be a long and exciting race that may eventually lead to the *Homo sapiens* creating a super species that far exceeds them in the evolutionary path in a controlled manner.

CRISPR is a series of short repeating DNA sequences with "spacers" separating them. The CRISPR technology harnesses an ancient bacteria-based defense system. Bacteria use these genetic sequences to "remember" the viruses that have attacked them by the simple mechanism of incorporating the virus' DNA into their own bacterial genome. The viral DNA thus resides as spacers in the CRISPR sequence as identification tags the bacteria can use to mount an attack if the virus attacks again. Accompanying the CRISPR are locally stationed genes called Cas (**C**rispr-**as**sociated) genes. Once activated, these genes produce enzymes that act as "molecular scissors" that can cut into DNA with specificity. The significance is that in subsequent virus attacks, the bacteria can recall the virus signature and send RNA and Cas to locate and destroy the virus. Among the Cas enzymes derived from bacteria, Cas9 is the best-known molecular scissors enzyme for cutting animal and human DNA. Although the CRISPR sequence was first discovered in 1987, its function was discovered only in 2012.

The ability to cut DNA allows one to either knock out, say, an unwanted disease-causing gene, or splice a "fixed" version of a gene into the DNA. This is analogous to the "Find & Replace" function in text editing software. Indeed, CRISPR technology has advanced so rapidly beyond the Find & Replace function that by December 2017, the Salk Institute had designed a version of the CRISPR-Cas9 system that could switch on or off a targeted gene without even editing the gene. The basic ingredients of gene editing are (1) a piece of RNA, called the guide RNA, that locates the targeted gene, (2) the scissors (the CRISPR-associated protein 9), and (3) the desired DNA segment for insertion after the break. Once the guide RNA locates the targeted gene, Cas9 makes a double-stranded break in the DNA carrying the targeted gene and replaces it with the desired DNA segment. A quick tutorial on CRISPR is available at [29].

CRISPR-based therapies are still nascent. As expected, single-gene disorders are among the best understood because of their simple inheritance patterns (recessive or dominant) and relatively simple genetic etiology (cause). Such disorders include cystic fibrosis, hemochromatosis, Tay-Sachs, and sickle cell anemia. For example, cure for sickle cell disease (an inherited form of anemia in which distorted red blood cells—rigid, sticky, and shaped like sickles—are present in such numbers as to prevent adequate oxygen supply throughout the body) has gained prominence because it is related to an abnormal hemoglobin molecule, which comes from a well-understood genetic mutation. Hence efforts are concentrated on creating therapeutic strategies for fixing the mutated gene. Online Mendelian Inheritance in Man® (OMIM®) provides an Online Catalog of Human Genes and Genetic Disorders, a comprehensive database provides information about the etiology, clinical symptoms, and a bibliography of thousands of genetic conditions.[4]

4.2 Artificial intelligence (AI)

> *The true test of intelligence is not how much we know how to do, but how we behave when we don't know what to do. [30]*

This behavior is a product of the brain-mind system an individual is born with and the environment it finds itself in. From conception to death, behavior and intelligence evolve through intimate interaction between the individual and the environment where the individual essentially tries to coexist with the environment by exploring networking strategies, *inter alia*, based on its information gathering and processing abilities (see Section 5.2). In the past few decades, in an ongoing process, the *Homo sapiens* using technology they have intelligently developed have already acquired massive amounts of information and placed it in easily accessible public repositories along with some sophisticated automated information processing services. This has happened unexpectedly, suddenly, and on a massive scale at an exponential rate in multiple disciplines (including molecular biology) due to breakthroughs in communication and computing technologies engineered by an exceptionally intelligent group of *Homo sapiens*. This development is well on its way to dwarfing the intellectual abilities of almost all *Homo sapiens*. In comparison, individual human brain capacity to understand, assimilate, create, and deal with knowledge appears pathetic and along with it, its ability to find gainful employment in the future. Machines are rapidly learning to create and deal with knowledge. On the positive side,

> *There is a paradox in the growth of scientific knowledge. As information accumulates in ever more intimidating quantities, disconnected facts and impenetrable mysteries give way to rational explanations, and simplicity emerges from chaos. [31]*

It is this scientific knowledge ferreted out by a few geniuses among the *Homo sapiens*, which has allowed the species to extend their life span and improve their lifestyle by not just adapting to an environment but also by aiding the environment to adapt to humans. Along the way, Claude Shannon provided a mathematical theory that highlighted an important aspect of how data can be condensed and communicated efficiently in binary bitstreams. This was an important

[4] "OMIM contain information on all known mendelian disorders and over 15,000 genes. OMIM focuses on the relationship between phenotype and genotype. It is updated daily, and the entries contain copious links to other genetics resources." http://omim.org/about

step in handling data by finding structure in data to reduce redundancy in data representation [32].

Big data revolution, development and deployment of wearable medical devices, and mobile health applications have provided new powerful tools to the biomedical community for applying AI and machine learning algorithms to vast amount of data. Its impact in predictive analytics, precision medicine, virtual diagnosis, patient monitoring, and drug discovery and delivery is already being felt. More powerful advances are anticipated in the near future. Even at this early stage, AI excels even human experts in certain well but narrowly defined tasks. AI is at a stage where basic building blocks are being built. Soon we will learn to network these blocks and build increasingly powerful systems and subsystems that will solve increasingly complex problems and even create new knowledge. We already have a glimpse of it in Alphabet's AlphaGo Zero's ability to learn complex decision-making from scratch [33, 34]. "Previous versions of AlphaGo initially trained on thousands of human amateur and professional games to learn how to play Go. AlphaGo Zero skips this step and learns to play simply by playing games against itself, starting from completely random play. In doing so, it quickly surpassed human level of play and defeated the previously published champion-defeating version of AlphaGo by 100 games to 0" [34]. It acquired this ability within 40 days of self-training in an essentially iterative manner. The key here is the iterative strategy it used. Indeed, *Homo sapiens* too acquire knowledge iteratively but slowly over years and generations, collaboratively across space and time with other *Homo sapiens*, by making conjectures and refutations. It is rather uncanny that the essence of the process and its unusual power is mathematically captured by the Mandelbrot set in fractal geometry (see Section 5.3).

Notwithstanding AlphaGo's success, many real-life problems are still far too difficult not just for current AI systems but also for the vast-vast majority of *Homo sapiens*. The competition is really between two classes of geniuses: *Homo sapiens* who create *ab initio* knowledge and *Homo sapiens* who develop AI. Eventually, the latter is expected to win even if they must create an artificial brain using synthetic biology and place it in a humanoid! The task is enormously complex but not out-of-reach, in principle. What is needed is the ability to automate the task of observing and collecting data about the world and about us, create categories, data structures, and algorithms that would enable the collected data to be condensed into a computer program that can calculate the observations. This necessarily means that the size of the computer program (say, as represented by a binary string) must be as compact as possible (an index of the AI system's intelligence) compared to the collected data (also represented by a binary string). Till this is accomplished, the collected data would remain incomprehensible, that is, algorithmically random, theory-less, unstructured, and irreducible [35]. This is what *Homo sapiens* in the genius class devote themselves to. As Oren Etzioni notes, machine learning is still 99% human work:

> *The equation for AI success is to take a set of categories (for example, cats and dogs) and an enormous amount of data (that is labeled as to whether it is a cat or a dog), and then feed those two inputs through an algorithm. That produces the models that do the work for us. All three of those elements—categories, data, algorithm—are created through manual labor. [36]*

The solution to eliminating manual labor may well be the creation of an artificial brain using synthetic biology. For the present, AI serves mainly by "augmenting human intelligence". But then automation too had begun by augmenting brawn (muscle) power to eventually become the superbrawn power during the industrial revolution. It only required the *Homo sapiens* to intelligently harness and control steam by first connecting water, heat, and work and then creating the thermodynamics, the science that would allow machines to make human brawn power look insignificant. Today's augmented intelligence appears destined to become super-intelligence. We have learnt to harness and control reasoning by first connecting logic, axiomatic systems and theorem proving. We are now advancing rapidly into understanding information theory so that quantum computers can become information engines to do intelligent work. It is interesting that the concept of entropy appears fundamental both in thermodynamics and information theory. Both are offsprings of rational thought in physics, and both are intimately related.[5]

4.3 Quantum computing will power synthetic biology and AI

Quantum mechanics deals with the world inhabited by photons, electrons, protons, atoms, molecules, etc. and how they interact among themselves to create larger matter entities. It is an incredibly mysterious world understood only in the language of advanced mathematics. This is the part of physics that tells us how atoms congregate into molecules by adjusting the electrons they carry into configurations that we call chemical bonds, how strong or weak those bonds will be or whether they will bond at all, what a congregation's physical and chemical properties will be. It has led to many technical innovations and many more are expected, for example, in synthetic biology. The success of quantum mechanics in using mathematical abstractions is such that to a lay person it appears mystical, which even religious mystics cannot understand! Its remarkable success comes even though we still do not know what is meant by measurement in the quantum world and how the measurement process captures the information it outputs and why it releases information in a randomized way. Yet its success is undeniably visible:

> *Quantum mechanics is an immensely successful theory. Not only have all its predictions been experimentally confirmed to an unprecedented level of accuracy, allowing for a detailed understanding of the atomic and subatomic aspects of matter; the theory also lies at the heart of many of the technological advances shaping modern society – not least the transistor and therefore all of the electronic equipment that surrounds us. [38, 39]*

Understanding quantum mechanics is out of reach except for a few thousand people in the world at any given time! This should immediately alert us to the fact that human intelligence needed to cope with AI-QC combination in the future will be very high and successor species of the *Homo sapiens* must evolve in the direction of better and smarter brains rather than any other physical trait. Computation, comprehension, and cognition are all a part of the brain's activity, and we may assume that a sharper brain will come with a sharper mind. And we may further assume that comprehension and cognition are driven by computation in addition to using intuition, serendipity, flashes of inspiration, and inputs from the environment, etc. The keys are computation, problem-solving algorithms, and rational decision-making processes. These can be simulated by a classical computer, which itself has an abstract mathematical description we call the universal Turing machine (UTM) [12].

Computing technology has now advanced to a stage where quantum computers can do everything that a UTM can do, and some more. A quantum computer's phenomenal computing power comes from the extraordinary laws of quantum

---

[5] This we know from the explanation of the Maxwell's demon paradox in thermodynamics. See, e.g., [37].

mechanics that include such esoteric concepts as superposition of quantum states, entanglement ("spooky action at a distance"), and tunneling through insulating walls, which, though highly counterintuitive, play extremely useful roles in understanding Nature at subatomic levels. However, it is not clear if these concepts can be ignored in biology and living processes in the way they are ignored in the design of cars and airplanes. May be not because there are areas in biology where quantum effects have been found, for example, in protein-pigment (or ligand) complex systems [40]. Thus, while the role of quantum mechanics is clear in quantum computing and hence in advancing both AI and synthetic biology research, it is not yet known if in the design of DNA, knowledge of quantum mechanics is required or that natural selection favors quantum-optimized processes. Essentially, we do not know if any cellular DNA maintains or can maintain sustained entangled quantum states between different parts of the DNA (even if it involves only atoms in a nucleotide). But we cannot rule out the possibility that sporadic random entanglements do occur that result in biological mutations or that researchers will not be able to achieve it in the laboratory and find novel uses for it in synthetic biology [41]. For example, in principle, it is possible to design molecular quantum computers, insert them in cells that can observe cellular activity, and activate select chemical pathways in the cell in a programmed manner. There is increasing speculation that some brain activity, for example, cognition, may be quantum mechanical [42].

5. Integrating the triad: mechanization of speciation

A combination of emerging technologies such as CRISPR, AI, and QC; new delivery models for products and services that form the core around which *Homo sapiens* organize themselves through collaborative division of labor; and talent migration, driven not by rote education but by innate creativity and global opportunities for employment open to them is disrupting and changing the character of the global talent pool that society needs today. Globalization has created opportunities for the talented to reach the skies, but in a resource-constrained world, it also means that many others must be or feel deprived. Sections 5.2 and 5.3 provide some glimpses of the dynamics of this situation captured in mathematics. Because mathematics is abstract, the depicted dynamics apply to entities and situations whether they are animate or inanimate. A resource-constrained world provides ample scope for adversarial dynamics in which some are predators and others are preys. Globalization has accentuated the problem at all levels of social structure, and since speciation is triggered by a changing environment, it affects the DNA. This has created survivability demands on the *Homo sapiens*. As this pressure mounts beyond endurance, *Homo sapiens* will face speciation by natural selection with uncertain outcomes. However, in the case of *Homo sapiens*, this process too may face a disruptive change because the highly intelligent among them may boldly initiate speciation using upcoming advances in synthetic biology, perhaps after perfecting their techniques by creating humanoids (a hybrid creation of life with embedded intelligent machinery). This will be a watershed event where a species takes on the task of speciation on itself. This remarkable possibility arises because *Homo sapiens* created and mastered mathematics, rational thought, computing machinery, and eventually deep data analytics so that life could be designed by them in the laboratory to create superior species.

Synthetic biology, using methods and rational knowledge of molecular biology, physical sciences, and engineering, aims to design and construct novel biological parts, artificial biological pathways, devices, organisms, and systems for useful purposes. This will also permit us, at all levels of the hierarchy of biological structures (molecules, cells, tissues, and organisms), to redesign existing natural biological systems and may even help us recreate certain extinct species (if we can also recreate the environment, they had adapted to). It is not surprising that an extinct species has never revived itself since speciation and environment go together. Successes of synthetic biology will change the face of human civilization and almost certainly bring in new elements into play when *Homo sapiens* eventually speciate by playing an active role in it.

Since the discovery of the double-helix structure of cellular DNA by James Watson and Francis Crick in 1953 [43] and its significance that the "precise sequence of the bases is the *code* which carries the genetical *information* ..." (emphasis added) [44], the jargon and theory of information has invaded molecular biology (see Section 3). This enriched biotechnology and computational biology with nomenclature, definitions, concepts, and meanings. This also facilitates integration of synthetic biology with AI and QC. DNA is an information-carrying polymer. It is an organized chemical information database that *inter alia* carries the complete set of instructions for making all the proteins a cell will ever need.

Just 20 years after Watson and Crick, in 1973 Cohen and Boyer published their pioneering work in recombinant DNA [45] and gave birth to genetic engineering and the biotechnology industry based on their patents [46] under liberal licensing terms. The next landmark was the creation of a bacterial cell controlled by a chemically synthesized genome by Craig Venter and his group in 2010 [47]. In 2014, Floyd Romesberg and colleagues [48] reported the creation of a semisynthetic organism with an expanded genetic alphabet by creating artificial nucleotides not found in Nature. Since its discovery in 2012 [49–51], CRISPR gene editing technology pioneered by Jennifer Doudna and Emmanuelle Charpentier, and Feng Zhang has come to occupy center stage in molecular biology as a new way of making precise, targeted changes to the genome of a cell or an organism. It has set the stage for major advances in synthetic biology (see Section 4.1). Another major advance was reported by Venter and his research group in March 2016 following their successful creation in 2010 of a bacterial cell controlled by a chemically synthesized genome noted above. In fact, they succeeded in creating a bacterium that contains the minimal genetic ingredients needed for free living. The genome of this bacterium consists of only 473 genes, including 149 whose precise biological function is unknown. It is a minimalist version of the genome of Mycoplasma mycoides [52, 53].

Synthesis capabilities have developed at a pace where DNA synthesis is now automated. All one needs to do is to provide the desired DNA sequence to a vendor. Researchers in synthetic biology are now inching toward anticipating and preempting evolutionary events that if left to themselves would perhaps take a few million years to occur, and of even resurrecting extinct species. The time is ripe to integrate synthetic biology with AI and QC with a common language to enable seamless communication among them, connect with, and discover conceptual similarities for consistent integration of subsystems and validation of the whole system. That common language is mathematics; it comes with the added benefit that it can be used to also communicate between humans and machines. It is fortuitous that the DNA serves as the "Book of Life" that appears to have structure and grammar amenable to translation into mathematics. Once translated, biologists will discover some amazing patterns that have a direct bearing on life at the molecular level. We introduce a few of these below in brief.

5.1 The molecular logic of the living state

All macromolecules are constructed from a few simple compounds comprising a few atoms. It appears paradoxical that the DNA that serves as the epitome of life is itself lifeless. The molecule conforms to all the physical and chemical laws that describe the behavior of inanimate matter. All living organisms extract, transform, and use energy by interacting with the environment. Unlike inanimate matter, a living cell has the unique capacity, using the genetic information contained completely within itself, to grow and maintain itself and do mechanical, chemical, osmotic, and other types of work. But its most unique attribute is its programmed capacity to self-replicate and self-assemble. The great mystery that engulfs molecular biology is: "How does life emerge from an interacting collection of inanimate molecules that constitute living organisms to maintain and perpetuate life?" Once this is understood, chemical engineers will create a new life industry and commoditize it! Imagine buying customized pets as starters.

As noted in Section 3, the mystery of life is almost certainly encoded in mathematics. The chemical basis of life is one indication because chemistry now has a strong mathematical foundation via quantum chemistry. Even more striking is the fact that all living organisms—bacterium, fish, plant, bird, animal—share common basic chemical features, for example, the same basic structural unit (the cell), the same kind of macromolecules (DNA, RNA (ribonucleic acids), and proteins) built from the same kind of monomeric subunits (nucleotides and amino acids), the same pathways for synthesis of cellular components, the same genetic code, and evolutionary ancestors. The monomeric subunits can be covalently linked in a virtually limitless variety of sequences just as the 26 letters of the English alphabet or the two binary numbers (0, 1) in binary arithmetic can be arranged into a limitless number of strings that stand for words, sentences, books, computer programs, etc.

Organic compounds of molecular weight less than about 500, such as amino acids, nucleotides, and monosaccharides, serve as monomeric subunits of proteins, nucleic acids, and polysaccharides, respectively. A protein molecule may have a thousand or more amino acids linked in a chain, and DNA typically has millions of nucleotides arranged in sequence. Only a small number of chemical elements from the periodic table of chemistry appear in biomolecules. The carbon atom dominates and, by virtue of its special covalent bonding properties, permits the formation of a wide variety of molecules by bonding with itself, and atoms of hydrogen, oxygen, nitrogen, etc. Nature has placed further constraints. DNA is constructed from only four different kinds of subunits, the deoxyribonucleotides; the RNA is composed from just four types of ribonucleotides; and proteins are put together using 20 different kinds of amino acids. The 8 kinds of nucleotides (4 for DNA and 4 for RNA) from which all nucleic acids are built and the 20 amino acids from which all proteins are built are identical in all living organisms. So, at this level, living organisms are remarkably alike in their chemical makeup. This by itself provides a tantalizing hope that the DNA may indeed be completely decipherable as to its grammar and information content.

The above observations strongly suggest the likelihood of an underlying, as yet undiscovered set of "axioms" of life that enforce emergent, organizing principles around which diverse life forms evolve and adapt to the environment at various levels, without transgressing any physical or chemical law. The organizing principles appear to include (1) Nature is red in tooth and claw (species are connected to each other in a predator-prey, food-chain relationship in a sparse resource matrix), (2) rules of genetic inheritance, (3) rules of environmental adaptation, and (4) rules of speciation. At each level, the rules are likely to appear stochastic given that there are innumerable interacting factors ranging from nature to nurture.

5.2 Law of network phase transition

In 1960, Erdős and Rényi [54, 55] proved a remarkable result in graph theory, which implies that when a large number of entities (e.g., men, machines, ideas, or arbitrary combinations of them represented by dots) begin to connect (link) randomly, a critical condition arises, following which a phase transition occurs in the way the entities form or reform into clusters of connected entities. The critical condition is reached when in a set of n dots, $n/2$ random links are made. The phase transition abruptly creates a giant connected component, while the next largest component is quite small. Such giant components then grow or shrink rather slowly with the number of dots as they continue to link or delink. Such behavior is observed in protein interaction networks, telephone call graphs, scientific collaboration graphs, and many others [56]. This immediately suggests an *involuntary* mechanism by which a society at various levels of evolution, by connections alone, spontaneously reorganizes itself as nodes (people, machines, resources, etc.) link or delink in apparent randomness. It is highly pronounced in an Internet of Things (IoT) connected world where the millennials spontaneously polarize on issue-based networks that concern them on social media.

Synthetic biologists must never forget that between the molecular and environmental levels, there are multiple intermediate levels through which regulated command and control communications pass. At all levels, level-related phase transitions and predatory fights for resources can occur and spread to other levels. In fact, the intimately coupled relationship between *Homo sapiens* and the environment is often overlooked. We rarely note what Richard Ogle has that

> *[I]n making sense of the world, acting intelligently, and solving problems creatively, we do not rely solely on our mind's internal resources. Instead, we constantly have recourse to a vast array of culturally and socially embodied idea-spaces that populate the extended mind. These spaces ... are rich with embedded intelligence that we have progressively offloaded into our physical, social, and cultural environment for the sake of simplifying the burden on our own minds of rendering the world intelligible. Sometimes the space of ideas thinks for us. [57]*

The deep significance of this intimate bonding between the *Homo sapiens* and the environment is that while they are adapting to the environment, they are also helping the environment to adapt to them. When entities connect, they also acquire emergent properties by virtue of the relationships they are bound by. Certain static group properties emerge based on the network's topology, while dynamic properties emerge depending on the rate at which entities make, break, or modify connections. The fluctuating dynamics witnessed in the social media, for example, is common among the millennials.

Rapidly increasing connectivity among men and machines has imposed upon the global socio-politico-economic structure, a series of issue-dependent phase transitions. More will occur in areas where massive connectivity is in the offing. Immediately before a transition, existing man-made laws begin to crack, and in the transition, they break down. Posttransition, new laws must be framed and enforced to establish order. Since such a phase transition is a statistical phenomenon, the only viable way of managing it is to manage groups by abbreviating individual rights. The emergence of strongman style of leadership and its contagious spreading across the world is thus to be expected because job-seeking millennials will expect them to destroy the past and create a new future over the rubble. It appears inevitable that many humans will perish during the transition for lack of jobs or their inability to adapt to new circumstances. Robots and humanoids will gain domination over main job clusters, while society undergoes radical structural changes. Ironically, robots neither need jobs, nor job satisfaction, nor a livelihood. There will be ruthlessness in the reorganization.

5.3 The logistic map and the Mandelbrot set

Consider the iteration $x_{n+1} = r\,x_n\,(1 - x_n)$, called the logistic map, and a number-pair (r, x_0) where $r > 0$ and $0 < x_0 < 1$, and plot the points $(r, x_{n \to \infty})$. Note our interest is only in the long-term trajectory of x_0 and not in its transitory phase. Note $x_n + (1 - x_n) = 1$. The plot (**Figure 3**) has numerous 2-pronged pitchforks and hence is called the bifurcation diagram. Depending on r, x_n may be settled as for $0 < r \leq 3$, and beyond $r = 3$ migrating from one prong to another of available pitchforks for a given r in the bifurcation diagram. At $r = 4$ and beyond, migration is chaotic. In between $r = 3.5$ and 4, there is an intuitively unexpected white band where migration options are few. Such and other unexpected (not discussed here) display of rich complexity tethered to r independent of x_0 (i.e., the starting state) caught researchers by great surprise.

There are countless situations for which the logistic map captures the essence of a situation. For example, in genetics it describes the change in gene frequency in time, or in epidemiology the fraction of the population infected at time t, or in economics it depicts the relationship between commodity quantity and price, or in theories of learning the number of bits of information one can remember after an interval, or in the propagation of rumors the number of people who have heard the rumor after time t, etc. The logistic map allows us to assess the volatility of an adversarial environment by assessing r, that is, the ferocity with which the predators and preys are battling for resources.

Now consider the following complex iteration. Given the complex variable $z = x + iy$, where $i = \sqrt{-1}$ and the complex constant $c = a + ib$, pick a value for c, and iterate with the seed $z_0 = 0$. If the iterations diverge, then c is not in the Mandelbrot set (it is in the escape set), otherwise (even when it is trapped in some repeating loop or is wandering chaotically), it is in the Mandelbrot set (black points in **Figure 4**) M. (Setting z_0 equal to any point in the set that is not a periodic point gives the same result.) This is perhaps the most famous mathematical object yet known. It is a fractal object, an object that is irregular or fragmented at all scales. It is a major discovery of the late 20th century. It cannot be replicated in Euclidean geometry.

In 1981–1982, Adrien Douady and John H. Hubbard [58] proved that the Mandelbrot set is connected. Quite astoundingly, the Mandelbrot set, when magnified enough, is seen to contain rough copies of itself, tiny bug-like objects (molecules) floating off from the main body, but no matter how great the magnification, none of these molecules exactly match any other (see **Figure 5** and follow the white-bordered square from left to right). The boundary of M is where a Mandelbrot set computer program spends most of its time deciding if a point belongs there or not.

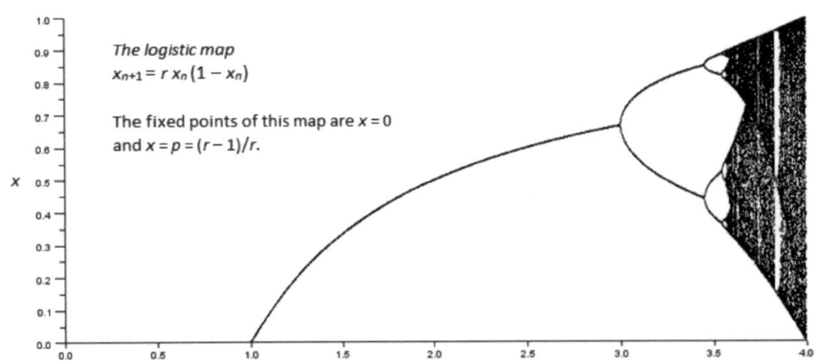

Figure 3.
The logistic map.

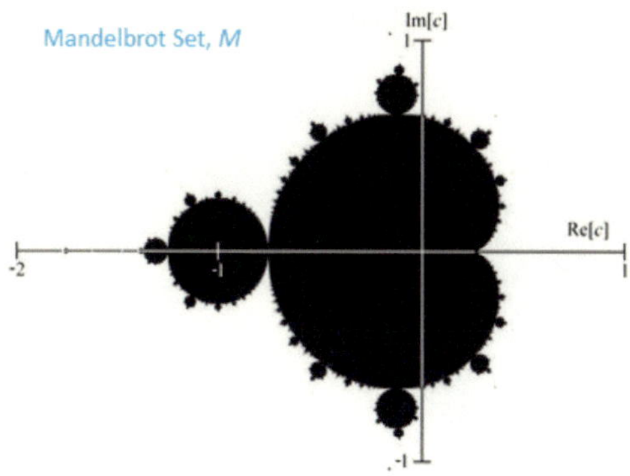

Figure 4.
Mandelbrot set.

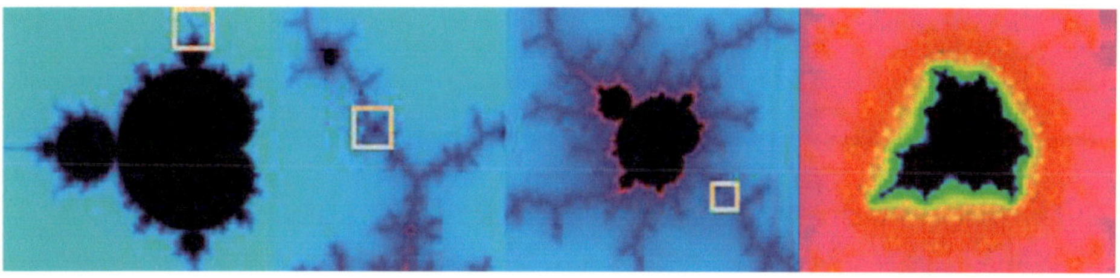

Figure 5.
Infinite variations of the Mandelbrot set are embedded in the set itself. Source: Ishaan Gulrajani, A zoom sequence of the Mandelbrot set showing quasi-self-similarity, 01 October 2011, https://commons.wikimedia.org/wiki/File:Blue_Mandelbrot_Zoom.jpg (Placed in public domain).

The simplicity of the iterative formula and the complexity of the Mandelbrot set leave one wondering how such a simple formula can produce a shape of great organic beauty and infinite subtle variation.

Since the logistic map and the Mandelbrot set map quadratic functions, and both represent behavior under iteration, it is not surprising that a one-to-one correspondence exists between the constants r and c and that the bifurcations created by r correspond to features that come with changes in c along the real axis where the Mandelbrot set compresses the information in the bifurcation diagram, that is, the map shows the points where the map converges to periodic oscillations and its periodicity, while the Mandelbrot set marks all the points, which end up oscillating, but the periodicity information is encoded in the bulbs of the set (see **Figure 6**).

It appears that the Mandelbrot set, *inter alia*, mimics the working of the mind. Its infinitely many variations embedded within itself seem to say that once the mind latches on to an idea and begins to deeply explore it, it does so by investigating its many variations, often in a random fashion (i.e., choosing c randomly), but does not abandon the core idea (the iterated function, equivalent of a law of Nature). On the other hand, if a mind randomly discovers a few of the dispersed similar looking sets, it begins a search for the mother set, M, itself. Is it then surprising that researchers often tackle new problems through random exploration based on a hunch (the iterated function), and if they are persistent enough, a solution finally emerges if the hunch is right? We see a game of conjectures and refutations at play here. On the other hand, the logistic map appears to work on a species scale where random interactions among minds lead to forming of societies (say, along the lines of the Erdős & Rényi theorem) functioning under constrained resources and an adversarial predator-prey law where the bifurcation points stand for points of speciation (measured in geological time scales).

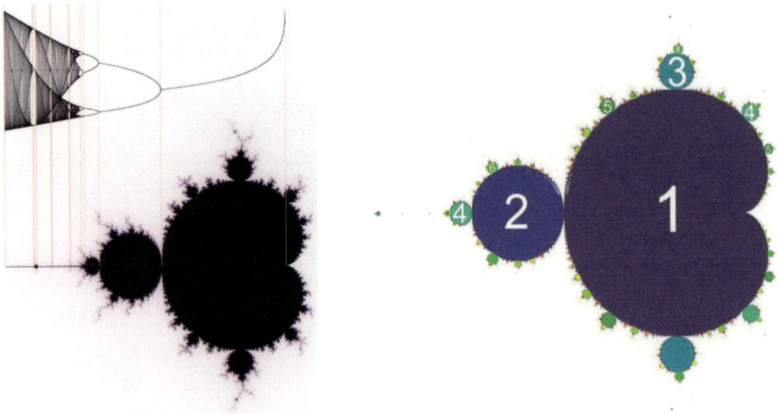

Figure 6.
(Left) Connection between the logistic map and the Mandelbrot set. (Public domain) Source: Georg-Johann Lay, 07 April 2008, at https://commons.wikimedia.org/wiki/File:Verhulst-Mandelbrot-Bifurcation.jpg. (Right) Frank Klemm, Mandelbrot set with periodicity of limiting sequences. 12 August 2017. https://commons.wikimedia.org/wiki/File:Mandelbrot_Set_%E2%80%93_Periodicities_coloured.png licensed under the Creative Commons Attribution-Share Alike 3.0 Unported.

The pace at which a system is driven through cyclic (iterative, also called self-referential) processes, that is, cycles of construction and destruction constrained by recyclable finite resources, has a profound effect on how the system evolves. A remarkably simple model as the logistic map shows an amazing variety of nonintuitive dynamics that a nonlinear system can display. It too provides a basic involuntary mechanism by which a society spontaneously reorganizes itself. In his seminal paper on the logistic map, Robert May, a theoretical ecologist and former President of the Royal Society (2000–2005) was so struck by the deep relationship between complexity and stability in natural communities that he exhorted:

> *Not only in research, but also in the everyday world of politics and economics, we would all be better off if more people realised that simple nonlinear systems do not necessarily possess simple dynamical properties. [59]*

What lessons can we draw from such simple mathematical models? For one, the logistic map indicates that the Earth's supply chain (the environment) has been grossly disrupted. In this predator-prey game where some *Homo sapiens* turn into predators and the rest into preys, a massive capture of supplies by predators results in a massive population of preys, and the preys must mutate or speciate to survive or die. The logistic map decides how the selfish genes play the game while the *Homo sapiens* mainly decide the value of r. The Mandelbrot set tells us that while the laws of Nature need not change for the environment to change, it does contain enough complexities in the form of fractal structures whereby the environment may change enough to force speciation to take place in niches. In the present innovation-driven environment, speciation will push to enhance the brain-mind system of the *Homo sapiens*. In the process, synthetic biology may discover life as we *do not* know it. The survival of the fittest is a statistical law and hence it rests on an ensemble being available. The world's current population certainly fulfills that.

In the present global environment, saturated by connectivity between humans, machines, and ideas, the largest component emerging in any socioeconomic context is populated by the deprived who cannot fend for themselves. *Inter alia*, this is highly visible at multiple scales of population size (global, national, provincial, urban, etc.) and context (employment, access to health care, education, skill development, etc.). A wide spectrum of power, opportunities, and assets are grabbed by a minority by simply ignoring the plight of the desperate. This alone enforces a massive decimation of the *Homo sapiens*' gene pool. Among the predators, many with inherited wealth (and hence generally lacking survival skills but not the means) too will become preys. In this planetary-scale debacle, a unique minority endowed with an exceptional brain-mind system, perhaps aided by AI and QC, will strive to improve their gene pool by artificial speciation[6] using synthetic biology and insulate themselves in an artificially created environment to improve their cognitive abilities, life span, and fecundity. A look at the logistic map shows that as the new species advance even more rapidly, increasingly wild fluctuations in their fortunes will take place within their insulated, resource-constrained environment unless they reduce r by allowing the environment to replenish itself.

In the absence of irreversible ecological damage, it is possible that, in the early stages, replenishment may happen by itself since Nature would have decimated a large component of the population from the less developed countries, thus presenting the survivors with a sudden increase in per capita resources. We may infer by analogy from the Mandelbrot set that once a new species survives long enough to avoid extinction (because it begins with a small population, which needs time to grow into adulthood), even if it is in some remote fringes of the set, it will likely someday reach the main (central) part of the set since the set is connected. Once this happens, the new species will likely continue for a very long time until it is decimated by the Sun entering its dying phase by turning into a giant red star. That will be a few billion years hence.

5.4 Creating novel DNA algorithmically

The way we acquire knowledge is iterative and nonlinear—we conjecture and put our conjectures on trial, that is, put them to severe critical tests (refutations). As the trial progresses, we edit, discard, refine, and add to our conjectures in a pseudorandom manner controlled by criticism, driven by instinct, hunches, inspiration, etc. Conjectures and refutations in scientific research are deemed self- and community-driven adversarial processes. We connect the dots. At every step of linking the dots, we consult the axioms (conjectures) and the rules for deriving conclusions (theorems) to ensure that we are within the axiomatic system we have put on trial. This means that the process leads us to understand the Universe solely based on our chosen beliefs (axiomatic system).

> *As we learn from our mistakes our knowledge grows, even though we may never know—that is, know for certain. Since our knowledge can grow, there can be no reason here for despair of reason. And since we can never know for certain, there can be no authority here for any claim to authority, for conceit over our knowledge, or for smugness. [1, Preface]*

As far as we can tell, creating an axiomatic system is a nonmathematical and a highly intelligent act. Developing a sequence of theorems with a specific nontrivial goal in mind (developing algorithms) is also a highly intelligent act. However, executing an algorithm, once developed, can be mechanized and does not require intelligence, in fact, none at all. If the most useful aspect of intelligence

[6] A controversial experiment to this effect seems to have been successfully conducted by He Jiankui who recently presented his work at the Second International Summit on Human Genome Editing in Hong Kong, November 27–29, 2018, http://www.nationalacademies.org/gene-editing/2nd_summit/index.htm [60, 61].

is algorithmic, then it must be mechanizable and converted into computation. We believe the DNA is a book of knowledge about the birth and death of life. In principle, it is in machine-readable form. AI and quantum computing are the most powerful tools we presently have to decipher it. When AI drives our lives, it is the algorithm that really drives us.

Some recent bold experiments using CRISPR gene editing have provided glimpses of DNA editing as a new source of creating a variety of biomatter and life forms. For example, experiments are in progress for producing meat (beef, pork, poultry, and sea food) without killing animals by growing meat in the laboratory from cultured stem cells by multiplying them dramatically and allowing them to differentiate into primitive fibers that then bulk up to form muscle tissue. This would substantially reduce environmental costs of meat production and eliminate much of the cruel and unethical treatment of animals [62]. Another example is producing offsprings from same-sex mice parents, again using stem cells and CRISPR gene editing technology [63].

In another development, till recently it was believed that mitochondrion DNA (mtDNA) in nearly all mammals (including humans) is inherited exclusively from the mother. However, recently, Luo et al. [64] have uncovered multiple instances of biparental inheritance of mtDNA "spanning three unrelated multiple generation families, a result confirmed by independent sequencing across multiple unrelated laboratories with different methodologies. Surprisingly, this pattern of inheritance appears to be determined in an autosomal dominant like manner." Given that the mitochondrion is an energy-producing organelle in the cell, this discovery will have profound implications in synthetic biology and in the design of new drugs.

Once humans master the art of designing DNA for self-replicating, multicellular organisms (we already know how to design cells not found in Nature and edit DNA), they will create living species of their own design. We also anticipate that when AI machines master the art of learning from mistakes (i.e., the art of making conjectures and refuting them in a spiraling process toward better knowledge, a possibility that mathematically exists), they would have taught themselves how to handily beat humans in intelligent activities and thereby break the human monopoly on intelligence. The seeds of this were sown when the AI program called AlphaGo decisively defeated the world's greatest Go players in 2016 [65, 66]. AlphaGo has achieved what many scientific researchers had dreamed of achieving. It means that a machine can teach itself in a tiny fraction of the time it takes humans to explore *ab initio* any axiomatic system. The last bastion of human supremacy over all other creatures on Earth in the form of intelligence has been cracked by AI machines. This is the world the millennials have stepped into. We have no idea how AI machines may organize themselves into networks and network with humans and *vice versa*. Will the future be written and created by humanoids with humans finding themselves relegated to footnotes and appendices once biotechnology and AI integrate? (See, e.g., [14].)

So, what comes after *Homo sapiens*? Given the accelerating march of AI and computing, everything points to the dominating power of algorithms created and executed by quantum computers. It is a matter of understanding how to create novel DNA sequences and creating an environment for it to thrive. It is about writing lengthy books of life using natural and artificial nucleotides. With AI-embedded quantum computers capable of surpassing human intelligence, and the smartest among them developing Godlike abilities, the raw material they will be hunting for is massive amounts of data and mining that data for usable information for the welfare of one or more new species to whom the *Homo sapiens* will be ancestors.

6. Conclusions

The stage appears set for some remarkable advances in synthetic biology including artificial speciation as an alternative to the natural evolution of species. *Homo sapiens* are now poised to change the evolutionary destiny of life forms (including their own) they choose to target and even design-to-order new life forms. The ramifications are far and wide (see, e.g., [67]). Creating species that can thrive on other planets, colonizing the Moon with single-celled life, etc. are no longer science fiction fantasies.

We, the *Homo sapiens*,[7] have been around for about 300,000 years [17, 18]. Records of our civilization date back approximately 6000 years. Since *Homo sapiens* are still evolving, speciation may yet produce superior creatures with new attributes that can give them superior knowledge of the Universe and its origin. After all, it is speciation that made the *Homo sapiens* overwhelmingly superior in intellect from the great apes and our cousins, the chimpanzees with whom we share 96% of our DNA sequence. "Darwin wasn't just provocative in saying that we descend from the apes—he didn't go far enough. We are apes in every way, from our long arms and tailless bodies to our habits and temperament."[8] Yet, at an intellectual level, within a span of few centuries, at the knee of the exponential curve that breathed energetic intellectual life into our neural and socioeconomic networks, we have attained such remarkable feats as formalizing and mechanizing axiomatic systems, discovering deep secrets of the Universe, partially mechanizing brain-mind activities, developing technologies that augment, supplement, and amplify our comparatively puny brain and brawn capacities. Within the past century or so, we have fathomed the power and limitations of rational thought and binary arithmetic to express it in, mechanized arithmetical calculations to unimaginable heights, and used this mechanization to develop robotics, 3D precision manufacturing, biotechnology, AI, QC, cloud computing, etc. These developments are now rapidly networking, the scale of which is such that we now see the combined effects of phase transition of graph theory in the Internet of Things (IoT) (creation and destruction of interlinked man-machine-idea components), of the logistic map in the rapidly changing socioeconomic scenarios that have increasingly made predicting the future at all levels of aggregating individuals a game of dice. The relationship between the logistic map and the Mandelbrot set implies that the future of *Homo sapiens* will indeed be so complex that a new species capable of handling that level of complexity must either evolve or be artificially created.

The raw physical limitations of the *Homo sapiens*' brain-mind system is distressingly visible in its waning ability to earn a living. Barring exceptional *Homo sapiens*, our search for meaning in life is now propelled by search engines roaming the Internet and not by our brains. The World Wide Web (WWW) has changed the way we think, what we think about, and how we communicate our thoughts. The millennials' cognitive abilities are very different from those they were born with and weaned on before the Internet invaded their lives. They are shaped not just by what they read but by how they read. Not only has their lifestyle changed but also has their thought style. All the work of the mind—deep thinking, exhaustive reading, deep analysis, introspection, etc.—is now delegated to AI machines. Humans have thus relinquished their right to control their individual lives and direct their souls (maybe deep inside they already know there is no soul!). If machines can outdo humans so easily without a soul, then perhaps the soul is holding humans back from

---

[7] The term *Homo sapiens* was coined by Carl Linnaeus in 1758.

[8] A quote from Frans de Waal, a primate scientist at Emory University in Atlanta, Georgia, as it appeared in [68].

reaching their potential. Perhaps it is time, AI machines became our role models and our mentors [14].

Modern computers have made increasingly powerful and compute intensive mathematical algorithms accessible to even those not trained in science and mathematics for solving complex problems. Rapid advances in artificial intelligence (AI) and quantum computing show an inevitable trend that a vast array of human activities that till now required intelligent *Homo sapiens* to perform and earn a livelihood will soon be performed by AI-enabled computers, including the design of cellular life forms. When this happens, can human-designed speciation of life forms, its DNA coded for superintelligence, and other designed characteristics be prevented by the *Homo sapiens*' instinct for survival? One day, nanotechnology will enable biocompatible, implantable, programmable quantum computers to be embedded into our organs or even introduce specialized new miniature organs, and we will be on our way to creating humanoids. We do not know how this will affect the speciation of the *Homo sapiens*. But before insight-driven complex experimentation aided by deep computing can happen; AI, new quantum algorithms, and embeddable quantum computers will have to evolve. Some early successes, for example, creation of artificial nucleotides, designed cells, attempts at resurrecting extinct species, etc. in molecular biology, indicate that once we master the biochemistry of very-very large molecules, for example, the DNA, RNA, proteins, by understanding their structure and their chemical-structural dynamics through quantum mechanical models, interactions between living and nonliving matter will undergo a sea change.

We therefore anticipate a forced speciation of the *Homo sapiens*. It will drastically reduce the emergence time for a new species to a few years compared to Nature's hundreds of millennia. Accelerated speciation by *Homo sapiens* via domestication, gene splicing, and gene drive mechanisms is now scientifically well understood. Synthetic biology can advance speciation far more rapidly using a combination of CRISPR technology, advanced computing technologies, and knowledge creation using AI. There is no reason why *Homo sapiens* themselves will not initiate their own speciation once synthetic biology advances to a level where it can safely modify the brain to temper emotion and enhance rational thinking as a means of competing against AI-embedded machines guided by quantum algorithms.

Rapidly advancing research in the life sciences, while promising tools to meet global challenges in health, agriculture, the environment, and economic development, some of which are already on the horizon, also raises the specter of new social, ethical, legal, and security challenges. These include the development of ethical principles for human genome editing, establishment of regulatory systems for the safe conduct of field trials of gene drive-modified organisms, and many others. Additional concerns arise since the knowledge, tools, and techniques resulting from such research could easily lead to the development of bioweapons, facilitate bioterrorism, and the extinction of the *Homo sapiens* themselves. All these concerns are global not merely national [69]. The subject of this chapter goes beyond such concerns because here the concern is the possibility of self-initiated speciation of the *Homo sapiens*. The ramification of such a self-referential (iterative) process akin to that of the logistic map and the Mandelbrot set involving, in addition, phase transitions seen in graph theory is unknown. The perspective presented in this chapter is vastly different from that of Erwin Schrödinger (among the pioneers of quantum mechanics) expressed in 1944 [70]. Much water has flown under the bridge since then. A decade later, in 1953, when the structure of the DNA and its role in replicating life was discovered by Watson and Crick [43, 44], molecular biology was born. That led to genetic engineering [45] and synthetic biology [47]. As we write, CRISPR-Cas9 has been used to alter the embryonic genes of twin girls born in December 2018 in China [60, 61], which has elicited deep concern in the scientific community and an immediate response from the WHO: "Gene editing may have unintended consequences, this is uncharted water and it has to be taken seriously ... WHO is putting together experts. We will work with member states to do everything we can to make sure of all issues—be it ethical, social, safety—before any manipulation is done" [71]. On the heels of this report comes the news that the world's first baby born via womb transplant from a dead donor has been successfully achieved in Brazil [72]. With CRISPR, AI, and QC, the *Homo sapiens* are now on the threshold of creating new life forms and initiating even their own speciation.

Author details

Rajendra K. Bera
Acadinnet Education Services India Pvt. Ltd., Bangalore, India

*Address all correspondence to: rajendrabera@yahoo.com

References

[1] Popper KR. Conjectures and Refutations: The Growth of Scientific Knowledge. London: Routledge; 1963. 412 p

[2] An Overview of the Human Genome Project. National Human Genome Research Institute. No date. Available from: https://www.genome.gov/12011239/a-brief-history-of-the-human-genome-project/ [Accessed: 01-12-2018]

[3] International Human Genome Sequencing Consortium Publishes Sequence and Analysis of the Human Genome. National Human Genome Research Institute. 2001. Available from: https://www.genome.gov/10002192/2001-release-first-analysis-of-human-genome/ [Accessed: 01-12-2018]

[4] The Human Cell Atlas. White Paper. The HCA Consortium. 2017. Available from: https://www.humancellatlas.org/files/HCA_WhitePaper_18Oct2017.pdf [Accessed: 01-12-2018]

[5] Major Brain Initiatives around the Globe. International Neuroinformatics Coordinating Facility. (No date). Available from: https://www.incf.org/about-us/major-brain-initiatives-around-the-globe [Accessed: 01-12-2018]

[6] Watts N et al. The 2018 report of the *Lancet* countdown on health and climate change: Shaping the health of nations for centuries to come. The Lancet. 2018;**Online**:1-36. DOI: 10.1016/S0140-6736(18)32594-7

[7] Reward Work, Not Wealth. Oxfam International. 2018. Available from: https://www.oxfam.org/en/research/reward-work-not-wealth [Accessed: 01-12-2018]

[8] Pimentel DAV, Aymar IA, Lawson M. Reward Work, Not Wealth. Oxfam International. 2018. Available from: https://d1tn3vj7xz9fdh.cloudfront.net/s3fs-public/file_attachments/bp-reward-work-not-wealth-220118-en.pdf [Accessed: 01-12-2018]

[9] Moyo D. The African Threat. Project Syndicate. 2018. Available from: https://www.project-syndicate.org/onpoint/the-african-threat-by-dambisa-moyo-2018-11 [Accessed: 01-12-2018]

[10] Ray Kurzweil Predicts Computers Will be as Smart as Humans in 12 Years. Fox News. 2017. Available from: http://www.foxnews.com/tech/2017/03/16/ray-kurzweil-predicts-computers-will-be-as-smart-as-humans-in-12-years.html [Accessed: 01-12-2018]

[11] Reedy C. Kurzweil Claims That the Singularity Will Happen by 2045. Futurism. 2017. Available from: https://futurism.com/kurzweil-claims-that-the-singularity-will-happen-by-2045/ [Accessed: 01-12-2018]

[12] Turing AM. On computable numbers, with an application to the entscheidungsproblem. Proceedings of the London Mathematical Society. 1937;**S2-42**(1):230-265. Available from: https://www.cs.virginia.edu/~robins/Turing_Paper_1936.pdf correction at: Turing AM. On computable numbers, with an application to the entscheidungsproblem. A Correction. 1938;S2-43(1):544-546. DOI: 10.1112/plms/s2-42.1.230

[13] Gödel K. Über formal unentseheidbare Sätze der Principia Mathematica und verwandter systeme I. Monatshefte für Mathematik und Physik. 1931;**38**:173-198. (On Formally Undecidable Propositions of Principia Mathematica and Related Systems I.) Available from: http://jacqkrol.x10.mx/assets/articles/godel-1931.pdf for an English translation by B. Meltzer [Accessed: 01-12-2018]

[14] Bera RK. AI Powered Society. SSRN. 2018. Available from: https://ssrn.com/abstract=3256873 [Accessed: 01-12-2018]

[15] Kurzweil R. How My Predictions are Faring. kurzweilai.net. 2010. Available from: http://www.kurzweilai.net/images/How-My-Predictions-Are-Faring.pdf [Accessed: 01-12-2018]

[16] Kennedy M. Best Futurists Ever: Ray Kurzweil's Predictions for the Future of Technology, Medicine, and A.I. RossDawson.com. 2018. Available from: https://rossdawson.com/futurist/best-futurists-ever/ray-kurzweil/ [Accessed: 01-12-2018]

[17] Hublin J-J et al. New fossils from Jebel Irhoud, Morocco and the Pan-African origin of *Homo sapiens*. Nature 2017;**546**:289-292. Available from: http://www.nature.com/articles/nature22336 [Accessed: 01-12-2018]

[18] Richter D et al. The age of the Hominin fossils from Jebel Irhoud, Morocco, and the origins of the Middle Stone Age. Nature. 2017;**546**:293-296. Available from: http://www.nature.com/articles/nature22335 [Accessed: 01-12-2018]

[19] Lehninger AL. Biochemistry. 2nd ed. New York: Worth Publishers; 1975

[20] Hofstadter DR. Gödel, Escher, Bach: An Eternal Golden Braid. New York: Vintage Books; 1989. xxi, 777 p

[21] Stewart I. Life's Other Secret: The New Mathematics of the Living World. New York: Wiley; 1999. 286 p

[22] Tegmark M. Our Mathematical Universe: My Quest for the Ultimate Nature of Reality. New York: Knopf; 2014. 432 p

[23] Feynman RP. The Character of Physical Law. New York: The Modern Library; 1994. (Originally published by BBC in 1965)

[24] Laplace PS. A Treatise of Celestial Mechanics. Dublin: Richard Milliken; 1822. Available from: https://archive.org/details/treatiseofcelest12lapl [Accessed: 01-12-2018]

[25] Ball WWR. A Short Account of the History of Mathematics. London: Macmillan; 1893. p. 423. Available from: https://archive.org/details/117770582 [Accessed: 01-12-2018]

[26] O'Neill S. How to 3D-print a living, beating heart. New Scientist. 2018. Available from: https://www.newscientist.com/article/mg24032040-400-how-to-3d-print-a-living-beating-heart/ [Accessed: 01-12-2018]

[27] Gilpin L. 3D 'bioprinting': 10 things you should know about how it works. TechRepublic. 2014. Available from: https://www.techrepublic.com/article/3d-bioprinting-10-things-you-should-know-about-how-it-works/ [Accessed: 01-12-2018]

[28] Bioprinted Human Tissue. Organo. 2018. Available from: https://organovo.com/science-technology/bioprinting-process/ [Accessed: 01-12-2018]

[29] Synthego. Everything You Need to Know About CRISPR-Cas9. CRISPER 101. 2018. Available from: https://www.synthego.com/learn/crispr [Accessed: 02-12-2018]

[30] Holt JC. How Children fail. Penguin Education; 1964, p. 163. Available from: http://www.schoolofeducators.com/wp-content/uploads/2011/12/HOW-CHILDREN-FAIL-JOHN-HOLT.pdf [Accessed: 02-12-2018]

[31] Alberts B et al. Molecular Biology of the Cell. 4th ed. New York: Garland Science; 2002. 3786 p. Available from: https://archive.org/details/AlbertsMolecularBiologyOfTheCell4thEd [Accessed: 01-12-2018] (In the Preface; as quoted from the Preface of the 1st ed. 1983)

[32] Shannon CE. A mathematical theory of communication. Reprinted with corrections from the Bell System Technical Journal. 1948:379-423, 623-656. Available from: https://www.cs.ucf.edu/~dcm/Teaching/COP5611-Spring2012/Shannon48-MathTheoryComm.pdf [Accessed: 02-12-2018]

[33] Silver D et al. Mastering the game of go without human knowledge. Nature 2017;**550**:354-359. Available from: http://www.nature.com/articles/nature24270 [Accessed: 02-12-2018]

[34] AlphaGo Zero: Learning from scratch. DeepMind.com. (no date). Available from: https://deepmind.com/blog/alphago-zero-learning-scratch/ Accessed: 02-12-2018

[35] Chaitin GJ. Leibniz, Information, math and physics. arXiv:math. 2003. Available from: http://arxiv.org/abs/math/0306303 [Accessed: 02-12-2018]

[36] National Academies of Sciences, Engineering, and Medicine. Artificial Intelligence and Machine Learning to Accelerate Translational Research: Proceedings of a Workshop—in Brief. Washington, DC: The National Academies Press. 2018. 9 p. DOI: 10.17226/25197

[37] Plenio MB, Vitelli V. The physics of forgetting: Landauer's erasure principle and information theory. Contemporary Physics.. 2001;**42**(1):25-60. Available from: https://pdfs.semanticscholar.org/d755/e42ff95317bd58f6815098a26df7cb4d1edc.pdf [Accessed: 02-12-2018]

[38] Zinkernagel H. Are we living in a quantum world? Bohr and quantum fundamentalism. In: Aaserud F, Kragh H, editors. One Hundred Years of the Bohr Atom: Proceedings from a Conference. Scientia Danica. Series M: Mathematica et Physica. Vol. 1. Copenhagen: Royal Danish Academy of Sciences and Letters; 2015. pp. 419-434. Available from: http://philsci-archive.pitt.edu/11785/1/BohrQuantumWorld.pdf [Accessed: 02-12-2018]

[39] Zinkernagel H. Niels Bohr on the wave function and the classical/quantum divide. Studies in History and Philosophy of Modern Physics. 2016;**53**:9-19. Available from: https://arxiv.org/abs/1603.00353 [Accessed: 02-12-2018]

[40] Brookes JC. Quantum effects in biology: Golden rule in enzymes, olfaction, photosynthesis and magnetodetection. Proceedings of the Royal Society A, Mathematical, Physical and Engineering Sciences. 2017;**473**:20160822. DOI: 10.1098/rspa.2016.0822

[41] Brooks M. Is quantum physics behind your brain's ability to think? New Scientist, 2015. Available from: https://www.newscientist.com/article/mg22830500-300-is-quantum-physics-behind-your-brains-ability-to-think/ [Accessed: 02-12-2018]

[42] Fisher MPA. Quantum cognition: The possibility of processing with nuclear spins in the brain. Annals of Physics. 2015;**362**:593-602. DOI: 10.1016/j.aop.2015.08.020

[43] Watson JD, Crick FHC. Molecular structure of nucleic acids. Nature. 1953;**171**(4356):737-738. Available from: http://www.nature.com/scitable/content/molecular-structure-of-nucleic-acids-a-structure-13997975 [Accessed: 02-12-2018]

[44] Watson JD, Crick FHC. Genetical implications of the structure of deoxyribonucleic acid. Nature. 1953;**171**(4361):964-967. Available from https://profiles.nlm.nih.gov/ps/access/SCBBYX.pdf [Accessed: 02-12-2018]

[45] Cohen SN, Chang ACY, Boyer HW, Helling RB. Construction of biologically

functional bacterial plasmids in vitro. Proceedings of the National Academy of Sciences of the United States of America. 1973;**70**(11):3240-3244. DOI: 10.1073/pnas.70.11.3240

[46] Bera RK. The story of the Cohen-Boyer patents. Current Science. 2009;**96**(6):760-763. Available from: http://www.currentscience.ac.in/Downloads/article_id_096_06_0760_0763_0.pdf [Accessed: 02-12-2018]

[47] Gibson D et al. Creation of a bacterial cell controlled by a chemically synthesized genome. Science. 2010;**329**(5987):52-56. DOI: 10.1126/science.1190719

[48] Malyshev DA et al. A semi-synthetic organism with an expanded genetic alphabet. Nature. 2014;**509**(7500):385-388. Available from: http://www.ncbi.nlm.nih.gov/pubmed/24805238 [Accessed: 02-12-2018]

[49] Jinek M et al. A programmable dual-RNA-guided DNA endonuclease in adaptive bacterial immunity. Science. 2012;**337**(6096):816-821. Available from: https://www.ncbi.nlm.nih.gov/pubmed/22745249 [Accessed: 02-12-2018]

[50] Cong L et al. Multiplex genome engineering using CRISPR/Cas systems. Science. 2013;**339**(6121):819-823. Available from: http://www.ncbi.nlm.nih.gov/pmc/articles/PMC3795411/ [Accessed: 02-12-2018]

[51] Sharlach M. CRISPR Pioneers Honored. The Scientist. 2014. Available from: http://www.the-scientist.com/?articles.view/articleNo/41455/title/CRISPR-Pioneers-Honored/ [Accessed: 02-12-2018]

[52] Hutchison III CA et al. Design and synthesis of a minimal bacterial genome. Science. 2016;**351**(6280):1414, aad6253-1-11. DOI: 10.1126/science.aad6253

[53] Saey TH. Scientists build minimum-genome bacterium. Science News. 2016. Available from: https://www.sciencenews.org/article/scientists-build-minimum-genome-bacterium [Accessed: 02-12-2018]

[54] Erdös P, Rényi A. On the evolution of random graphs. Publications of the Hungarian Academy of Sciences. 1960;**5**(1):17-61. Available from: https://users.renyi.hu/~p_erdos/1960-10.pdf [Accessed: 02-12-2018]

[55] Krivelevich M, Sudakov B. The Phase Transition in Random Graphs—A Simple Proof. arXiv: 1201.6529v4 [math.CO]. 2012. Available from: https://arxiv.org/pdf/1201.6529v4.pdf [Accessed: 02-12-2018]

[56] Bollobas B, Janson S, Riordan O. The Phase Transition in Inhomogeneous Random Graphs. arXiv:math/0504589 [math.PR]. 2007. Available from: https://arxiv.org/abs/math/0504589 [Accessed: 02-12-2018]. Also as: Random Structures and Algorithms. 2007;**31**:3-122

[57] Ogle R. Smart World: Breakthrough Creativity and the New Science of Ideas. Boston, Massachusetts: Harvard Business School Press; 2007. 303 p

[58] Douady A, Hubbard JH. Exploring the Mandelbrot set. The Orsay Notes. 2009. Available from: http://pi.math.cornell.edu/~hubbard/OrsayEnglish.pdf [Accessed: 03-12-2018]

[59] May RM. Simple mathematical models with very complicated dynamics. Nature. 1976;**261**:459-467. Available from: http://abel.harvard.edu/archive/118r_spring_05/docs/may.pdf [Accessed: 03-12-2018]

[60] Wilson C. Scientists are now very sure that the babies really were gene-edited. New Scientist. 2018. Available from: https://www.newscientist.com/

article/2186956-scientists-are-now-very-sure-that-the-babies-really-were-gene-edited/ [Accessed: 03-12-2018]

[61] Le Page M. CRISPR Babies: More Details on the Experiment that Shocked the World. New Scientist. 2018. Available from: https://www.newscientist.com/article/2186911-crispr-babies-more-details-on-the-experiment-that-shocked-the-world/ [Accessed: 03-12-2018]

[62] Schaefer G. Lab-Grown Meat. Scientific American. 2018. Available from: https://www.scientificamerican.com/article/lab-grown-meat/ [Accessed: 03-12-2018]

[63] Maron DF. Same-sex mice parents give birth to healthy brood. Scientific American. 2018. Available from: https://www.scientificamerican.com/article/same-sex-mice-parents-give-birth-to-healthy-brood/ [Accessed: 03-12-2018]

[64] Luo S et al. Biparental inheritance of mitochondrial DNA in humans. In: Proceedings of the National Academy of Sciences. 2018. DOI: 10.1073/pnas.1810946115

[65] Gibney E. Google masters go. Nature. 2016;**529**:445-446. Available from: http://www.nature.com/polopoly_fs/1.19234!/menu/main/topColumns/topLeftColumn/pdf/529445a.pdf [Accessed: 03-12-2018]

[66] Gibney E. Google secretly tested AI bot. Nature. 2017;**541**:142. Available from: http://www.nature.com/polopoly_fs/1.21253!/menu/main/topColumns/topLeftColumn/pdf/nature.2017.21253.pdf [Accessed: 03-12-2018]

[67] Doudna JA, Sternberg SHA. Crack in Creation: Gene Editing and the Unthinkable Power to Control Evolution. New York: Houghton Mifflin Harcourt; 2017. 307 p

[68] Lovgren S. Chimps, Humans 96 Percent the Same, Gene Study Finds. National Geographic News. 2005. Available from: https://news.nationalgeographic.com/news/2005/08/0831_050831_chimp_genes.html [Accessed: 03-12-2018]

[69] Revill J, Husbands J, Bowman K, Rapporteurs. Governance of Dual Use Research in the Life Sciences: Advancing Global Consensus on Research Oversight: Proceedings of a Workshop. Washington, DC: The National Academies Press; 2018. Available from: http://nap.edu/25154 [Accessed: 04-12-2018]

[70] Schrödinger E. What is life? The physical aspect of the living Cell. 1944. Available from: http://www.whatislife.ie/downloads/What-is-Life.pdf [Accessed: 04-12-2018]

[71] Nebehay S. WHO Looks at Standards in 'Uncharted Water' of Gene Editing. Reuters. 2018. Available from: https://www.reuters.com/article/us-china-health-who/who-looks-at-standards-in-uncharted-water-of-gene-editing-idUSKBN1O227Q [Accessed: 05-12-2018]

[72] Kelland K. World's First Baby Born via Womb Transplant from Dead Donor. Reuters. 2018. Available from: https://www.reuters.com/article/us-health-womb-transplant/worlds-first-baby-born-via-womb-transplant-from-dead-donor-idUSKBN1O32WS [Accessed: 05-12-2018]

Chapter 3

Construction and Analysis of Metagenome Library from Bacterial Community Associated with Toxic Dinoflagellate *Alexandrium tamiyavanichii*

Muhd Danish-Daniel, Mohd Ezhar Mohd Noor, Yik Sung Yeong, Tan Min Pau and Gires Usup

Abstract

Previous studies have suggested that a specific community of bacteria coexists within the phycosphere of marine dinoflagellates. In order to better understand the dinoflagellate-bacteria relationships, a fosmid clone library was constructed from the metagenome DNA and analyzed. Some of the fosmid clones were end-sequenced. A total of 1501 fosmid clones with insert sizes of 30–40 Kbp were produced. End sequencing of 238 clones showed that 55% of the genes had known functions, 11% were of putative function and 34% were genes of unknown function or had no match in Genbank. There were approximately 14% sequences with no classification and could potentially represent novel genes. Analysis of these partial sequences also revealed some promising enzymes that possess various potential industrial applications such as chitinases, kinases, agarases and oxygenases. The results also showed that the bacterial flora of the Alexandrium tamiyavanichii culture was dominated by the Alpha-proteobacteria, followed by Bacteroidetes and Gamma-proteobacteria. The findings in this study suggested that the bacterial community may play various role in the association with dinoflagellate. This study had also shown that dinoflagellate-associated bacterial community is a valuable source for discovery of novel genes and gene products.

Keywords: metagenomic, fosmid library, bacterial community, toxic dinoflagellate, genes discovery

1. Introduction

Microalgae are the major producers of biomass and organic compounds in the ocean. More than 5000 species of marine microalgae are known to date and are separated into six major divisions: *Chlorophyta* (green algae), *Ochrophyta* (yellow algae, golden brown and diatoms), *Haptophyta* (coccolithophorids), *Pyrrhophyta* (dinoflagellates), *Euglenophyta* and *Cyanophyta* (blue-green algae) [1]. Among the 5000 species about 300 can proliferate in high numbers to form the so-called red tide and brown tide phenomena [1, 2].

Many planktonic organisms can form mass occurrences in the water column. When the cell densities reach values considerably higher than their general background distribution, they are called blooms [3]. Blooms can be almost mono specific, others are formed by a combination of species [4, 5]. Many prominent blooms can be traced back to high nutrient loads [6–8], but they can occur whenever a species is able to outgrow its competitors while partially reducing grazer pressure [9].

Microscopic marine algae can be vectors of microbial communities because they are universally associated in the ocean. In nature, most microbial communities are found adhered to microalgae, organism and inanimate surfaces. These interactions are dynamic and are important factors in microbial proliferation and survival. Aquatic algae in situ as well as in laboratory culture condition are often found to be associated with a variety of bacterial strains [10]. Bacteria community can be defined as multi – species of bacteria assemblages in which organisms live together in a contiguous environment (host) and interact with other [11]. Bacteria reproduce asexually, are sized between 0.1 to 20 μm, and can be rod, cocci or comma shaped.

For marine microorganisms (bacterioplankton), there are approximately 10^6 bacterial cells per ml of surface seawater throughout the world's oceans [12]. While this number has been known for at least 30 years, how many bacterial species are actually present in the bacterioplankton are still unknown. Bacterioplankton commonly found in marine environment are mainly from bacteria group of Proteobacteria, Cytophaga-Flexibactar-Bacteroides (CFB), marine Archaea and other groups of bacteria, where bacteria group from Proteobacteria is the largest. Proteobacteria group are divided to some class, which are Alpha (α-), Beta (β-), Delta (δ-), Epsilon (ε-) and Gamma (γ-) Proteobacteria [13]. Up until now, the estimated abundance and genetic diversity of bacterioplankton are based on the data in the GenBank database. Hagström et al. [14] had analyzed on all of the 16S rDNA sequences sent to GenBank to get the estimation of marine bacterioplankton species that were available in the GenBank database. Their studies show that the richness of marine bacterioplankton species in the GenBank database was low relatively.

The ecology of bacterioplankton and phytoplankton is widely recognized to be tightly coupled. Interactions between bacteria and phytoplankton such as dinoflagellates may play an important role in regulating dinoflagellate toxin production. Previous studies on the interactions between bacteria and dinoflagellates have been shown to be highly variable and are sometimes specific. Effects of bacteria on toxic dinoflagellates include negative effects such as cell lysis and death [15] and positive effects such as growth enhancement with an addition of bacteria to cultures [16]. Examples of factors which may cause stimulation or inhibition by bacteria include production of co-factors and secretion of signaling molecules controlling cellular processes of dinoflagellates [17]. In addition, bacterial influences on nutrient availability may result in stimulation or inhibition of the growth or toxin production of dinoflagellates. Both toxin production by dinoflagellates and bacteria associated with toxic or non-toxic dinoflagellates have been documented. For example, Gallacher et al. [18] described evidence of paralytic shellfish toxin (PST) production by bacteria associated with dinoflagellates cultures.

Cultures of dinoflagellates contain a considerable amount of bacteria which probably accompanied the dinoflagellates in the original sample. Bacterial assemblage found in the phycosphere of dinoflagellates may play an important role in regulating dinoflagellate toxin production. While several studies have suggested that bacteria-phytoplankton interactions have the potential to dramatically influence harmful algal bloom dynamics, little is known about how bacteria and phytoplankton communities interact at the species composition level. Other studies have indicated that inside a phytoplankton bloom, α-Proteobacteria overwhelm the free-living bacterioplankton, while microorganisms connected to phytoplankton are basically distinguished as fitting in with (CFB), γ-Proteobacteria, and Planctomycetes groups [19, 20].

At present the precise association of bacteria with cultured dinoflagellates is still not well understood. Moreover, current estimates indicate that more than 99% of the microorganisms present in many natural environments are not readily culturable and therefore not accessible for biotechnology or basic research [21]. Technology to access the genomic DNA or RNA of microorganisms, directly from environmental samples without prior cultivation, has opened new ways of understanding microbial diversity and functions. Thus, this present study is an important step towards understanding bacteria-dinoflagellate interactions.

Metagenomics has become a powerful tool to investigate the biodiversity of complex microbial communities and for studying its metabolic pathways. This technique can be considered as a revolutionary approach to study the microbial community that is unapproachable by available conventional methods and this approach also can capture the total genomes that present in a community of interest. According to Schloss and Handelsman [22], metagenomics was builds on advances in microbial genomics and in the polymerase chain reaction (PCR) amplification and cloning of genes. The field of metagenomics has played a pivotal role for significant progress in microbial ecology, evolution, and diversity over the past years. This approach has allowed researchers to elucidate some possible mechanisms governing ecosystem function and diversity.

2. Methodology

Dinoflagellate Culture. Clonal culture of *Alexandrium tamiyavanichii* were obtained from UKM Microalgae Culture Collections and maintained in ES-DK medium [23] and growth in a light–dark cycle (14:10 hour) incubator at 26°C (model 2015 Shelab, USA).

DNA Extraction. Bulk genomic DNA were directly extracted from a 2.0 L of mid exponential growth phase dinoflagellate [24]. Firstly, culture medium was filtered through 0.2 μm nitrate cellulose membrane (Whatmann, England). Cell pellets were then concentrated and resuspended in buffer (100 mM EDTA, 10 mM Tris–HCl [pH 8.0]) and treated with proteinase K (0.5 mg/mL)-1% sodium dodecyl sulfate (SDS) for 1 h at 37°C. Lysates were further treated by CTAB extraction (0.5 M NaCl, 1% CTAB) for 10 min at 65°C. Then, DNA was extracted once with equal volume of chloroform-isoamyl alcohol (24:1) and phenol-chloroform-isoamyl alcohol (25:4:1) and spin at 21000 x g for 5 min at 4°C. After that, DNA was precipitated with 0.6 volume of isopropanol by centrifugation at 21000 x g for 15 min. The DNA pellet was then washed with one volume of 70% ethanol and spin at 21000 x g for 10 min. Finally, DNA was resuspended in 50 μL of ddH_2O and stored at −20°C.

Metagenomic Library Construction and End-sequences Analysis. Sheared DNA with sizes ranged from 30 kilo bases to 40 kilo bases were used to construct the metagenomic library. Metagenomic library was constructed using CopyControl pCC1FOS library construction kit (Epicenter, USA) following the manufacturer's protocol and fosmids were then purified using Millipore 96-well prep BAC purification kit (Millipore, USA) following the manufacturer's protocol and end-sequenced using T7 universal primer (5′- TAATACGACTCACTATAGGG-3′). End-sequences were edited by using Staden Package software [25]. Low quality DNA sequences were identified and trimmed using Pregap4. The resulting high-quality sequences were assembled into contigs by using Gap4. All dataset was then analyzed by BLASTX [26]. The taxonomical analysis of sequence matches was performed using MEGAN version 4.0 [27] and gene ontology analysis was carried out using Blast2GO suite [28].

3. Results and Discussion

About 4–6 x 10^{30} microbes exist on this earth [29]. They form the foundation of the biosphere, regulate the biogeochemical cycle and influence geology, hydrology, local and global climate. Furthermore, microorganisms have the potential to produce beneficial products to humans such as bioactive compound products, enzymes and polymers. Research on microbial interactions in a natural environment allows us to better understand complex global issues such as greenhouse gases, biodegradation of harmful compounds and enable us to discover new natural products such as antibiotics. However, it is estimated that 99% of the microbes are "viable but nonculturable" [21, 30]. In the meantime, the function and role of the majority of microbes present in the natural environment are still not well understood. Furthermore, they are a valuable resource in biotechnology applications and new product discoveries. The design of metagenomic techniques has allowed us to study in-depth interactions and the role of microbial communities in a natural environment without the need for culturing [31].

The metagenomic approach to studying the bacterial community has begun about more than 20 years ago. Since then, the analysis of bacterial communities using this technique has been widely reported. However, most metagenomic studies have been carried out on bacterial communities from seawater samples, sediments, freshwater. Some metagenomic studies on bacterial communities associated with other organisms were also reported such as from the marine sponges [32], beetle [33], polychetes [34] and tubeworm [35]. However, the analysis of bacterial communities associated with HAB by using metagenomic methods is still poorly reported.

A total of 1501 fosmid clones with insert sizes of 30 kbp to 40 kbp were selected for amplification. Sequences of 80 bp to 550 bp in length were obtained from 238 clones. BLASTX results showed that 23% of the sequences had no match with GenBank data at e-value $>10^{-4}$, 11% were functionally unknown and 11% were putative (**Figure 1**). **Figure 2** shows the functional classification of significant sequences. Most of the sequences could be functionally categorized into a metabolism cluster (37%). There were approximately 14% sequences with no classification and could potentially represent novel genes. Analysis of these partial sequences also revealed some promising enzymes that possess various potential industrial applications such as chitinases, kinases, agarases and oxygenases.

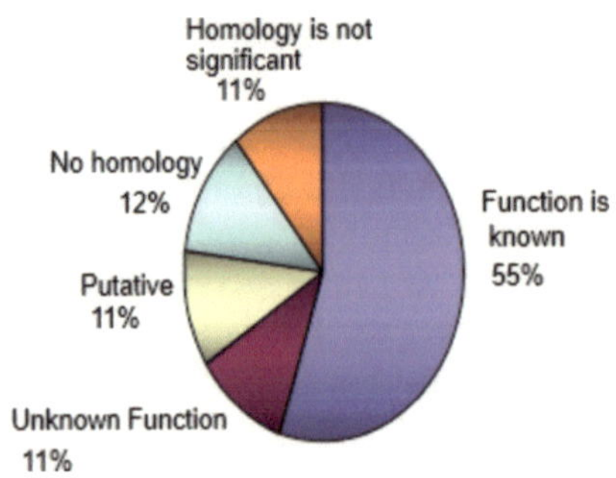

Figure 1.
Distribution of fosmid end sequences based on BLASTX results.

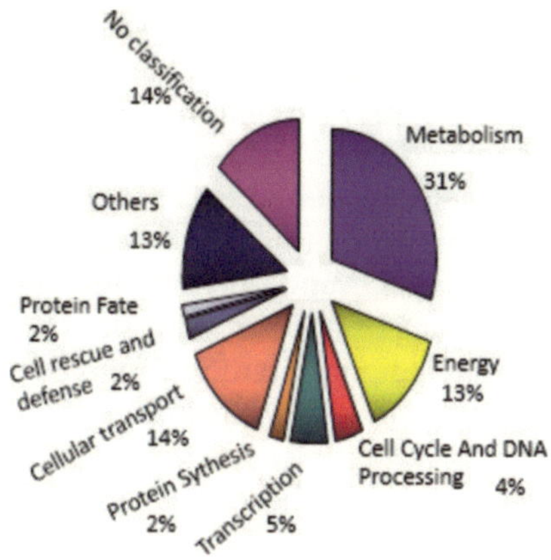

Figure 2.
Classification of significant sequences into the functional categories.

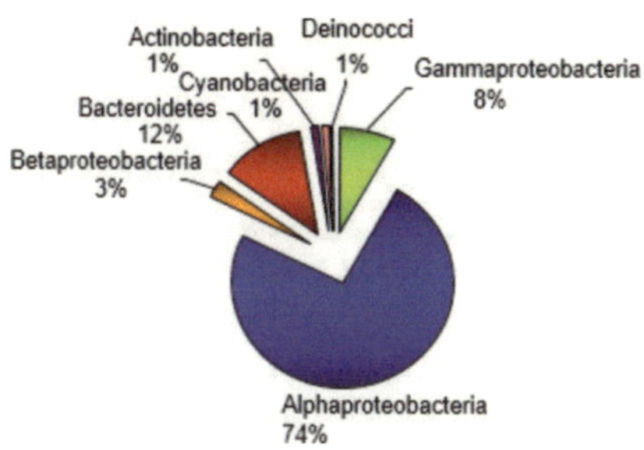

Figure 3.
Classification of sequences into bacteria divisions.

The results also showed that the bacterial flora of the *Alexandrium tamiyavanichii* culture was dominated by the Alpha-proteobacteria, followed by Bacteroidetes and Gamma-proteobacteria (**Figure 3**). This is similar to the findings of Hold *et al.* [36] and Green *et al.* [37]. Alpha-proteobacteria is the largest group in the proteobacteria clade and many members under these taxa are as yet uncultivated bacteria. In this study some of the partial sequences matched those of as yet uncultivable bacteria species. These results suggested that bacteria associated with dinoflagellates are a valuable source for metagenomic studies. Such studies could yield products useful for environmental monitoring, bioremediation and biodegradation [38].

Fosmid end-sequencing has been done to assess the diversity of gene reservoirs in the constructed metagenomic fosmid library. The nucleotide sequence analysis obtained from 238 fosmid clones showed that most of the sequences are still functionally unknown and are believed to represent most of the undiscovered proteins and potentially to provide important new information or pathways if analyzed more deeply. The analysis of the fosmid end sequences also revealed that the majority of the sequences have similarities with the sequence of the Proteobacteria phylum. Some studies also showed that microflora around the marine dinoflagelate phycosphere was dominated by the Proteobacteria phylum [36, 37, 39]. We also found that part of the sequences was matched with genes derived from Roseobacter-Sulfitobacter-Silicibacter clade. Many *Roseobacter* species have been shown to utilize dimethyl sulfoniopropionate (DMSP) as both a carbon source and a sulfur source, and it is likely DMSP metabolism is important in *Roseobacter*-phytoplankton interactions [40].

Analysis of these partial sequences also revealed some genes that might be important in bacteria-algal interactions. One of the contigs was similar to the response regulator of the LuxR family protein from *Roseovarius* sp. This protein is known to be responsible for a variety of biological processes in the natural environment, including the quorum sensing and production of toxins [41]. In a complex community like during an algal bloom, this protein may play a significant role in determining the population structure and function through signaling or inducing the production of certain proteins [42]. Thus, it is believed that bacteria use this type of protein to adapt to the changing conditions around the phycosphere of dinoflagellate such as changes in nutrients, cell densities, and increasing concentration of PSP toxins.

The end-sequences obtained can not be used to describe the metabolic activity of each bacterial taxon involved but the analysis of the nucleotide sequences has shown that the constructed metagenomic library has great potential as a source to study the physiology and function of the bacterial community involved.

4. Conclusion

The advantage of metagenomic method is that it allows us to study the genome of the bacterial community directly from the natural environment in which the function and role of certain bacteria on the environment can be determined. Studies have shown that metagenomics are a very useful technology in finding genes that can be applied in industrial, biotechnology, pharmaceutical and medical fields such as esterase, lipase, agarase, polymerase, polyketide synthases, chitinase and so on. Some potentially uncultured microbes and new genes were discovered through this study. In this study, metagenomic libraries using fosmid vectors were constructed from the bacterial community associated with A. tamiyavanichii. A total of 1501 fosmid clones ranging from 30 to 40 Kbp have been obtained and this is equivalent to 13 bacterial genomes. Finally, to our knowledge, the metagenomic library in this study was the first being constructed from the bacterial communities associated with toxic marine dinoflagellate. This collection of libraries can be used as a major source for finding new genes or pathways for biosynthesis and to study the interactions of dinoflagelates more profoundly, especially in the production of the saxitoxins as there is a hypothesis that the toxins produced by dinoflagelates are derived from bacteria.

Acknowledgements

We thank all the people involved directly or indirectly in this study especially staffs from the School of Fisheries and Aquaculture Sciences, Universiti Malaysia Terengganu and Bachok Marine Research Station, University of Malaya.

Conflict of interest

The authors declare no conflict of interest.

Author details

Muhd Danish-Daniel[1,2*], Mohd Ezhar Mohd Noor[1], Yik Sung Yeong[2], Tan Min Pau[1,2] and Gires Usup[3]

1 School of Fisheries and Aquaculture Sciences, Terengganu, Malaysia

2 Institute of Marine Biotechnology, Terengganu, Malaysia

3 University College Sabah Foundation, Kota Kinabalu, Sabah, Malaysia

*Address all correspondence to: mdda@umt.edu.my

References

[1] Hallegraeff GM. Harmful algal blooms: A global overview. In: Hallegraeff GM, Anderson DM, Cembella AD, editors. Manual on Harmful Marine Microalgae. Vol. 33. UNESCO; 1995. pp. 1-22

[2] Daranas AH, Norte M, Fernandez JJ. Toxic marine microalgae. Toxicon. 2001;**39**:1101-1132. DOI: 10.1016/S0041-0101(00)00255-5

[3] Smayda TJ. What is a bloom? A commentary. Limnology and Oceanography. 1997;**42**(5part2):1132-1136. DOI: 10.4319/lo.1997.42.5_part_2.1132

[4] Garcés E, Vila M, Masó M, Sampedro N, Giacobbe MG, Penna A. Taxon-specific analysis of growth and mortality rates of harmful dinoflagellates during bloom conditions. Marine Ecology Progress Series. 2005;**301**:67-79. DOI: 10.3354/meps301067

[5] Popovich CA, Spetter CV, Marcovecchio JE, Freije RH. Dissolved nutrient availability during winter diatom bloom in a turbid and shallow estuary (Bahía Blanca, Argentina). Journal of Coastal Research. 2008:95-102. DOI: 10.2112/06-0656.1

[6] Hallegraeff GM. A review of harmful algal blooms and their apparent global increase. Phycologia. 1993;**32**(2):79-99. DOI: 10.2216/i0031-8884-32-2-79.1

[7] Hwang DF, Lu YH. Influence of environmental and nutritional factors on growth, toxicity, and toxin profile of dinoflagellate *Alexandrium minutum*. Toxicon. 2000;**38**(11):1491-1503. DOI: 10.1016/S0041-0101(00)00080-5

[8] Yentsch CS, Lapointe BE, Poulton N, Phinney DA. Anatomy of a red tide bloom off the southwest coast of Florida. Harmful Algae. 2008;**7**(6):817-826. DOI: 10.1016/j.hal.2008.04.008

[9] Irigoien X, Flynn KJ, Harris RP. Phytoplankton blooms: A 'loophole' in microzooplankton grazing impact? Journal of Plankton Research. 2005;**27**(4):313-321. DOI: 10.1093/plankt/fbi011

[10] Berland BR, Bonin DJ, Maestrini SY. Study of bacteria associated with marine algae in culture. Marine Biology. 1970;**5**(1):68-76. DOI: 10.1007/BF00352494

[11] Konopka A. What is microbial community ecology? The ISME Journal. 2009;**3**:1223-1230. DOI: 10.1038/ismej.2009.88

[12] Ducklow H. Bacterial production and biomass in the oceans. Microbial Ecology of the Oceans. 2000;**1**:85-120

[13] Hagström Å, Pinhassi J, Zweifel UL. Biogeographical diversity among marine bacterioplankton. Aquatic Microbial Ecology. 2000;**21**(3):231-244. DOI: 10.3354/ame021231

[14] Hagström Å, Pommier T, Rohwer F, Simu K, Stolte W, Svensson D, et al. Use of 16S ribosomal DNA for delineation of marine bacterioplankton species. Applied and Environmental Microbiology. 2002;**68**(7):3628-3633. DOI: 10.1128/AEM.68.7.3628-3633.2002

[15] Lovejoy C, Bowman JP, Hallegraeff GM. Algicidal effects of a novel marinepseudoalteromonas isolate (Class Proteobacteria, Gamma Subdivision) on harmful algal bloom species of the generachattonella, gymnodinium, and heterosigma. Applied and Environmental Microbiology. 1998;**64**(8):2806-2813

[16] Ferrier M, Martin JL, Rooney-Varga JN. Stimulation of *Alexandrium fundyense* growth by bacterial assemblages from

the Bay of Fundy. Journal of Applied Microbiology. 2002;**92**(4):706-716. DOI: 10.1046/j.1365-2672.2002.01576.x

[17] Gallacher S, Smith EA. Bacteria and paralytic shellfish toxins. Protist. 1999;**150**(3):245-255. DOI: 10.1016/S1434-4610(99)70027-1

[18] Gallacher S, Flynn KJ, Franco JM, Brueggemann EE, Hines HB. Evidence for production of paralytic shellfish toxins by bacteria associated with *Alexandrium* spp.(Dinophyta) in culture. Applied and Environmental Microbiology. 1997;**63**(1):239-245

[19] DeLong EF, Franks DG, Alldredge AL. Phylogenetic diversity of aggregate-attached vs. free-living marine bacterial assemblages. Limnology and Oceanography. 1993;**38**(5):924-934. DOI: 10.4319/lo.1993.38.5.0924

[20] González JM, Moran MA. Numerical dominance of a group of marine bacteria in the alpha-subclass of the class Proteobacteria in coastal seawater. Applied and Environmental Microbiology. 1997;**63**(11):4237-4242

[21] Amann RI, Ludwig W, Schleifer KH. Phylogenetic identification and in situ detection of individual microbial cells without cultivation. Microbiology and Molecular Biology Reviews. 1995;**59**(1):143-169

[22] Schloss PD, Handelsman J. Biotechnological prospects from metagenomics. Current Opinion in Biotechnology. 2003;**14**(3):303-310. DOI: 10.1016/S0958-1669(03)00067-3

[23] Kokinos JP, Anderson DM. Morphological development of resting cysts in cultures of the marine dinoflagellate *Lingulodinium polyedrum* (= L. machaerophorum). Palynology. 1995;**19**(1):143-166. DOI: 10.1080/01916122.1995.9989457

[24] Danish-Daniel M, Ahmad A, Usup G. Microbial communities associated with some harmful dinoflagellates from Malaysian waters revealed by culture-independent and culturedependent approaches. Aquaculture, Aquarium, Conservation & Legislation. 2016;**9**(5):976-984

[25] Staden R. The Staden sequence analysis package. Molecular Biotechnology. 1996;**5**(3):233. DOI: 10.1007/BF02900361

[26] Altschul SF, Madden TL, Schäffer AA, Zhang J, Zhang Z, Miller W, et al. Gapped BLAST and PSI-BLAST: A new generation of protein database search programs. Nucleic Acids Research. 1997;**25**(17):3389-3402. DOI: 10.1093/nar/25.17.3389

[27] Huson DH, Auch AF, Qi J, Schuster SC. MEGAN analysis of metagenomic data. Genome Research. 2007;**17**(3):377-386. DOI: 10.1101/gr.5969107

[28] Götz S, García-Gómez JM, Terol J, Williams TD, Nagaraj SH, Nueda MJ, et al. High-throughput functional annotation and data mining with the Blast2GO suite. Nucleic Acids Research. 2008;**36**(10):3420-3435. DOI: 10.1093/nar/gkn176

[29] Johri BM. Microbial diversity. Current Science. 2005;**89**:3-4

[30] Colwell RR, Grimes DJ. Semantics and strategies. In: Nonculturable Microorganisms in the Environment. Boston, MA: Springer; 2000. pp. 1-6. DOI: 10.1007/978-1-4757-0271-2_1

[31] Rondon MR, August PR, Bettermann AD, Brady SF, Grossman TH, Liles MR, et al. Cloning the soil metagenome: A strategy for accessing the genetic and functional diversity of uncultured microorganisms. Applied and Environmental

Microbiology. 2000;**66**(6):2541-2547. DOI: 10.1128/AEM.66.6.2541-2547.2000

[32] Fieseler L, Quaiser A, Schleper C, Hentschel U. Analysis of the first genome fragment from the marine sponge-associated, novel candidate phylum Poribacteria by environmental genomics. Environmental Microbiology. 2006;**8**(4):612-624. DOI: 10.1111/j.1462-2920.2005.00937.x

[33] Piel J. A polyketide synthase-peptide synthetase gene cluster from an uncultured bacterial symbiont of *Paederus* beetles. Proceedings of the National Academy of Sciences. 2002;**99**(22):14002-14007. DOI: 10.1073/pnas.222481399

[34] Campbell BJ, Stein JL, Cary SC. Evidence of chemolithoautotrophy in the bacterial community associated with *Alvinella pompejana*, a hydrothermal vent polychaete. Applied and Environmental Microbiology. 2003;**69**(9):5070-5078. DOI: 10.1128/AEM.69.9.5070-5078.2003

[35] Hughes DS, Felbeck H, Stein JL. A histidine protein kinase homolog from the endosymbiont of the hydrothermal vent tubeworm *Riftia pachyptila*. Applied and Environmental Microbiology. 1997;**63**(9):3494-3498

[36] Hold GL, Smith EA, Rappë MS, Maas EW, Moore ER, Stroempl C, et al. Characterisation of bacterial communities associated with toxic and non-toxic dinoflagellates: *Alexandrium* spp. and *Scrippsiella trochoidea*. FEMS Microbiology Ecology. 2001;**37**(2):161-173. DOI: 10.1111/j.1574-6941.2001.tb00864.x

[37] Green DH, Llewellyn LE, Negri AP, Blackburn SI, Bolch CJ. Phylogenetic and functional diversity of the cultivable bacterial community associated with the paralytic shellfish poisoning dinoflagellate *Gymnodinium catenatum*. FEMS Microbiology Ecology. 2004;**47**(3):345-357. DOI: 10.1016/S0168-6496(03)00298-8

[38] Dennis P, Edwards EA, Liss SN, Fulthorpe R. Monitoring gene expression in mixed microbial communities by using DNA microarrays. Applied and Environmental Microbiology. 2003;**69**(2):769-778. DOI: 10.1128/AEM.69.2.769-778.2003

[39] Babinchak JA, Doucette GJ. Isolation and characterization of the bacterial flora associated with PSP- related dinoflagellate species. In: VIII International conference on Harmful algae-Abstracts and Posters Classification. vp; 1997

[40] Jasti S, Sieracki ME, Poulton NJ, Giewat MW, Rooney-Varga JN. Phylogenetic diversity and specificity of bacteria closely associated with *Alexandrium* spp. and other phytoplankton. Applied and Environmental Microbiology. 2005;**71**(7):3483-3494. DOI: 10.1128/AEM.71.7.3483-3494.2005

[41] Fuqua WC, Winans SC, Greenberg EP. Quorum sensing in bacteria: The LuxR-LuxI family of cell density-responsive transcriptional regulators. Journal of Bacteriology. 1994;**176**(2):269. DOI: 10.1128/jb.176.2.269-275.1994

[42] Parsek MR, Greenberg EP. Acyl-homoserine lactone quorum sensing in gram-negative bacteria: A signaling mechanism involved in associations with higher organisms. Proceedings of the National Academy of Sciences. 2000;**97**(16):8789-8793. DOI: 10.1073/pnas.97.16.8789

Section 2

Molecular Cloning

Chapter 4

Applied Molecular Cloning: Present and Future for Aquaculture

Tapas Chakraborty, Sipra Mohapatra, Chimwar Wanglar and Dipak Pandey

Abstract

With the grim picture of millions of people living in poverty and hunger, there is also an international alarm over future world food supply. This global concern of food scarcity has established the need to not only increase the production of traditional staples but also fisheries and aquaculture. Genetically, physiologically and phenotypically, fish are the most diverse group of livings. Similar to mammals, molecular biology is being extensively used in aquaculture, be it in disease management, or growth and reproduction enhancement. In this chapter we aim to discuss the molecular methodologies applied to uplift and attain sustainability in aqua farming.

Keywords: aquaculture, fish, disease diagnosis, genome editing, genomic marker

1. Introduction

Agriculture, livestock (bird, cattle, pig, etc.) farming and fish rearing are traditionally used to cater the nutritional requirement since ages. Evidence of agriculture, including meat farming, can be found as far back as the end of the Pleistocene Era, roughly around 12,000 years ago. In contrast, fish have only been farmed in aquaculture setting for over 2000 years [1]. Our world roughly comprises of 70% water and majority of them are unutilized due to inadequate knowledge and resources. Additionally, the availability of terrestrial space of agriculture and livestock farming are now on a decline. The lower FCR values of various aquaculturable species (e.g., cobia 0.96–1.50:1) than various terrestrial animals (e.g., cattle 5.15–6.95:1; poultry 2.13–2.61:1) [2, 3] are not only important for reducing the production cost but also have less environmental burden to bear. However, aquaculture, the farming of fish and aquatic plants, is the fastest growing food sector in the world, recently (since 1970s) growing exponentially to meet the increasing population and declining wild fish stock availability. The aquaculture industry's contribution to the total food supply has increased dramatically since 2000–2012 by 6.2% [4], and it is expected that by 2030, 60% of the total fish supply intended for direct human consumption will be produced by the aquaculture industry [5]. With the development of new and environment friendly Silvofisheries (fish integrated with mangroves), Aquaponics and IMTA (integrated multitrophic aquaculture), etc., the probability of sustainable growth of aquaculture has been raised several folds. But, unlike agriculture and livestock farming, aquaculture has lot of geographical restriction, such as in North America and Europe, clams, oysters, and other shellfish are the main species being farmed, while in Japan, edible seaweed, marine shrimp, and yellowtail are the desired species for culture. Likewise, carps in India, freshwater prawns in Hawaii, and eels in Taiwan are the preferred culturable species [1]. Although numerous species (>694) have made their way into aquaculture and have international consumer market, only the Norwegian salmon has gained commercially popularity in recent years. If we analyze deeply, it is clear that it is neither the geographical restriction nor the consumer demand, but rather the huge industrial success of this specific salmon is related to meticulous research, better strain availability through years of selective breeding, authenticated and steady high quality seed availability and one stop consultancy [6].

Molecular biology and cloning set sailed its journey with the DNA molecule in 1950s and encountered several breakthrough including RNA and restriction endonucleases, however in reality, the recombinant DNA technology has made a revolution in modern molecular biology. Through this technique, large quantities of proteins present in trace amount, as well as other biologically active substances, could be generated through biotechnology and these genetically engineered macromolecules have very little side effects. Emerging technologies promise even greater possibilities, such as enabling researchers to seamlessly stitch together multiple DNA fragments and transform the resulting plasmids into bacteria in under 2 h, or the use of swappable gene cassettes, which can be easily moved between different constructs, to maximize speed and flexibility. During the past 2–3 decades, fish molecular biology has been intensively investigated in all aspects of fisheries, including diseases, genetics, nutrition, and ecology. Molecular tools are used to investigate changes in the DNA, RNA or proteins to detect certain genetic or biochemical changes that are associated with certain disease-causing pathogens [7–9]. Another advantage of molecular tools is that the analysis can be done on stored specimens and abundance of genetic information in the database. In recent years, great advances have been made to simplify the techniques and reduce the cost without compromising on the sensitivity. In this chapter we will discuss about the issues of aquaculture, and the potential of molecular cloning/biology in fish.

2. Aquatic animal and molecular cloning

2.1 Major hurdles of aquaculture

Fish live in a complex 3D environment, so whether it is the density of the fish, or extra feed given by farmer, or local environment and water quality, everything impacts the aquaculture output. Although new concepts like precision fish farming are emerging, the following categories still are a cause of major concern.

2.1.1 Adequate disease diagnosis and health management

Diseases are the major constricting factor for expansion of aquaculture industry, and they potentially cost the sector nearly $6 billion in yield loss each year [10]. Aquatic environments impose a constant risk of exposure to disease-causing pathogens and poor knowledge of background microbial "diversity" in aquatic farm systems often leads to frequent emergence of previously unknown diseases. Healthy looking fish can carry pathogens without a clinical sign and disease become evident only under stressful conditions. Therefore, disease management and assessment of cultured fish is a major concern to commercial aquaculturists. The ability to identify the presence or absence and concentration of a pathogenic organism in fish would have significant economic benefits. Statistically, relevant disease surveillance and monitoring requires testing large numbers of fish as it increases the probability of detecting pathogen from clinically normal fish. Reliable detection of fish pathogens in a fish population is difficult if fish with disease are not available or only a low percentage of the fish is infected. To detect pathogen carrying fish, a cost effective, sensitive, and specific system is required for surveillance and monitoring of fish population. Traditionally, the diagnosis and management of diseases is carried out by culture dependent methods which are slow, require skill, and only selective organism can be detected [11]. Potentially faster, more sensitive diagnostic techniques for identification and characterization of pathogens, even from asymptomatic carrier fish, are of utmost necessary.

2.1.2 Maintenance of the environment and biodiversity

Since farmed fish are selected and bred for certain genetic criteria like size, quick growth and hardiness, escaped species can become invasive and pose a massive threat to global biodiversity. The ever-growing aquaculture industries also have to bear the public concern in regard to pollution and other environmental effects and thus maintaining and sustaining the environment is of paramount importance. Attention to genetic variability and biodiversity in aquaculture development, proper stock maintenance and aquatic resource management are therefore crucial elements for sustainable environment. In this sense, traceability tools are essential to assess the impact of aquaculture escapees in natural populations or distinguish the farmed and wild specimens.

2.1.3 Reproductive medley

Reproduction is crucial for steady and quality seed supply and hence of utmost importance for aquaculture sustainability. Fish gonadal development is influenced by intrinsic (genetics, growth, behavior, etc.), and extrinsic (temperature, hormone, environmental pollution, etc.) factors. Though, large diversity of aqua animals has its own advantages, each species has distinct reproductive and embryonic development biology that hinders the timely breeding and smooth progression of commercial aquaculture. For instance, some gonochoristic fish harbors sex chromosome while others do not, and several commercially lucrative fish sequentially changes their sex. Moreover, some hybrids tend to grow bigger with the expense of reproductive unfitness (e.g., hybrids of Atlantic and pacific salmon).

2.1.4 Improper growth

Fish growth largely depends on feeding, environment and genetic background. For example, farmed Atlantic salmon tend to grow faster than wild ones, and genetically modified (GM) farmed salmons are even better. Though FDA recently approved GM salmon, till date it is not ethically preferable to use GM fish for commercial aquaculture. There are few more success stories of using myostatin knockout to improve growth of tilapia, red sea bream and common carp; however, yellow catfish [12] did not display similar results, suggesting functional variation among species.

2.2 Application of molecular cloning in aquaculture

2.2.1 Restriction enzyme/endonuclease digestion

Restriction enzymes (or restriction endonucleases, RE) are enzymes or better known as "molecular scissors" that recognize and cleave the DNA into fragments at or near specific "recognition" sites. The DNA fragments are observed by gel electrophoresis and the pattern of bands are used to generate the "fingerprint" of a particular DNA molecule. The cut DNA can be observed by gel electrophoresis and the pattern of bands compiled to create a restriction enzyme map [13]. This map is useful to identify and characterize a particular DNA region and analyze genetic variation. Restriction enzymes are used to manipulate DNA and are vital tools in molecular cloning. They form the basis for several diagnostic tools like RFLP, AFLP, Southern blotting, etc. For instance, RFLP recognizes size variations, and in combination with PCR can be used to reduce the labor-intensive DNA isolation for RFLP analysis [14]. SNPs (single-nucleotide polymorphism) or INDELs change the restriction endonuclease recognition sites that cause differences in restriction fragment lengths. AFLP technique is based on cutting with two Res (one average (e.g., EcoRI), and another rare (e.g., MseI) cutter), ligation of adapters to these restriction fragments and followed by a PCR-based selective amplification with adapter-specific radioactive or fluorescent-labeled primers.

2.2.2 Random amplified polymorphic DNA (RAPD)

RAPDs are DNA fragments that are amplified using short random primers (~10 bp) and are used to detect polymorphisms. RAPDs are randomly distributed throughout the genome and have high abundance. This technique is quick and easy and requires low quantity of DNA. Fish pathogens have been studied using RAPD, but problems with reproducibility and risks of contamination render the method unsuitable as a stand-alone method of diagnosis. However, RAPD can be a useful technique as a first step in the development of specific primers or probes and has been used in such a way in the study of bacteria.

2.2.3 Polymerase chain reaction (PCR)

The polymerase chain reaction is a robust technique used to produce large copies of the target DNA sequence by amplifying the specific region of interest. The reaction includes template DNA, primers, polymerase enzyme to catalyze creation of new copies of DNA, and nucleotides to form the new copies. The template DNA can be collected from sample tissue, blood, serum, fluid, mucus or can be a purified DNA. The principle of PCR is based on the repetitive cycling of denaturation, annealing and extension. Each copy of the DNA then serves as another template for further amplification and copy number of PCR products then doubles in each cycle. After "n" rounds of replication, 2^n copies of the target sequence are theoretically produced. After thirty cycles, PCR can produce 2^{30} or more than ten billion copies of a single target DNA sequence. The PCR product can be detected by gel electrophoresis. The whole process just needs 2–5 h depending on the number and types of nucleotide. PCR has distinct advantages over conventional microbiological diagnostic methods as it can detect slow growing and unculturable pathogens. PCR is faster, extremely efficient and sensitive and can be used to amplify sequences from wide variety of samples even if they only have a small amount of DNA. Some of the shortcomings of PCR are the false positive results from DNA contamination, limited detection platform for simultaneous identification of multiple samples, etc.

In most cases, the target DNA sequence is the rRNA operon and in bacteria, the most frequently used is the variable region of the evolutionary conserved 16S rRNA gene. Nevertheless, other types of genes or sequences of unknown sequences can also be used.

To overcome the shortcoming and to increase the diagnostic capacity of conventional PCR, multiplex PCR was developed to simultaneously amplify several target sequences by using more than one pair of primers. It can detect multiple pathogens, which save time and cost without compromising test utility, but might require further analysis such as DNA sequencing to confirm the identity of the species.

Nested PCR, which uses two pairs of primers and two successive PCR run, was developed to increase specificity and sensitivity of conventional PCR. The first set of primers is used to amplify target sequence in first run and the PCR products are used as template for the second run and amplification is conducted with the second set of primers. Though, it is popular for unknown/homologous gene identification, due to the lengthy process and complexity, this type of PCR is limited to cases where single PCR is not sufficient to identify pathogen.

Though DNA is reliable, RNA is often a more accurate indicator of viable microorganism. Therefore, Reverse Transcription-Polymerase Chain Reaction (RT-PCR) was developed to first synthesize cDNA from RNA by reverse transcription (RT) and later amplify the cDNA by PCR. However, for effective detection, sufficient amount of detectable RNA concentrations is required, and the RNA sample should be free of genomic DNA to avoid false positive results.

Most recently, real time PCR is used to detect, confirm and quantify PCR products at "real time" during the amplification process using Fluorescent dyes. Two types of dyes are generally used; one is the use of non-sequence specific dyes like SYBR green I or ethidium bromide and the second is the use of fluorescently labeled internal probe like TaqMan, FRET (fluorescence resonance energy transfer), etc. The real time PCR has three novel features—temperature cycling occurs considerable faster than in standard PCR assays, hybridization of specific DNA probes occurs continuously during the amplification and the dye fluoresces only when hybridization takes place. This technique is quick and convenient, and with the recent introduction of multiplex real time PCR, detection of multiple targets in a single reaction can be achieved at cheaper cost, shorter time and faster diagnosis.

2.2.4 Loop-mediated isothermal amplification (LAMP)

It is a novel nucleic acid amplification method that amplifies DNA with high specificity, efficiency and rapidity under isothermal conditions. This method employs a DNA polymerase and a set of four specially designed primers to recognize six distinct regions of the target DNA. Unlike PCR, LAMP is carried out in constant temperature (60–65°C) using an auto-cycling strand displacement DNA synthesis and does not require thermal cycler. The amplified product can be detected as white precipitate or yellow green color solution after addition of SYBR Green. It is cost effective and when combined with reverse transcription, this method can also amplify RNA sequences with high efficiency. It can be used to detect the identification of genus and species-specific parasites. However, this technique is not effective for detection of different pathogens simultaneously.

2.2.5 Fluorescence in situ hybridization (FISH)

In situ hybridization refers to detection of DNA or RNA on actual tissues, cells, or any biological sample in their natural positions within a chromosome, by using a complementary probe. *ISH* correlates DNA localization and mRNA expression with morphological findings [15]. Most current *in situ* hybridization methods use *FISH* [16, 17] in which fluorescent labeled pieces of DNA or RNA (probe) hybridize to target nucleic acid in cells under appropriate conditions. These labeled cells can then be visualized by flow cytometry or fluorescence microscopy. *FISH* can be used on formalin fixed paraffin embedded tissues, frozen tissues, etc. The technique has also been used to detect bacterial and viral DNA in an infected cell. Since the probe has to reach the target inside the cells, only probes that are small (~300 bases) can be used for tissue penetration, hence sensitivity is limited to the accessibility of the target in the cell.

2.2.6 Molecular padlock probes (MPP)

Padlock probes (PLPs) are single stranded long oligonucleotides whose 5′ and 3′ ends are complementary to two immediately adjacent target sequences. Upon hybridization to the target, the two ends are brought into contact, effectively circularizing the probe with a nick. DNA ligase is added to convert this linear PLP into a covalently closed circular molecule. Single strand specific DNA exonucleases can be used to "chew up" the linear strands and only make available the intact circular molecules. PLPs provide extremely specific target recognition, which is followed by universal amplification and microarray. However, synthesis of long probes can be little expensive as compared to short primers for PCR. At present, the most common application for PLPs is the detection of single nucleotide polymorphisms (SNPs) and multiplex pathogen detection assays.

2.2.7 Rolling circle amplification (RCA)

RCA is an isothermal enzymatic process where short DNA/RNA primer amplified to form a long single stranded DNA/RNA using a circular DNA template and special DNA/RNA polymerases. The product is a concatemer containing tens to hundreds of tandem repeats that are complementary to the circular template. By manipulating the circular template, RCA can be employed to generate complex DNA nanostructures such as DNA origami, nanotubes, nanoribbons and DNA based metamaterials which can be used for bio-detection, drug delivery, etc. Millard et al. [18] combined RCA, MPP and hyperbranching (Hbr) to develop a multiplex detection assay for IHNV and ISAV.

2.2.8 Microarray

This technology is used to assess expression rate of thousands of genes and identify wide range of pathogens from complex samples in one single reaction. This technique usually involves hybridization of DNA with large number of probes and can overcome the shortcomings of multiplex PCR, which can detect only a maximum of six pathogens at a time. There are two types of DNA microarrays that are widely used—cDNA microarrays and oligonucleotide/DNA chips. There are a number of ways of using DNA microarrays. One method is the use of fluorescent labeled DNA sequences that are hybridized to the microarray slide. The data is detected by fluorescent array detection and analyzed by computer programs. The second and more practical method is the use of fluorescent labeled competitor oligonucleotide. When target DNA does not hybridize to the tethered oligonucleotide in the microarray, fluorescent labeled competitor oligonucleotide will bind to the tethered oligonucleotide on the chip and displace the test DNA. Then the fluorescent microarray detector and computer program will analyze the fluorescent array for the presence or absence of the species/strain specific DNA sequence. Microarray does not require clear length differences between PCR products and therefore, PCR assays can be designed to generate smaller sized amplicons that can improve efficiency and probability of template recovery from degraded DNA and reduces PCR template biasedness. Compared to traditional nucleic acid hybridization with membranes, microarrays offer the additional advantages of high density, high sensitivity, rapid detection, lower cost, automation, and low background levels. Since most of the pathogens genetic sequences are known, oligonucleotide probes complementary to all pathogens can be used for microarray. Although the set-up cost for the use of DNA microarrays is high, once the equipment is available and microarrays are prepared, cost per unit of sample analyzed becomes low. In the post-genome sequencing era, microarrays have been developed from model and non-model fish and have the possibility of heterologous application. Though majority of them are publicly available, however, they vary in type, size, complexity, methodological development and motivation and degree of annotation, so it is advisable to carefully select the array beforehand [19].

2.2.9 DNA sequencing

DNA sequencing is used to determine the four chemical blocks—adenine, guanine, thymine and cytosine, that make up the DNA molecule. The sequence information can help determine changes in the gene that may cause disease. First generation sequencing techniques include the Sanger method and the Maxam-Gilbert techniques. Maxam-Gilbert are based on chemical modification of DNA and subsequent cleavage at specific bases while Sanger method requires that each read start be cloned for production of single-stranded DNA. Maxam–Gilbert sequencing is less popular due to its technical complexity. The chain-terminator method or Frederick Sanger method, which uses dideoxynucleotide triphosphates (ddNTPs) as DNA chain terminators, became a popular method of DNA sequencing due to its greater efficiency, use of fewer toxic chemicals and lower amounts of radioactivity than Maxam-Gilbert method. Second generation sequencing includes technologies such as Illumina and Ion Torrent that produce massive parallel sequencing of short read length of reads of DNA (150–400 bp), which require extensive assembly. Third generation sequencing method includes PacBio and ONT and involves sequencing through extended repetitive regions in the genome to produce much longer reads (6–20 kb) but far fewer reads per run (typically hundreds of thousands). The second and third generation sequencing methods, collectively known as the next generation sequencing (NGS) or high throughput sequencing allows the sequencing of DNA and RNA more quickly and cheaply. The goal of NGS is to investigate functional genome, epigenome and transcriptome elements in cells and tissues, and their temporal expression, which permits the definition of variation in gene expression among the different types of tissue, organs or life stages of the target organism. Over the past decade, the cost of NGS has decreased significantly, making it possible to use non-model fish species to investigate emerging environmental issues, understand the cell-cell interactions, and whole organismal physiology. To cope with it, bioinformatics is also rapidly evolving and new algorithms are being published. It is expected that NGS with bioinformatics is the way to revolutionize the field of fisheries and might also help clarify the previous findings and dogmas prevalent in aquaculture and biology.

2.2.10 RAD sequencing

Restriction-site associated DNA sequencing (RAD sequencing or RAD-Seq) combine the use of genome complexity reduction with REs and the high sequencing output of NGS technologies. Original RAD-Seq was first described by Baird et al. [20] and several variants of this methodology have been described since then [21]. But, only the original RAD-Seq [20], 2b-RAD and ddRAD are extensively used in aquaculture research. In aquaculture, RAD-Seq has been used in genetic mapping [22], reference genome assembly sex determination loci mapping [23–26], etc. Some of the main reasons for its instant success is that RAD-Seq does not require any prior genomic knowledge, it allows generation of population-specific genotype data (i.e., no ascertainment bias) and it offers flexibility in terms of desired marker density across the genome. The use of different REs or innovative modifications to the base technique allows a high level of control over the number of markers obtained for a specific study. RAD-Seq and similar techniques are also amenable tools for aquaculture breeding, where genetic markers have typically been used in family assignment and pedigree reconstruction [27]. Mass spawning species are common in aquaculture, where mixed rearing and unknown parental contribution necessitate the use of genotyping for family-based breeding. RAD-Seq potentially facilitates a single experiment whereby pedigrees are reconstructed, genetic diversity is quantified, QTL are mapped, and genomic breeding values calculated [28].

2.2.11 Genomic marker development

Most of the genetic improvement in fish and shellfish species to date has been made through the use of traditional selective breeding of Atlantic salmon, Rainbow trout, tilapia and many other fish [29]. Notably, spontaneous mutations in the genome create genetic variability (or polymorphism) and this variability can be an effective means to analyze fish trait and geological pedigree. Boom in whole genome sequencing technology, though still costly, encourage fish researchers to investigate genomic marker's potential in selective breeding and aquaculture production. There are several available markers for fish research: AFLP, RAPD, etc., but most prevalent ones are microsatellite and SNPs. Microsatellite markers, identified using microsatellite sequence enriched genomic library or Expressed tagged sequence library, are simple tandem sequence repeats scattered across the genome and used increasingly in aquaculture species [29]. SNPs are generally identified using in depth genome sequencing and require huge financial and bioinformatical investment. MAS (marker assisted selection) is useful for traits that are difficult to measure on breeding candidates, particularly when they are largely linked to QTL (quantitative trait loci). With the help of MAS and GS (genomic selection), several studies have demonstrated increased accuracy of breeding value predictions in growth and disease resistance in yellowtail and Atlantic salmon [30–33]. Nevertheless, this approach requires a great amount of detailed information in order to choose which gene explains the greatest effect and to have sufficient power to detect the association.

2.2.12 Metagenomics

There are two main methods for studying the microbiome using high-throughput sequencing: marker-gene studies and whole-genome-shotgun (WGS) metagenomics. While marker-gene studies, amplify a particular gene (16S rRNA for bacteria/archaea, 18S for fungi), metagenomics refer to the sequencing of DNA from the entire genome of samples obtained directly from the environment (water, soil) or tissues. Advances in metagenomics have themselves been driven by advances in second- and third-generation sequencing technologies, which are now capable of producing hundreds of gigabases of DNA sequenced data at a very low cost [34]. Unlike bacteria that use the 16S ribosomal RNA as a common gene for their identification, viruses lack a single common gene for their identification which makes it difficult to monitor their population dynamics in different aquatic environments [35]. Metagenomics also holds the promise of revealing the genomes of the majority of microorganisms that cannot be readily obtained in pure culture [36]. Breitbart et al. [37] have shown that it is possible to sequence entire genomes of uncultured marine viruses using metagenomics. For metagenomic sequences linked to novel diseases, there is need to isolate the virus involved followed by verification using conventional diagnostic approaches such as cell culture to exhibit the cytopathic effect (CPE), morphological characterization using electron microscopy, and molecular characterization using PCR ([38], **Table 1**).

2.2.13 DNA vaccines

DNA vaccines are composed of bacterial plasmids which has two units-antigen expressing unit that comprises of promoter/enhancer sequences, antigen coding and polyadenylation sequences; and the production unit comprising of sequences necessary for plasmid amplification and selection [39]. The vaccine inserts are constructed by molecular cloning and transformed into bacterial cells, and the purified plasmid DNA is injected into fish. Hansen et al. [40] first introduced vaccination in fish by injecting plasmid constructs encoding viral glycoprotein directly into skeletal muscle of common carp that resulted in efficient protection of the fish against rhabdoviruses. More than 20 different virus DNA vaccines have been developed experimentally for prophylactic use in fish targeting viruses such as rhabdoviridae, orthomyxoviridae, togaviridae and nodaviridae [41, 42]. However, despite this huge prospect, DNA vaccines for farmed animals remain at the moment experimental. DNA vaccines seem to be more harmless and more stable than ordinary vaccines [42]. Plasmids are non-viable and do not multiply, and therefore have a low risk of developing secondary disease and infection. The main concern about the potential DNA vaccines is that they might integrate into the host genome and generate immune responses. However, extensive surveys have found little evidence of integration, and the merger risk appears to be less than normal mutation. Significant advantages of these vaccines include cheapness, simplicity of

Pathogens	Detection method
V. vulnificus, *L. anguillarum*, *P. damselae*, *V. parahaemolytocus*	Multiplex PCR, DNA microarray
Y. ruckeri, *A. salmonicida*, *F. psychrophilum*	Multiplex PCR
Infectious salmon anemia virus (ISAV)	RT PCR
Myxobolus cerebralis	Real time PCR
Edwardsiella tarda	LAMP
Infectious hematopoietic necrosis virus (IHNV) & ISAV	Molecular padlock
R. salmoninarum, *A. salmonicida*, *E. ictaluri*, *F. columnare*, *F. psychrophilum*, *Y. ruckeri*, *P. salmonis*, *T. maritimum*	DNA microarray
A. salmonicida, *E. ictaluri* and *F. psychrophilum*	PCR and DNA microarrays
Aeromonas (*A. hydrophila*, *A. sobria*, *A. caviae* and *A. veronii*)	Multiplex PCR
P. salmonis (Salmonid Rickettsial Septicaemia)	PCR-RFLP

Table 1.
Prevalent examples of established disease diagnostics in aquaculture.

production and consumption, transport and higher resistance. The other important feature of these vaccines is the ability to put several antigens in the plasmid, resulting in immunization against all agents [43]. In 2005, APEX-IHN (Novartis/Elanco) became the first DNA vaccine licensed for commercial use in aquaculture for protection of Atlantic salmon against Infectious Hematopoietic Necrosis Virus (IHNV) in British Colombia. In 2017, the European Commission through the European Medicines Agency (EMA) granted marketing authorization of CLYNAV (Elanco), a polyprotein-encoding DNA vaccine against Salmon Pancreas Disease Virus (SPDV) infection in Atlantic salmon (*Salmo salar*) for use within the EU. However, administration of vaccines typically requires individual handling and treatment of all production fish, which can be expensive and impractical in a large-scale production environment.

2.2.14 Transgenesis

Transgenics are those genetically engineered organisms which have heterologous DNA (transgene) integrated stably into their genome through artificial means like microinjection, electroporation, sperm mediated transfer, lipofection, retrovirus, etc. The transgene construct carries a target gene, encoding product of interest and regulatory elements that regulate the expression of the gene in a spatial, temporal and developmental manner [44]. Since the development of the first transgenic fish in 1984, a wide number of transgenic fish species have been produced (**Table 2**) to improve growth, disease resistance, cold resistance, etc. [45].

2.2.15 Gene therapy

In the mid-twentieth century, researcher demonstrated that the rate of mutagenesis could be enhanced with radiation or chemical treatment [46, 47]. Later with the help of transposons, targeted genomic changes were made in various model organism including medaka and zebrafish [48–50]. But due to prevalence of transposon machinery in these fish, longer time requirement for generating particular line and

Species	Foreign gene	Desired effect
Striped bass (*Morone saxatilis*)	Insect genes	Disease resistance
Common carp (*Cyprinus carpio*)	Salmon and human GH; rainbow trout GH	Improved disease resistance
Grass carp (*Ctenopharyngodon idellus*)	hLF hLF + common carp β-actin promoter	Increased disease resistance to bacterial pathogen Increased disease resistance to grass carp hemorrhage virus
Channel catfish (*Ictalurus punctatus*)	Silk moth (*Hyalophora cecropia*) cecropin genes	Enhance bactericidal activity
Japanese Medaka (*Oryzias latipes*)	Insect cecropin or pig cecropin-like peptide genes + CMV	Enhanced bactericidal activity against common fish pathogens
Atlantic Salmon (*Salmo salar*)	Mx genes	Potential resistance to pathogens following treatment with poly I:C
Nile Tilapia (*O. niloticus*) and Redbelly Tilapia (*Tilapia zillii*)	Shark (*Squalus acanthias* L.) IgM genes	Enhanced immune response

Table 2.
Transgenesis in aquaculture.

DOI: http://dx.doi.org/10.5772/intechopen.88197

concerns about transgenics associated wild genepool contamination and biodiversity degradation has led aquaculture researchers to focus on other knockdown and knockout technologies.

In fish, antisense morpholinos, small interfering RNA (siRNA) and PNAs (peptide nucleic acid) are widely used to transiently interfere with gene function. Morpholinos are typically 25 bp long oligos that specifically interfere with gene function based on their complementarity to the target sequence either by blocking translation initiation or by interfering with splicing. The non-ribose-based backbone renders morpholinos insensitive to enzymatic degradation. PNAs have a higher affinity for RNA, yet they are less soluble and therefore the *in vivo* use is limited. Dorn et al. [51] changed the chemical composition of the PNA backbone to increase solubility and showed efficient knockdown of the *six3* gene in medaka. In most cases, the chemical/RNA is micro-injected or electroporated into fertilized eggs at early cleavage stages to ensure a ubiquitous distribution to all cells of the developing embryo. If thus applied, they interfere with gene function during early development. To study gene function during later stages, morpholinos can be activated conditionally by light-induced uncaging. However, recent results in zebrafish indicate that morpholino-based gene knockdown often results in unspecific off-target effects [52].

To overcome abovementioned complications advanced genome editing techniques were developed, in which, no genetic material from another species is introduced and thus the genome remains untainted. Although tilling (target induced local lesion in genome) was first of this kind, it mostly creates single point mutation and requires large screening. Some of the next generation gene editing tools used in fish are zinc finger nucleases (ZFNs), transcription activator like effector nucleases (TALENs) and CRISPR/Cas system. Mutations can be achieved by introducing double strand breaks into the target gene and non-homologous end joining (NHEJ) repair mechanism is used to produce insertions or deletions in a site-specific manner resulting in permanent disruption of the function of the target gene. On the other hand, exogenous gene sequence can be introduced into the genome by co-delivering the targeted nucleases along with a target vector containing the DNA homologous to the break site for gene correction (**Figure 1**).

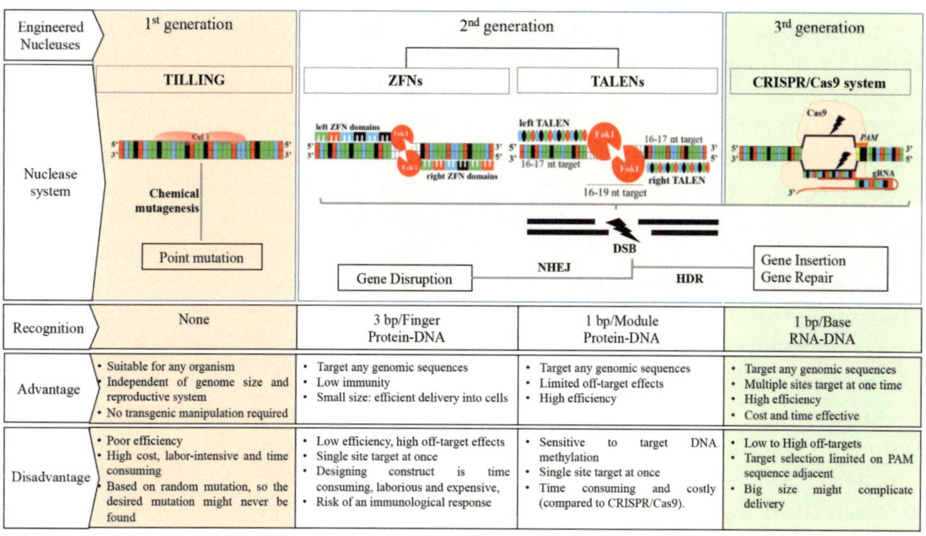

Figure 1.
Comparative evaluation of various knockout technologies used in fish manipulation.

Fishes	Genes (method)	Fishes	Genes (method)
Atlantic salmon	*dnd*, *tyr*, *slc24a5* (C) [60, 61]	Sturgeon	*dnd* (C) [62]
Atlantic killifish	*ahr2* (C) [63]	Tilapia	*fox12a*, *cyp19a1a*, *dmrt1*, *nanos*, *gsdf*, *sf-1/nr5a*, *mstn* (C); *rspo1*, *fox12a*, *cyp19a1a* (T) [64–69]
Cavefish	*oca2* (T) [70]		
Channel catfish	*lh* (Z) [71]		
Chinese lamprey	*slc24a5* (C) [72]	Yellow catfish	*mstn* (Z) [12]
Common carp	*sp7a/b*, *runx2*, *bmp2a*, *opg & mstn* (T & C) [73]	Zebrafish	*dnd* (M); *ntl*, *slc24a5*, *kdr1*, *prl*, (Z); *gria3a*, *hey2*, *cyp19a1a*, *ryr3*, *ryr1a*, *tbx6*, *slc24a*, *slc45a2*, *fsh*, *lh*, *fshr*, *ihcgr*, *pgr*, *rb1*, *bmp15*, *mesp*, *gnrh3*, *zap70*, *nrld1*, *leg1a*, *mstn*, *rnf213a*, *mpl*, *dmrt1*, *cyp17a1*, *stat3*, *kiss1/2 & kissr1/2*(T); *mitfa*, *ddx19*, *slc24a5*, *slc45a2*, *seta/b*, *nrg1-I*, *stxbp1*, *nERs*, *gspt11*, *fus*, *akt2*, *atp6v1h*, *cyp19a1a* (C) [62, 74–108]
Japanese anchovy	*mstn* (T & C) [109]		
Medaka	*dnd* (M); *fox13*, *dmy*, *dmc1*, *fshb*, *gnrh1* (T); *gsdf* (Z) [110–114]		
Red sea bream	*mstn* (C) [115]		
Rice field eel	*dmrt1*, *foxl2*, *cyp19ala* (T) [116]		
Rohu	*tlr22* (C) [117]		
Starlet and sturgeon	*Ntl*, *dnd* (T & C) [118, 119]		

M, morpholino; Z, zinc finger nuclease (ZFN); T, transcription activator-like effector nucleases (TALEN), C, clustered regularly interspaced short palindromic repeats (CRISPR).

Table 3.
Genome editing using ZFN, TALEN and CRISPR system in varies model and non-model fish species.

Theoretically, ZFN is an ideal tool for inducing mutations at target DNA sites in any organisms [53]. However, its application has been constrained by limitations in zinc finger domain design and construction as well as low efficiency [54]. Compared with ZFN, the recently emerged TALEN provides us a more advanced approach for genome editing; it is much easier to construct plasmids for expressing TALE proteins, making this technology easily available to most molecular biology laboratories. Because of this and its high specificity and efficiency, TALEN has quickly replaced ZFN as a dominant platform for genome editing since its establishment in 2011 [55]. Unlike ZFN and TALEN, the nuclease Cas9 is guided towards the target DNA site by a small guide RNA followed by random cleavage of the DNA. Particularly, the rapid emergence of CRISPR/Cas9 caused a paradigm shift in the research community [56]. There is complementary usage of these two technologies in recent years, as CRISPR/Cas9 works as monomer, it consists of protein and RNA and produces blunt end, while TALEN works as dimer, it consists of protein only and produces cohesive ends [57]. Although each one has its associated pros and cons [58], TALENs and CRISPR technologies have comparatively high specificity and efficiency with low off target effect [59]. Not only the methodology, but selection of delivery methodology (microinjection, electroporation, etc.), target tissue, and host is critical for ensured success in aquaculturable strain production. Numerous genes are being knocked out using various techniques and some of them are already adapted for commercial aquaculture (**Table 3**).

3. Conclusions

With the continual growth of global aquaculture, fish production continues to grow globally and till date only a small proportion of the aquatic animals come from managed breeding especially through applied molecular cloning and genomics (**Table 4**). The molecular biology of aquatic organisms offers many opportunities for rapid genetic gains as new genetic techniques make the improvement feasible in a wider range of model and non-model species. The future of molecular biology in aquaculture is bright with the technologies mentioned above being cheaper than ever, widely available and easily applicable in laboratories. However, the results obtained from these methods should not be conclusive without additional information, such as clinical diagnosis, as the mere detection of a certain pathogen does not

Category	Type of approach	Popular methods
Genomics	High throughput analysis	Microarray, NGS, whole genome bisulfate sequencing
	Marker based analysis	Rad sequencing, microsatellite, SNP, AFLP, RAPD, RFLP
Forward genetics	Chemical mutagenesis	ENU mutagenesis
	Transposon mutagenesis	Sleeping beauty, AcDs, Tol2, EnSpm-N6
Reverse genetics	Antisense and small RNA	Morpholino, PNA, SiRNA, shRNA
	Micro RNA	miRNA sponges, miRNA knockdown, miRNA mimics
	Conditional knockdown	Tet on/off
	Tilling	ENU mutagenesis
	Genome editing	ZFN, CRISPR/Cas9, TALEN
Transgenesis	Meganuclease	ISecI
	Transposon	Sleeping beauty, AcDs, Tol2, EnSpm-N6
	Recombinases (site specific)	PhiC3, Cre-loxP, BAC, Fosmid, YAC
Molecular genetics	Reporter cell line	Promoter analysis,
	Cell lineage	Gaudi toolbox
	Transactivation	LexPR, Gal4, tet on/off, heat shock protein
Transcriptomics	RNA detection	In situ hybridization, expressed sequence tagging, CDNA library, RNA-seq, microarray, QPCR, PCR
Proteomics	Protein detection	Antibody based analysis, chromatography and spectrophotometry

Table 4.
Summary of molecular biology application in fish.

imply necessarily that it is responsible for or even involved in a disease. Effective use of these techniques will reduce economic losses as well as risk of infection among wild fish species. Taking advantage of the numerous tissue specific sequence information available in the database, predictions of gene function by bioinformatics tools such as *in silico* and *in vitro* can be employed to identify candidate genes responsible for diseases or disease resistance that will reduce labor and cost of diagnosis and treatment. *In silico* approaches use computational tools to analyze raw DNA sequence data to simulate and predict the function and structural features of protein. In addition, the use of *in vitro* organoid models that refer to growing stem cells in 3D to generate cellular units that mimic an organ in both structure and function, is advancing rapidly. This method can also be applied in fish to study organ development, reproductive enhancement, fast tract selective breeding, disease and drug interactions as well. The new diagnostic techniques like, droplet digital PCR, Hybrid fusion FISH might improve the credibility and cost effectiveness of disease diagnosis.

Genome editing though has the advantage over traditional selective breeding and a trait can be introduced in a single generation without disrupting a favorable genetic background. Many traits of great significance in aquaculture could be targets for improvement by genome editing, including growth and reproductive performance, disease resistance, feed conversion efficiency, and tolerance to environmental stressors (temperature, salinity and oxygen). Keeping the animal welfare issues of "genetically modified organisms" in mind, fish that carry more muscle mass have also been produced by the disruption of a single gene (Myostatin, an inhibitor of skeletal muscle growth) in Common carp, Tilapia, Red sea bream and Japanese anchovy [74, 75, 82, 91]. But still the key question is whether the precise natural genome modifications will find greater public acceptance and make a way to commercial aquaculture. The long-term impacts of these non-transgenic GMOs on wild biodiversity and environment are an uncharted area too. So, in the coming era, we must rethink to what extent we can and should use these molecular advancements for aquaculture betterment.

Acknowledgements

This work was in part supported by Grants from Ministry of Education, Culture, Sports, Science and Technology (MEXT), Japanese Society for the Promotion of Science (JSPS) Kakenhi, Grant Nos. 16H04981, 18 K14520 and 19H03049; Sumitomo Grant No. 180959.

DOI: http://dx.doi.org/10.5772/intechopen.88197

Author details

Tapas Chakraborty[1]*, Sipra Mohapatra[1], Chimwar Wanglar[2] and Dipak Pandey[1]

1 South Ehime Fisheries Research Center, Ehime University, Ainan, Japan

2 College of Fisheries, Central Agricultural University, Imphal, India

*Address all correspondence to: tchakraborty83@gmail.com

References

[1] Nash CE. The History of Aquaculture. Ames Iowa: Wiley-Blackwell; 2011. 227 pp. ISBN: 978-0-8138-2163-4

[2] Smith P, Christofilogiannis P. Application of normalised resistance interpretation to the detection of multiple low-level resistances in strains of vibrio anguillarum obtained from Greek fish farms. Aquaculture. 2007;**272**(1):223-230

[3] Grace S. Lessons for aquaculture from agriculture: Selected comparisons of fish and animal farming. Masters thesis. University of Miami; 2014

[4] FAO Statistical Yearbook. Asia and the Pacific Food and Agriculture. 2014. Available from: http://www.fao.org/3/a-i3590e.pdf

[5] The World Bank annual report. End extreme poverty, promote shared prosperity. 2013. Available from: http://documents.worldbank.org/curated/en/947341468338396810/Main-report

[6] Houston RD, Macqueen DJ. Atlantic salmon (*Salmo salar* L.) genetics in the 21st century: Taking leaps forward in aquaculture and biological understanding. Animal Genetics. 2019;**50**(1):3-14

[7] Mialhe E, Bachère E, Boulo V, Cadoret JP. Strategy for research and international cooperation in marine invertebrate pathology immunology and genetics. Aquaculture. 1995;**132**:33-41

[8] Abollo E, Ramilo A, Casas SM, Comesaña P, Cao A, Carballal MJ, et al. First detection of the protozoan parasite Bonamia exitiosa (Haplosporidia) infecting flat oyster Ostrea edulis grown in European waters. Aquaculture. 2008;**274**:201-207

[9] Grijalva-Chon JM, Castro-Longoria R, Enriquez-Espinoza TL, Maeda-Martinez AN, Mendoza-Cano F. Molecular evidence of the protozoan parasite Marteilia refringens in Crassostrea gigas and Crassostrea corteziensis del Golfo de California. Latin American Journal of Aquatic Research. 2015;**43**:776-780

[10] Stentiford GD, Sritunyalucksana K, Flegel TW, Williams BAP, Withyachumnarnkul B, Itsathitphaisarn O, et al. New paradigms to help solve the global aquaculture disease crisis. PLoS Pathogens. 2017;**13**(2):e1006160

[11] Proxton IR. Molecular techniques in the diagnosis and management of infectious diseases: Do they have a role in bacteriology? Medical Principles and Practice. 2005;**14**(1):20-26

[12] Dong Z, Ge J, Li K, Xu Z, Liang D, et al. Heritable targeted inactivation of myostatin gene in yellow catfish (*Pelteobagrus fulvidraco*) using engineered zinc finger nucleases. PLoS One. 2011;**6**:e28897

[13] Grizzle JM, Altinok I, Fraser WA, Francis-Floyd R. First isolation of largemouth bass virus. Diseases of Aquatic Organisms. 2002;**50**:233-235

[14] Heppell J, Berthiaume L, Tarrab E, Lecomte J, Arella M. Evidence of genomic variations between infectious pancreatic necrosis virus strains determined by restriction fragment profiles. Journal of General Virology. 1992;**73**:2863-2870

[15] Radinsky R, Bucana CD, Ellis LM, Sanchez R, Cleary KR, Brigati DJ, et al. A rapid colorimetrie in situ messenger RNA hybridization technique for analysis of epidermal growth factor receptor in paraffin-embedded surgical specimens of human colon carcinomas. Cancer Research. 1993;**5**:937-943

[16] Trask BJ. Human cytogenetics: 46 chromosomes 46 years and counting. Nature Reviews Genetics. 2002;**3**:769-778

[17] Speicher MR, Carter NP. The new cytogenetics: Blurring the boundaries with molecular biology. Nature Reviews Genetics. 2005;**6**:782-792

[18] Millard PJ, Bickerstaff LE, LaPatra SE, Kim CH. Detection of infectious haematopoietic necrosis virus and infectious salmon anemia virus by molecular padlock amplification. Journal of Fish Diseases. 2006;**29**:201-213

[19] Miller KM, Maclean N. Teleost microarrays: Development in a broad phylogenetic range refleting diverse application. Journal of Fish Biology. 2008;**72**:2039-2050

[20] Baird NA, Etter PD, Atwood TS, Currey MC, Shiver AL, Lewis ZA, et al. Rapid SNP discovery and genetic mapping using sequenced RAD markers. PLoS One. 2008;**3**:e3376

[21] Andrews KR, Good JM, Miller MR, Luikart G, Hohenlohe PA. Harnessing the power of RADseq for ecological and evolutionary genomics. Nature Reviews Genetics. 2016;**17**:81-92

[22] Gonen S, Bishop SC, Houston RD. Exploring the utility of cross-laboratory RAD-sequencing datasets for phylogenetic analysis. BMC Research Notes. 2015;**8**:299

[23] Palaiokostas C, Bekaert M, Davie A, Cowan ME, Oral M, Taggart JB, et al. Mapping the sex determination locus in Atlantic halibut (*Hippoglossus hippoglossus*) using RAD sequencing. BMC Genomics. 2013;**14**:566

[24] Palaiokostas C, Bekaert M, Khan MG, Taggart JB, Gharbi K, McAndrew BJ, et al. A novel sex-determining QTL in Nile tilapia (*Oreochromis niloticus*). BMC Genomics. 2015;**16**:171

[25] Palaiokostas C, Bekaert M, Taggart JB, Gharbi K, McAndrew BJ, Chatain B, et al. A new SNP-based vision of the genetics of sex determination in European sea bass (*Dicentrarchus labrax*). Genetics Selection Evolution. 2015;**47**:68

[26] Wang W, Hu Y, Ma Y, Xu L, Guan J, Kong J. High-density genetic linkage mapping in turbot (*Scophthalmus maximus* L.) based on SNP markers and major sex- and growth-related regions detection. PLoS One. 2015;**13**:e0120410

[27] Vandeputte M, Haffray P. Parentage assignment with genomic markers: A major advance for understanding and exploiting genetic variation of quantitative traits in farmed aquatic animals. Frontiers in Genetics. 2014;**5**:432

[28] Palaiokostas C, Ferraresso S, Franch R, Houston RD, Bargelloni L. Genomic prediction of resistance to pasteurellosis in gilthead sea bream (*Sparus aurata*) using 2b-RAD sequencing. G3 (Bethesda). 2016;**6**:3693-3700

[29] Martnez V. Marker assisted selection in fish and shellfish breeding schemes. In: Guimarães E, Ruane J, Scherf B, Sonnino A, Dargie J, editors. Marker-Assisted Selection: Current Status and Future Perspectives in Crops Livestock Forestry and Fish. Rome, Italy: Electronic Publishing Policy and Support Branch Communication Division FAO; 2007. pp. 329-362

[30] Tsai HY, Hamilton A, Tinch AE, Guy DR, Gharbi K, Stear MJ, et al. Genome wide association and genomic prediction for growth traits in juvenile farmed Atlantic salmon using a high density SNP array. BMC Genomics. 2015;**16**:969

[31] Nguyen HN, Rastas PMA, Premachandra HKA, Knibb W. First high-density linkage map and single

nucleotide polymorphisms significantly associated with traits of economic importance in Yellowtail Kingfish *Seriola lalandi*. Frontiers in Genetics. 2018;**2018**:9-127

[32] Bangera R, Correa K, Lhorente JP, Figueroa R, Yanez JM. Genomic predictions can accelerate selection for resistance against Piscirickettsia salmonis in Atlantic salmon (*Salmo salar*). BMC Genomics. 2017;**18**:121

[33] Robledo D, Matika O, Hamilton A, Houston RD. Genome-wide association and genomic selection for resistance to amoebic gill disease in Atlantic salmon. G3. 2018;**8**:1195-1203

[34] Watson M. Illuminating the future of DNA sequencing. Genome Biology. 2014;**15**:108

[35] Munang'andu HM. Environmental viral metagenomics analyses in aquaculture: Applications in epidemiology and disease control. Frontiers in Microbiology. 2016;**7**:1986

[36] Hugenhotlz P. Exploring prokaryotic diversity in the genomic era. Genome Biology. 2002;**3**:reviews0003.1

[37] Breitbart M, Salamon P, Andresen B, Mahaffy JM, Segall AM, Mead D, et al. Genomic analysis of uncultured marine viral communities. Proceedings of the National Academy of Sciences of the United States of America. 2002;**99**:14250-14255

[38] Bibby K. Metagenomic identification of viral pathogens. Trends in Biotechnology. 2013;**31**:275-279

[39] Schirmbeck R, Reimann J. Revealing the potential of DNA-based vaccination lessons learned from the hepatitits B virus surface antigen. Biological Chemistry. 2001;**382**:543-552

[40] Hansen E, Fernandes K, Goldspink G, Butterworth P, Umeda PK, Chang KC. Strong expression of foreign genes following direct injection into fish muscle. FEBS Letters. 1991;**290**:307-312

[41] Dalmo RA. DNA vaccines for fish: Review and perspectives on correlates of protection. Journal of Fish Diseases. 2018;**41**:1-9

[42] Yoshikawa T, Kawamura Y, Ohashi M. Universal varicella vaccine immunization in Japan. Vaccine. 2016;**34**(19):1965-1970

[43] Soltani S, Farahani A, Dastranj M, Momenifar N, Mohajeri P, Emamie DA. DNA vaccine: Methods and mechanisms. Advances in Human Biology. 2018;**8**:132-139

[44] Chen TT, Lu JK, Fahs II R. Transgenic fish technology and its application in fish production. In: Altman A, editor. Agricultural Biotechnology. Marcel Dekker, Inc.; 1998. pp. 527-547

[45] Beardmore JA, Porter JS. Genetically modified organisms and aquaculture. FAO Fisheries Circular NO 989. Rome FAO 38. 2003

[46] Muller HJ. Artificial transmutation of the gene. Science. 1927;**66**:84-87

[47] Auerbach C, Robson JM, Carr JG. Chemical production of mutations. Science. 1947;**105**:243-247

[48] Rothstein RJ. One-step gene disruption in yeast. Methods in Enzymology. 1983;**101**:202-211

[49] Scherer S, Davis RW. Replacement of chromosome segments with altered DNA sequences constructed in vitro. Proceedings of the National Academy of Sciences of the United States of America. 1979;**76**:4951-4955

[50] Thomas KR, Folger KR, Capecchi MR. High frequency targeting of genes to specific sites in the mammalian genome. Cell. 1986;**44**:419-428

[51] Dorn S, Aghaallaei N, Jung G, Bajoghli B, Werner B, et al. Side chain modified peptide nucleic acids (PNA) for knock-down of six3 in medaka embryos. BMC Biotechnology. 2012;**12**:50

[52] Kok FO, Shin M, Ni CW, Gupta A, Grosse AS, et al. Reverse genetic screening reveals poor correlation between morpholino-induced and mutant phenotypes in zebrafish. Developmental Cell. 2014;**32**(1):97-108

[53] Gupta RM, Musunuru K. Expanding the genetic editing tool kit: ZFNs TALENs and CRISPR-Cas9. The Journal of Clinical Investigation. 2014;**124**:4154-4161

[54] Urnov FD, Rebar EJ, Holmes MC, Zhang HS, Gregory PD. Genome editing with engineered zinc finger nucleases. Nature Reviews. Genetics. 2010;**11**:636-646

[55] Miller JC, Tan S, Qiao G, Barlow KA, Wang J, Xia DF, et al. A TALE nuclease architecture for efficient genome editing. Nature Biotechnology. 2011;**29**:143-148

[56] Sakuma T, Yamamoto T. CRISPR/Cas9: The leading edge of genome editing technology. In: Yamamoto T, editor. Targeted Genome Editing Using Site-Specific Nucleases. Tokyo: Springer; 2015. pp. 25-41

[57] Sakuma T, Yamamoto T. Acceleration of cancer science with genome editing and related technologies. Cancer Science. 2018;**109**:3679-3685

[58] Zhu B, Wei G. Genome editing in fishes and their application. General and Comparative Endocrinology. 2018;**257**:3-12

[59] Wright DA, Li T, Yang B, Spalding MH. TALEN-mediated genome editing: Prospects and perspectives. The Biochemical Journal. 2014;**482**:15-24

[60] Wargelius A, Leininger S, Skaftnesmo KO, Kleppe L, Andersson E, Taranger GL, et al. Dnd knockout ablates germ cells and demonstrates germ cell independent sex differentiation in Atlantic salmon. Scientific Reports. 2016;**6**:21284

[61] Edvardsen RB, Leininger S, Kleppe L, Skaftnesmo KO, Wargelius A. Targeted mutagenesis in Atlantic salmon (*Salmo salar* L.) using the CRISPR/Cas9 system induces complete knockout individuals in the F0 generation. PLoS One. 2014;**9**:e108622

[62] Solin SL, Shive HR, Woolard KD, Essner JJ, McGrail M. Rapid tumor induction in zebrafish by TALEN-mediated somatic inactivation of the retinoblastoma1 tumor suppressor rb1. Scientific Reports. 2015;**5**:13745

[63] Aluru N, Karchner SI, Franks DG, Nacci D, Champlin D, Hahn ME. Targeted mutagenesis of aryl hydrocarbon receptor 2a and 2b genes in Atlantic killifish (*Fundulus heteroclitus*). Aquatic Toxicology. 2015;**158**:192-201

[64] Baloch AR, Franek R, Tichopad T, Fucikova M, Rodina M, Psenicka M. Dnd1 knockout in sturgeons by CRISPR/Cas9 generates germ cell free host for surrogate production. Animals. 2019;**9**(4):174

[65] Li MH, Yang HH, Li MR, Sun YL, Jiang XL, Xie QP, et al. Antagonistic roles of Dmrt1 and Foxl2 in sex differentiation via estrogen production in tilapia as demonstrated by TALENs. Endocrinology. 2013;**154**:4814-4825

[66] Li M, Yang H, Zhao J, Fang L, Shi H, Li M, et al. Efficient and heritable gene targeting in tilapia by CRISPR/Cas9. Genetics. 2014;**197**:591-599

[67] Jiang DN, Yang H, Li MH, Shi HJ, Zhang XB, Wang DS. Gsdf is a downstream gene of dmrt1 that functions in the male sex determination pathway of the Nile tilapia. Molecular Reproduction and Development. 2016;**83**:497-508

[68] Wu L, Yang P, Luo F, Wang D, Zhou L. R-spondin1 signaling pathway is required for both the ovarian and testicular development in a teleosts Nile tilapia (*Oreochromis niloticus*). General and Comparative Endocrinology. 2016;**230-231**:177-185

[69] Xie QP, He X, Sui YN, Chen LL, Sun LN, Wang DS. Haploinsufficiency of SF-1 causes female to male sex reversal in Nile tilapia *Oreochromis niloticus*. Endocrinology. 2016;**157**:2500-2514

[70] Ma L, Jeffery WR, Essner JJ, Kowalko JE. Genome editing using TALENs in blind Mexican cavefish Astyanax mexicanus. PLoS One. 2015;**10**:e0119370

[71] Qin Z, Li Y, Su B, Cheng Q, Ye Z, Perera DA, et al. Editing of the luteinizing hormone gene to sterilize channel catfish *Ictalurus punctatus* using a modified zinc finger nuclease technology with electroporation. Marine Biotechnology (New York, N.Y.). 2016;**18**:255-263

[72] Zu Y, Zhang XS, Ren JF, Dong XH, Zhu Z, Jia L, et al. Biallelic editing of a lamprey genome using the CRISPR/Cas9 system. Scientific Reports. 2016;**6**:23496

[73] Zhong Z, Niu P, Wang M, Huang G, Xu S, Sun Y, et al. Targeted disruption of sp7 and myostatin with CRISPR-Cas9 results in severe bone defects and more muscular cells in common carp. Scientific Reports. 2016;**6**:22953

[74] Yeh YC, Kinoshita M, Ng TH, Chang YH, Maekawa S, Chiang YA, et al. Using CRISPR/Cas9-mediated gene editing to further explore growth and trade-off effects in myostatin mutated F4 medaka (*Oryzias latipes*). Scientific Reports. 2017;**7**:11435

[75] Doyon Y, McCammon JM, Miller JC, Faraji F, Ngo C, Katibah GE, et al. Heritable targeted gene disruption in zebrafish using designed zinc-finger nucleases. Nature Biotechnology. 2008;**26**:702-708

[76] Siegfried KR, Nusslein-Volhard C. Germ line control of female sex determination in zebrafish. Developmental Biology. 2008;**324**:277-287

[77] Sander JD, Cade L, Khayter C, Reyon D, Peterson RT, Joung JK, et al. Targeted gene disruption in somatic zebrafish cells using engineered TALENs. Nature Biotechnology. 2011;**29**:697-698

[78] Dahlem TJ, Hoshijima K, Jurynec MJ, Gunther D, Starker CG, Locke AS, et al. Simple methods for generating and detecting locus-specific mutations induced with TALENs in the zebrafish genome. PLoS Genetics. 2012;**8**:e1002861

[79] Jao LE, Wente SR, Chen W. Efficient multiplex biallelic zebrafish genome editing using a CRISPR nuclease system. Proceedings of the National Academy of Sciences of the United States of America. 2013;**110**:13904-13909

[80] Irion U, Krauss J, Nusslein-Volhard C. Precise and efficient genome editing in zebrafish using the CRISPR/Cas9 system. Development. 2014;**141**:4827-4830

[81] Chu L, Li J, Liu Y, Hu W, Cheng CH. Targeted gene disruption in zebrafish reveals non canonical functions of LH signaling in reproduction. Molecular Endocrinology. 2014;**28**:1785-1795

[82] Chu L, Li J, Liu Y, Cheng CH. Gonadotropin signaling in zebrafish ovary and testis development: Insights from gene knockout study. Molecular Endocrinology. 2015;**29**:1743-1758

[83] Zhang Z, Lau SW, Zhang L, Ge W. Disruption of zebrafish follicle-stimulating hormone receptor (fshr) but not luteinizing hormone receptor (lhcgr) gene by TALEN leads to failed follicle activation in females followed by sexual reversal to males. Endocrinology. 2015;**156**:3747-3762

[84] Zhang Z, Zhu B, Ge W. Genetic analysis of zebrafish gonadotropin (FSH and LH) functions by TALEN-mediated gene disruption. Molecular Endocrinology. 2015;**29**:76-98

[85] Tang HP, Liu Y, Luo DJ, Ogawa S, Yin YK, Li SS, et al. The kiss/kissr systems are dispensable for zebrafish reproduction: Evidence from gene knockout studies. Endocrinology. 2015;**156**:589-599

[86] Shu Y, Lou Q, Dai Z, Dai X, He J, Hu W, et al. The basal function of teleost prolactin as a key regulator on ion uptake identified with zebrafish knockout models. Scientific Reports. 2016;**6**:18597

[87] Dranow DB, Hu K, Bird AM, Lawry ST, Adams MT, Sanchez A, et al. Bmp15 is an oocyte-produced signal required for maintenance of the adult female sexual phenotype in zebrafish. PLoS Genetics. 2016;**12**:e1006323

[88] Yabe T, Hoshijima K, Yamamoto T, Takada S. Quadruple zebrafish mutant reveals different roles of Mesp genes in somite segmentation between mouse and zebrafish. Development. 2016;**143**:2842-2852

[89] Spicer OS, Wong TT, Zmora N, Zohar Y. Targeted mutagenesis of the hypophysiotropic gnrh3 in zebrafish (*Danio rerio*) reveals no effects on reproductive performance. PLoS One. 2016;**11**(6):e0158141

[90] Moore JC, Mulligan TS, Torres Yordan N, Castranova D, Pham VN, Tang Q, et al. T cell immune deficiency in zap70 mutant zebrafish. Molecular and Cellular Biology. 2016;**23**:2868-2876

[91] Huang G, Zhang F, Ye Q, Wang H. The circadian clock regulates autophagy directly through the nuclear hormone receptor Nr1d1/Rev-erb and indirectly via Cebpb/(C/ebp.) in zebrafish. Autophagy. 2016;**12**:1292-1309

[92] Hu M, Bai Y, Zhang C, Liu F, Cui Z, Chen J, et al. Liver-enriched gene 1 a glycosylated secretory protein binds to FGFR and mediates an anti-stress pathway to protect liver development in zebrafish. PLoS Genetics. 2016;**12**:e1005881

[93] Gao Y, Dai Z, Shi C, Zhai G, Jin X, He J, et al. Depletion of Myostatin b promotes somatic growth and lipid metabolism in zebrafish. Frontiers in Endocrinology. 2016;**7**:88

[94] Wen J, Sun X, Chen H, Liu H, Lai R, Li J, et al. Mutation of rnf213a by TALEN causes abnormal angiogenesis and circulation defects in zebrafish. Brain Research. 1644;**2016**:70-78

[95] Serifi I, Tzima E, Soupsana K, Karetsou Z, Beis D, Papamarcaki T. The zebrafish homologs of SET/I2PP2A oncoprotein: Expression patterns and insights into their physiological roles during development. The Biochemical Journal. 2016;**473**:4609-4627

[96] Samsa LA, Ito CE, Brown DR, Qian L, Liu J. IgG-containing isoforms of neuregulin-1 are dispensable for cardiac trabeculation in zebrafish. PLoS One. 2016;**11**:e0166734

[97] Grone BP, Marchese M, Hamling KR, Kumar MG, Krasniak CS, Sicca F, et al. Epilepsy behavioral abnormalities and physiological comorbidities in syntaxin-binding protein 1 (STXBP1) mutant zebrafish. PLoS One. 2016;**11**:e0151148

[98] Lau ES, Zhang Z, Qin M, Ge W. Knockout of zebrafish ovarian aromatase gene (cyp19a1a) by TALEN and CRISPR/Cas9 leads to all-male offspring due to failed ovarian differentiation. Scientific Reports. 2016;**6**:37357

[99] Lin Q, Zhang Y, Zhou R, Zheng Y, Zhao L, Huang M, et al. Establishment of a congenital amegakaryocytic thrombocytopenia model and a thrombocyte-specific reporter line in zebrafish. Leukemia. 2017;**31**:1206-1216

[100] Webster KA, Schach U, Ordaz A, Steinfeld JS, Draper BW, Siegfried KR. Dmrt1 is necessary for male sexual development in zebrafish. Developmental Biology. 2017;**422**:33-46

[101] Zhai G, Shu TT, Xia YG, Jin X, He JY, Yin Z. Androgen signaling regulates the transcription of anti-Mullerian hormone via synergy with SRY-related protein SOX9A. Scientific Bulletin. 2017;**62**:197-203

[102] Lu H, Cui Y, Jiang L, Ge W. Functional analysis of nuclear estrogen receptors (nERs) in zebrafish reproduction by genome editing approach. Endocrinology. 2017;**158**:2292-2308

[103] Wang H, Luo L, Yang D. Loss of Gspt1l disturbs the patterning of the brain central arteries in zebrafish. Biochemical and Biophysical Research Communications. 2017;**486**:156-162

[104] Xiong ST, Wu JJ, Jing J, Huang PP, Li Z, Mei J, et al. Loss of stat3 function leads to spine malformation and immune disorder in zebrafish. Scientific Bulletin. 2017;**62**:185-196

[105] Lebedeva S, de Jesus Domingues AM, Butter F, Ketting RF. Characterization of genetic loss-of-function of Fus in zebrafish. RNA Biology. 2017;**14**:29-35

[106] Zhang D, Wang J, Zhou C, Xiao W. Zebrafish akt2 is essential for survival growth bone development and glucose homeostasis. Mechanisms of Development. 2017;**143**:42-52

[107] Liu Y, Tang HP, Xie R, Li SS, Liu XC, Lin HR, et al. Genetic evidence for multifactorial control of the reproductive axis in zebrafish. Endocrinology. 2017;**158**:604-611

[108] Zhang Y, Huang H, Zhao G, Yokoyama T, Vega H, Huang Y, et al. ATP6V1H deficiency impairs bone development through activation of MMP9 and MMP13. PLoS Genetics. 2017;**13**:e1006481

[109] Sakaguchi K, Yoneda M, Sakai N, Nakashima K, Kitano H, Matsuyama M. Comprehensive experimental system for a promising model organism candidate for marine teleosts. Scientific Reports. 2019;**9**:4948

[110] Kurokawa H, Saito D, Nakamura S, Katoh-Fukui Y, Ohta K, Baba T, et al. Germ cells are essential for sexual dimorphism in the medaka gonad. Proceedings of the National Academy of Sciences of the United States of America. 2007;**104**:16958-16963

[111] Nishimura T, Sato T, Yamamoto Y, Watakabe I, Ohkawa Y, Suyama M, et al. foxl3 is a germ cell-intrinsic factor involved in sperm-egg fate decision in medaka. Science. 2015;**349**:328-331

[112] Luo D, Liu Y, Chen J, Xia X, Cao M, Cheng B, et al. Direct production of XYDMY− sex reversal female medaka (*Oryzias latipes*) by embryo

microinjection of TALENs. Scientific Reports. 2015;**5**:14057

[113] Chen J, Cui XJ, Jia ST, Luo DJ, Cao MX, Zhang YS, et al. Disruption of dmc1 produces abnormal sperm in medaka (*Oryzias latipes*). Scientific Reports. 2016;**6**:30912

[114] Zhang X, Guan G, Li M, Zhu F, Liu Q, Naruse K, et al. Autosomal gsdf acts as a male sex initiator in the fish medaka. Scientific Reports. 2016;**6**:19738

[115] Takahashi A, Kanda S, Abe T, Oka Y. Evolution of the hypothalamic-pituitary-gonadal axis regulation in vertebrates revealed by knockout medaka. Endocrinology. 2016;**157**:3994-4002

[116] Kishimoto K, Washio Y, Yoshiura Y, Toyoda A, Ueno T, Fukuyama H, et al. Production of a breed of red sea bream *Pagrus major* with an increase of skeletal muscle mass and reduced body length by genome editing with CRISPR/Cas9. Aquaculture. 2018;**495**:415-427

[117] Feng K, Luo H, Li Y, Chen J, Wang Y, Sun Y, et al. High efficient gene targeting in rice field eel *Monopterus albus* by transcription activator-like effector nucleases. Science Bulletin. 2017;**62**:162-164

[118] Chakrapani V, Patra SK, Panda RP, Rasal KD, Jayasankar P, Barman HK. Establishing targeted carp TLR22 gene disruption via homologous recombination using CRISPR/Cas9. Developmental and Comparative Immunology. 2016;**61**:242-247

[119] Chen J, Wang W, Tian Z, Dong Y, Zhu H, Zhu HH, et al. Efficient gene transfer and gene editing in Sterlet (*Acipenser ruthenus*). Frontiers in Genetics. 2018;**9**:117

Chapter 5

Molecular Cloning of Genic Male-Sterility Genes and Their Applications for Plant Heterosis via Biotechnology-based Male-sterility Systems

Xiangyuan Wan and Suowei Wu

Abstract

In this chapter, we summarize the strategies about molecular cloning and functional confirmation of plant genic male-sterility (GMS) genes and their applications for hybrid breeding and seed production via biotechnology-based male-sterility (BMS) systems in crop plants. The main content includes four sections: (1) GMS gene cloning strategies, including forward genetic approaches (e.g., map-based cloning, T-DNA or transposon tagging, and MutMap method) and reverse genetic approaches (e.g., homology-based cloning, anther-specific expression gene screening, and other reverse genetic methods); (2) functional confirmation methods of GMS genes, including transgenic complementation, targeted mutagenesis, allelic mutant test and sequencing, anther spatiotemporal expression analysis, and cytological observation; (3) application value assessment of GMS genes and mutants, such as genetic stability analysis of male sterility controlled by GMS genes under different genetic backgrounds and multiple environments, and genetic effects driven by GMS genes on plant heterosis and analysis of potential linkage with bad traits; (4) development and application of BMS systems based on GMS genes and/or their mutants, including transgenic construct-driven non-transgenic seed systems (e.g., seed production technology (SPT) and multi-control sterility (MCS)), and transgenic male-sterility systems (e.g., roundup hybridization systems (RHS1 and RHS2) and Barnase/Barstar system). Finally, we summarize and provide our perspectives on the studies of GMS genes and development of cost-effective and environment-friendly BMS systems in crop plants.

Keywords: gene cloning, genic male sterility (GMS), biotechnology-based male sterility (BMS), heterosis application, genetically modified plants

1. Introduction

The demand for food supply is increasing exponentially with the human population continuously growing. According to a report, the world population is predicted to increase by 34% by 2050 [1], whereas the area of land for agriculture practices is decreasing consistently over the last few decades because of urbanization and land degradation. Therefore, it is necessary to increase the food production per unit area as cultivated lands are limited [2].

IntechOpen

Hybrid vigor (or heterosis) is the superior performance of the heterozygous hybrid progeny over both homozygous parents. Most crops show hybrid vigor, such as maize, rice, wheat, sorghum, rapeseed, and sunflower, but commercial production of hybrids is only feasible if a reliable and cost-effective pollination control system is available. In cereal crops, maize is a monoecious and diclinous species, which makes it very successful in heterosis utilization with relatively feasible emasculation. The emasculation, namely, the physical removal of the male floral structure, usually includes manual and mechanical detasseling. However, emasculation is not only time-consuming, labor-intensive, and expensive but also detrimental to plant growth, thus reducing the yield of hybrid seed. At the same time, it is unfeasible for the crops that have small, bisexual flowers, such as rice, wheat, and barley. Therefore, it is an ideal alternative to use male-sterile line for pollination control in these cereal crops [3, 4].

Male sterility (MS) refers to cases in which viable male gametes (i.e., pollen) are not produced, while female gametes are fully fertile. Male sterility can be generated by either cytoplasmic or nuclear genes. Cytoplasmic male sterility (CMS) is caused by mitochondrial genes together with nuclear genes and has been used in commercial hybrid production in crops (such as maize, rice, and oilseed rape), but this method suffers from the poor genetic diversity, increased disease susceptibility, and unreliable restoration of CMS lines [5]. Genic male sterility (GMS) is caused by nuclear genes alone, and the use of GMS can overcome these drawbacks, but it is difficult to obtain a pure and large-scale increase of male-sterile female lines through self-pollination. Fortunately, with the rapid development of GMS gene isolation methods, plant-transformation techniques, and other new biotechnologies, many efforts have been made to identify and utilize GMS genes and ultimately develop more efficient biotechnology-based male sterility (BMS) systems in crop plants [3, 4, 6].

In this chapter, we systemically described the molecular cloning methods, functional confirmation approaches, application value assessment of GMS genes, as well as the strategies and comprehensive evaluation of BMS systems based on elite GMS genes in cereal crops (**Figures 1** and **2**). This will provide a guideline and shed light on GMS gene cloning and application in hybrid seed breeding and production via BMS systems in major cereal crops.

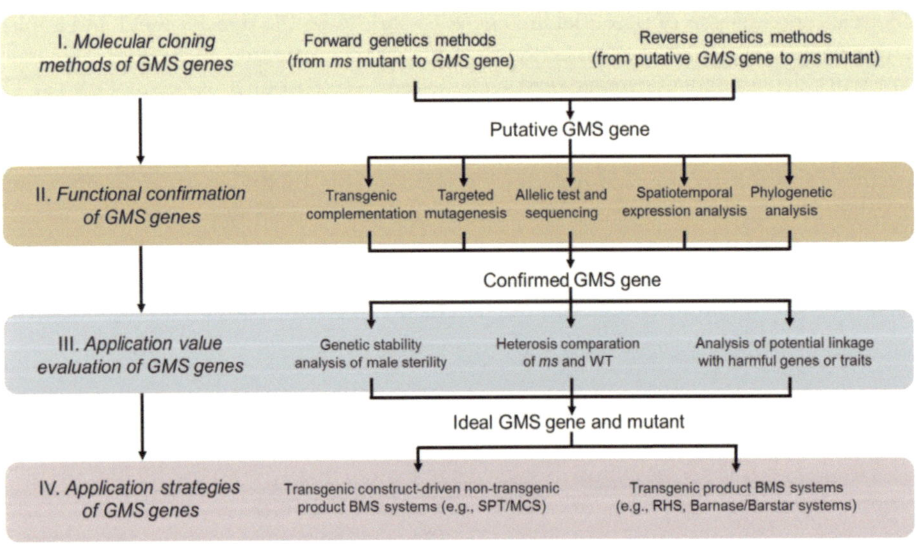

Figure 1.
The technology workflow of cloning methods and application strategies of GMS genes in crop plants.

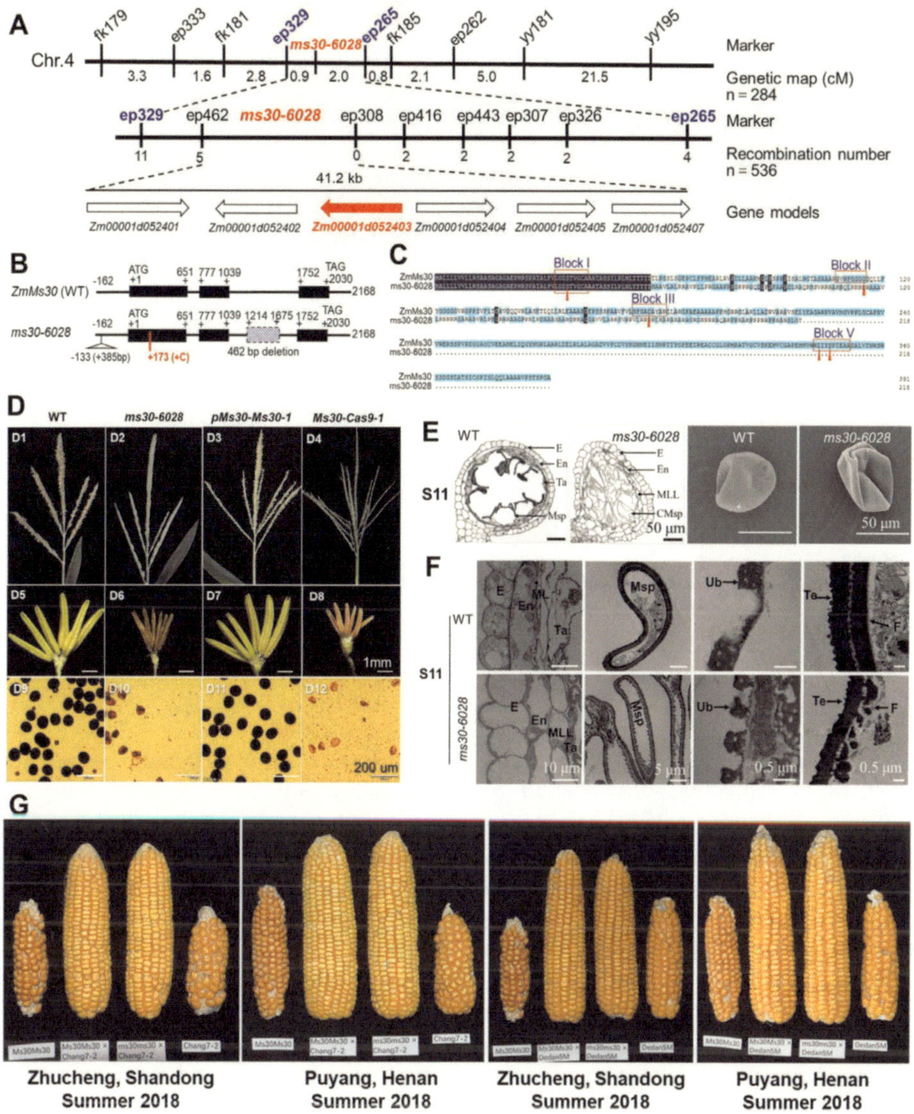

Figure 2.
A typical example of maize ZmMs30 *gene: from map-based cloning and functional confirmation to application value assessment (adapted from Ref. [18]). (A) Map-based cloning of* ZmMs30 *gene; (B) gene structure and mutation site comparison between WT and* ms30-6028 *mutant; (C) predictive protein sequence comparison of ZmMs30 between WT and* ms30-6028 *mutant; (D) transgenic complementation and CRISPR-Ca9-targeted mutagenesis confirmation of ZmMs30 gene in maize; (E and F) cytological observation of anther and pollen development in WT and* ms30-6028 *mutant at stage 11 (S11) by using transverse section light microscopy, SEM (E) and TEM (F); (G) heterosis comparison of WT and* ms30-6028 *mutant by using two representative hybrid combinations with male lines Chang 7-2 and Dedan5M in two locations, respectively.*

2. Molecular cloning strategies of GMS genes in crop plants

There are basically two ways to clone GMS genes in crops: forward and reverse genetics. Forward genetic approaches require the cloning of sequences underlying the male-sterile phenotype, such as map-based cloning, T-DNA or transposon tagging, and MutMap method (**Figure 3**), whereas reverse genetic strategies seek to identify and select mutations in a known sequence, such as homology-based cloning, anther-specific expression gene screening, and other reverse genetic cloning strategies.

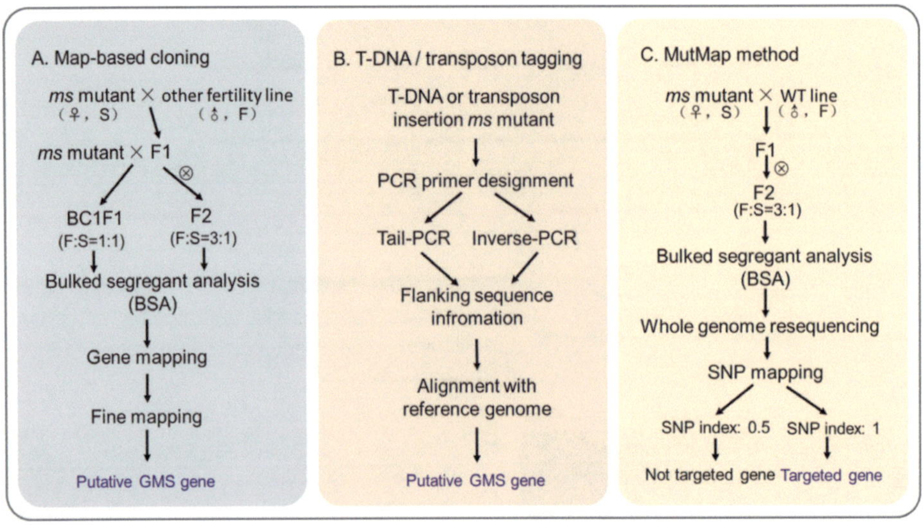

Figure 3.
The forward genetic approaches of GMS gene cloning in crop plants.

2.1 Forward genetic approaches

2.1.1 Map-based cloning

Map-based cloning or positional cloning is a classical forward genetic strategy of GMS gene cloning. Map-based cloning strategy relies on linkage disequilibrium between markers and the gene of interest, that is, as distances between the gene of interest and the analyzed markers decrease, so does the frequency of recombination. In general, the procedure of map-based cloning method includes the following steps (**Figure 3A**). First is the construction of segregating population of F_2 or BC_1F_1 by crossing male-sterile mutant with a distant male-fertile line followed by self-pollination or backcrossing with the male-sterility mutant line. Second is primary mapping of GMS gene based on bulked segregant analysis (BSA) and molecular marker (such as SSR, SNP, and INDELs) linkage analysis using the F_2 or BC_1F_1 segregating populations which have high levels of linkage disequilibrium. Third is fine mapping of GMS gene by developing more polymorphic markers and enlarging the segregating population. Finally, the GMS gene will be narrowed down to a small interval on the targeted chromosome. Under the help of bioinformatic analysis, the putative GMS gene will be identified.

So far, there are at least 38 GMS genes in major cereal crops that have been cloned via map-based cloning strategy, including 20, 15, and 3 GMS genes reported in rice, maize, and wheat, respectively (**Table 1**). As the genome sequence information of more crop plants is available, there will be more GMS genes isolated by map-based cloning strategy in crop plants.

2.1.2 T-DNA or transposon tagging

T-DNA or transposon tagging are efficient and straightforward approaches for GMS gene cloning based on the T-DNA or transposon insertion male-sterile mutants (**Figure 3B**), PCR, and bioinformatic analysis. If the male-sterile mutant comes from a T-DNA or transposon insertion, rapid identification of the GMS gene is at least theoretically possible by locating the sequence tag and analyzing its neighboring sequences by using thermal asymmetric interlaced (TAIL) PCR,

No.	Cloning strategy	GMS genes	Crops	Functional confirmation methods*	Application value evaluation	References
1	Map-based cloning	*ZmMs7*	Maize	1, 3, 4, 5	MCS system	[9]
		ZmMs8	Maize	4	No data	[10]
		ZmMs9	Maize	3, 4	No data	[11]
		ZmMs10/ APV1	Maize	3, 4	No data	[12]
		ZmMs22/ MSCA1	Maize	1, 3, 4, 5	No data	[13, 14]
		ZmMs23	Maize	3, 4, 5	No data	[15]
		ZmMs26	Maize	1, 2, 3, 4	SPT system	[16, 17]
		ZmMs30	Maize	1, 2, 3, 4	MCS, sterility stability, and heterosis analysis	[18]
		ZmMs32	Maize	3, 4, 5	No data	[19]
		ZmMs33	Maize	1, 2, 3, 4, 5	MCS, MAS	[20, 21]
		Zmms44	Maize	4	Maize SPT-like	[22]
		ZmMs6021	Maize	1, 3, 4, 5	No data	[23]
		IG1	Maize	3, 4	No data	[24]
		MAC1	Maize	2, 3, 4	No data	[25]
		IPE1/ ZmMs20	Maize	3, 4	No data	[26, 27]
		MIL1	Rice	1, 4	No data	[28]
		MIL2	Rice	3, 4	No data	[29]
		TIP2/ bHLH142	Rice	1, 4, 5	No data	[30, 31]
		TIP3	Rice	1, 2, 3, 4	No data	[32]
		CYP704B2	Rice	1, 4, 5	No data	[33]
		CYP703A3	Rice	4, 5	No data	[34]
		PTC1	Rice	1, 4, 5	No data	[35]
		TDR	Rice	1, 4, 5	No data	[36]
		OsNP1	Rice	1, 4, 5	No data	[37]
		OsGPAT3	Rice	1, 3, 4, 5	No data	[38]
		DPW	Rice	1, 4, 5	No data	[39]
		DPW2	Rice	1, 3, 4	No data	[40]
		OsDEX1	Rice	1, 3, 4, 5	No data	[41]
		CSA	Rice	1, 4	No data	[42]
		OsABCG26	Rice	1, 2, 4, 5	No data	[43]
		OsPKS2	Rice	1, 4, 5	No data	[44]
		EAT1	Rice	1, 3, 4, 5	No data	[45]
		PDA1/ OsABCG15	Rice	3, 4, 5	No data	[46]
		MTR1	Rice	1, 4	No data	[47]
		OsERS1	Rice	1, 4	No data	[48]
		TaMs1	Wheat	1, 2, 3, 4	Wheat SPT-like	[49]
		TaMs2	Wheat	1, 2, 3, 4	No data	[50, 51]
		TaMs5	Wheat	1, 2, 3, 4	No data	[52]

No.	Cloning strategy	GMS genes	Crops	Functional confirmation methods*	Application value evaluation	References
2	T-DNA tagging	*bHLH142*	Rice	1, 4, 5	No data	[31]
		OsAPI5	Rice	1, 3, 4	No data	[53]
		OsGT1	Rice	3, 4	No data	[54]
		UDT1	Rice	3, 4, 5	No data	[7]
		RIP1	Rice	2, 3, 4	No data	[55]
		WDA1	Rice	2, 3, 4, 5	No data	[56]
		OsCP1	Rice	4,	No data	[57]
		GSL5	Rice	2, 3, 4, 5	No data	[58]
		DTM1	Rice	3, 4	No data	[59]
		DTC1	Rice	3, 4	No data	[60]
3	Transposon tagging	*ZmMs45*	Maize	1, 2, 3	STP system	[8, 61, 62]
		OCL4	Maize	2, 3, 4	No data	[63]
		OsGAMYB	Rice	1, 3, 4, 5	No data	[64]
		MSP1	Rice	1, 4, 5	No data	[65]
		CAP1	Rice	1, 4, 5	No data	[66]
4	MutMap cloning	*OsLAP6/ OsPKS1*	Rice	2, 3, 4, 5	No data	[67]
		OsABCG26	Rice	1, 2, 4, 5	No data	[68]
		OsNP1	Rice	1, 2, 3, 4, 5	Rice SPT-like	[69]
		TaMs1	Wheat	1, 2, 3, 4	No data	[70]
5	Homology-based cloning	*OsTDF1*	Rice	1, 2, 4, 5, 6	No data	[71]
		OsACOS12	Rice	1, 3, 4, 5, 6	No data	[72]
		OsIG1	Rice	2, 3, 4, 5, 6	No data	[24, 73]
		OsCER1	Rice	2, 3, 4, 5, 6	No data	[74]
		OsRAFTIN	Rice	2, 4, 5, 6	No data	[75]
		TaMs45	Wheat	1, 2, 3, 4, 5	No data	[76]
		TaMs26	Wheat	1, 2, 4, 5, 6	No data	[77]
6	Anther-specific expression gene screening	*OsC6*	Rice	2, 4, 5, 6	No data	[78]
		OsG1	Rice	2, 4, 6	No data	[79]
		OsADF	Rice	2, 4, 6	No data	[80]
		OsUAM3	Rice	2, 4, 6	No data	[81]
		TaRAFTIN	Wheat	2, 4, 5, 6	No data	[75]
7	Other reverse genetic cloning	*OsSTRL2*	Rice	2, 4, 5, 6	No data	[82]
		OsFTIP7	Rice	2, 3, 4	No data	[83]
		OsTGA10	Rice	2, 3, 4, 5, 6	No data	[84]
		OsAGO2	Rice	2, 3, 4, 6	No data	[85]

*Notes: *(1) functional complementation, (2) knockout by using CRISPR-Cas9 or knockdown by using RNAi, (3) allelism test and allelic mutant sequencing, (4) anther-specific expression analysis, (5) phylogenetic analysis and orthologous analysis with known GMS gene, (6) cytological observation*

Table 1.
Cloning, functional confirmation, and application value evaluation of GMS genes in crops.

inverse PCR, and genomic PCR methods. There are at least 10 GMS genes cloned by using T-DNA tagging in rice, such as *API5*, *bHLH142*, *OsGT1*, *UDT1*, *RIP1*, *WDA1*, *OsCP1*, *GSL5*, *DTM1*, and *DTC1* (**Table 1**). For instance, rice *UDT1* (*Undeveloped Tapetum1*) gene was isolated from a T-DNA insertional rice male-sterile mutant by using T-DNA tagging method [7]. The flanking region of the inserted T-DNA in mutant line was amplified by TAIL–PCR. Sequence analysis of that region revealed that T-DNA was inserted into a gene located on chromosome 7. BLAST analysis indicated that the most similar proteins are the *Brassica napus* bHLH transcription factor CAD54298 and the *Arabidopsis* bHLH protein AMS (At2g16910), each of which shares 32% overall identity with the rice protein. These results indicated that *UDT1* encodes a putative bHLH transcription factor in rice [7].

In addition, there are at least two and three GMS genes cloned via transposon tagging in maize (*Ms45* and *OCL4*) and rice (*OsGAMYB*, *MSP1*, and *CAP1*), respectively (**Table 1**). For example, maize *Ms45* gene is isolated by an activator transposon tagging, the tassel-specific transcription of *Ms45* gene is shown by RNA hybridization analysis, and genetic transformation of *ms45* mutant with a copy of *Ms45* gene can restore the fertility phenotype in maize [8].

2.1.3 MutMap method

MutMap method is based on whole-genome sequencing of pooled DNA from a segregating population of plants that show a useful phenotype [86], for example, male sterility resulted from ethyl methanesulfonate (EMS) mutagenesis (**Figure 3C**). In classic MutMap method, a GMS mutant is crossed directly to the original wild-type line; the resulting F_1 is self-pollinated to obtain F_2 progeny segregating for the GMS mutant and wild-type phenotypes. DNA of F_2 displaying the mutant phenotype is bulked and subjected to whole-genome sequencing followed by alignment to the reference sequence. SNPs with sequence reads composed only of mutant sequences (SNP index of 1; SNP index is defined as the ratio between the number of reads of a mutant SNP and the total number of reads corresponding to the SNP) are closely linked to the causal SNP for the mutant phenotype [86]. The MutMap method was used for rice GMS gene cloning, e.g., *OsLAP6/OsPKS1* [67]. Recently, a modified MutMap method was developed in rice male-sterility gene (*OsMs55/MER3*) cloning [87]. Different from the original MutMap method that aligns the mutant pool DNA sequence with the assembled WT genome, the modified MutMap method was to align the re-sequencing data of the mutant pool DNA and WT DNA with the Nipponbare reference genome. The resulting SNPs of mutant/Nipponbare and WT/Nipponbare were further compared to determine the candidate mutant gene. This modified method does not need an assembled WT genome as reference and thus is more cost-effective and widely applicable. The modified MutMap method was used for GMS gene cloning in rice and wheat, such as *OsABCG26* [68], *OsNP1* [69], and *TaMs1* [70] (**Table 1**). As the next-generation sequencing technology advances and cost of sequencing decreases rapidly, the MutMap method will be applicable for more crop plants except for rice and wheat.

2.2 Reverse genetic approaches

Reverse genetic approach means from gene to phenotype and relies upon sequence information as retrieved from genome, cDNA library, and/or expressed sequence tag (EST) sequencing. The scientist starts with the selection of a specific sequence and tries to gain insight into the underlying function by selecting for mutations that disrupt the sequence and thereby its function. The reverse genetic approaches for GMS gene cloning include homology-based cloning, anther-specific expression gene screening, and other methods.

2.2.1 Homology-based cloning

Homology-based cloning is a simple and straightforward method of GMS gene cloning, and it relies on the conservation in sequence and function of the reference GMS gene among different species, mainly through the sequence alignment and phylogenetic analysis of the related GMS genes. As a lot of GMS genes have been cloned in model plants and the genome sequencing information become available for most important crops [88], there are several GMS genes that have been identified through homology-based cloning approach, such as *OsTDF1*, *OsACOS12*, *OsCER1*, *OsIG1*, *OsRAFTIN*, *TaMs26*, and *TaMs45* (**Table 1**). In *Arabidopsis* and rice, the molecular, genetic, and biochemical pathways regulating anther and pollen development have been extensively studied [89, 90], revealing the same number of developmental stages (14) and relatively conserved regulatory pathways in both species [91, 92]. The information about GMS obtained in *Arabidopsis* and rice provides opportunities to identify and utilize male sterility in economically important crops such as maize, barley, and wheat where GMS systems are not as well characterized [88, 93]. Based on this gene cloning strategy, about 62 putative maize GMS genes have been predicted and analyzed recently [3], and this will greatly enlarge the GMS gene number after functional confirmation via multiple methods (refer to Section 3).

2.2.2 Anther-specific expression gene screening

Given that most of GMS genes show anther-specific expression pattern, some putative GMS genes can be isolated by differential screening of the anther cDNA library, such as the GMS genes *OsC6*, *OsG1*, *OsADF*, and *OsUAM3* in rice and *TaRAFTIN* in wheat (**Table 1**). *OsC6*, encoding a lipid transfer protein, was reported to be abundantly expressed in tapetal cells of the anther and played a crucial role in the development of lipidic orbicules and pollen exine during another development in rice [78, 94]. *OsG1* was originally cloned from a rice anther cDNA library, encoding a β-1,3-glucanase and belonging to the defense-related subfamily A. *OsG1* was essential for callose degradation in tetrad dissolution, and its silencing results in male sterility [79]. *OsADF*, encoding an anther development F-box protein, was obtained from a rice panicle cDNA clone and played a critical role in rice tapetum cell development and pollen formation [80]. *OsUAM3* (UDP-arabinopyranose mutase 3) was identified by screening the expression patterns of the *OsUAM* genes in various vegetative and reproductive tissues and found to be a unique gene required for pollen wall morphogenesis in reproductive development [81]. *TaRAFTIN* was identified from an anther cDNA library of hexaploid wheat and cloned by using the RACE-PCR method, encoding a sporophytically produced structural protein that is essential for pollen development [75].

2.2.3 Other reverse genetic approaches

Once a GMS gene is cloned and characterized, its interaction protein or targeted gene may be involved in male-sterility regulation, too. Therefore, some of the GMS genes could be isolated by other reverse genetic approaches, such as chromatin immunoprecipitation sequencing (ChIP-Seq), genome-wide expression analysis of a specific gene family, targeted mutagenesis of candidate GMS genes, etc. For example, *OsTGA10* encoding a bZIP transcription factor was identified as a target of the MADS box protein OsMADS8 by using the ChIP-seq technique, and mutation of OsTGA10 resulted in male sterility [84]. *OsSTRL2* was identified based on the genome-wide expression analysis of rice STR-like (*OsSTRL*) gene family and its anther-specific expression pattern [82]. *OsFTIP7* was identified as GMS gene through targeted mutagenesis of the rice genes encoding multiple C2 domain and transmembrane region proteins (MCTPs) using the clustered regularly interspaced short palindromic repeats (CRISPR)—CRISPR-associated nuclease 9 (Cas9) technology and targeted mutation of *OsFTIP7* lead to complete male-sterility phenotype in rice [83].

3. Functional confirmation methods of GMS genes in crop plants

As described above, once the putative GMS gene has been cloned, it should be tested by using a series of experiments, including transgenic complementation, targeted mutagenesis, allelism test and allelic mutant sequencing, anther-specific expression analysis, phylogenetic analysis, and cytological observation (**Figure 4**).

3.1 Transgenic complementation

Transgenic complementation is an essential tool and an effective way to confirm the function of a putative GMS gene. Based on the difference of transformation receptors, it includes two ways. The first one is transformation of the male-sterile mutants from which the GMS gene has been cloned, and then observation of the male-fertility phenotype in transgenic plant. For example, maize *ZmMs7* gene was confirmed by the transformation of *proZmMs7-ZmMs7* construct into maize Hill hybrid line.

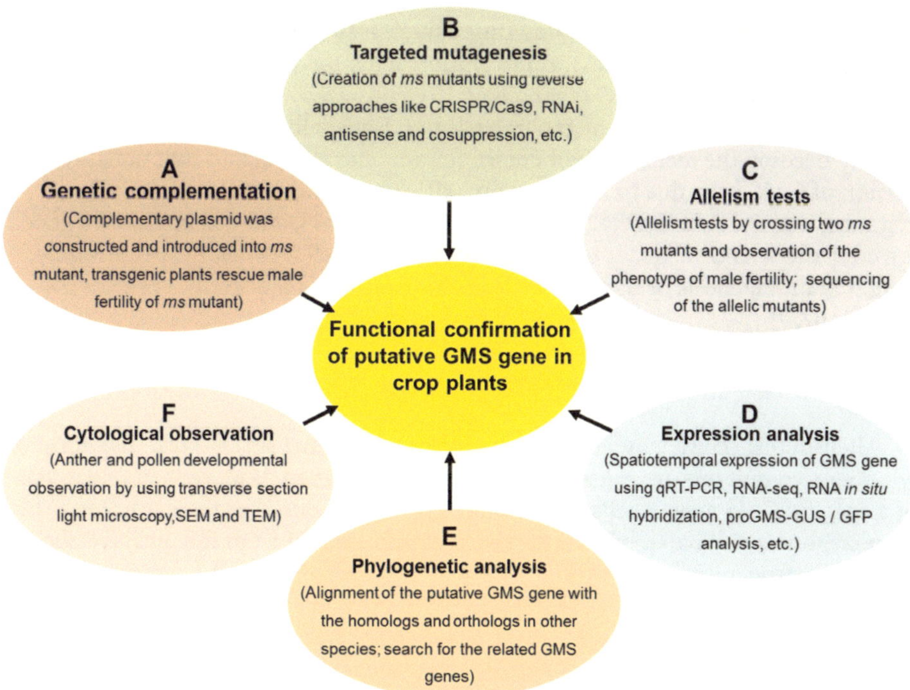

Figure 4.
The functional confirmation approaches of GMS genes in crop plants.

The transgenic plants were then crossed with the *ms7-6007* mutant, and transgenic plant in the *ms7-6007* homozygous mutant background can rescue the male-sterility defect of *ms7-6007* mutant and recovered the fertility phenotype (**Table 1**) [9]. The second one is transformation of the corresponding heterozygous male-sterility mutants with the orthologous GMS gene in model plants (such as *Arabidopsis*) and segregation analysis of complementation by the transgene. The putative GMS ortholog needs to be fused to a promoter to drive its expression in the *Arabidopsis* mutant, either by a constitutive, overexpression promoter, or via the *Arabidopsis* native gene-specific promoter. Although the first option is usually quicker, the results are not always satisfactory, due to the temporal and cell-specific regulation observed in some genes. For instance, anther and pollen transcription factors such as *AtMs1* orthologs in rice (*PTC1*) and barley (*HvMs1*) did not recover *Arabidopsis ms1* mutant fertility when driven by the CaMV35S overexpression promoter. However, once the rice and barley ortholog genes were fused to the *Arabidopsis AtMs1* native promoter, fertility was restored in the *ms1* homozygous mutant [35, 93].

3.2 Targeted mutagenesis

Targeted mutagenesis of the putative GMS gene includes two ways: knockdown and knockout approaches. Knockdown strategy, such as RNA interference (RNAi) silencing, is very helpful to those genes in which null mutant is lethal. RNAi silencing is a useful technique to characterize gene function; however, this approach may not generate clear phenotypes due to the threshold level needed for effective silencing [61]. RNAi target genes generally have reduced expression rather than being fully silenced; thus enough transcript may remain to maintain wild-type function. This partial reduction in gene expression was seen in several GMS gene RNAi silencing [63, 73, 80, 81, 93], where pollen development was affected by the silencing and showed a partial male-sterility phenotype. In addition, RNAi silencing has been shown to be unreliable after successive generations [95].

Knockout strategies, such as zinc finger nucleases (ZFNs), customized homing endonucleases (meganucleases), transcription activator-like effector nucleases (TALENs), and CRISPR-Cas9 technology, have been shown to significantly increase the frequency and precision of genome editing. Especially, CRISPR-Cas9 has quickly become the technology of choice for genome editing and functional confirmation of GMS gene due to its simplicity, efficiency, and versatility [96]. For instance, rice *OsLAP6/OsPKS1*, maize *ZmMs30*, *ZmMs33*, and wheat *TaMs45* gene are confirmed as GMS genes by using the CRISPR-Cas9 technology, respectively. Targeted mutagenesis of these genes leads to complete male-sterility phenotype [18, 20, 67, 76].

3.3 Allelism test and allelic mutant sequencing

Allelism test (complementation test for functional allelism) is a test to determine whether two mutants are caused by the same gene. If there is more than one mutant of a specific GMS gene, allelism test should be carried out. A male-sterile (*ms*) homozygote is pollinated by a fertile heterozygote (*+/ms*) from the putative allelic line. If the progeny exhibits a fertile/ sterile segregation ratio of 1:1, the two mutants are allelic with each other. If all the progenies display male fertile, suggest that the two mutations complement each other and they are not allelic. Furthermore, the allelic mutant gene can be confirmed based on sequencing and alignment with each other. If different *ms* mutants come from the mutation of the same GMS gene, the GMS gene function in male-sterility will be confirmed. For instance, the function of maize *ZmMs33* has been confirmed by allelism test and sequencing of several *ms33* allelic mutants, such as *ms33-6019*, *ms33-6029*, *ms33-6024*, *ms33-6038*, and *ms33-6052* [20, 97]. Most of the cloned GMS genes have allelic mutants and are confirmed by allelic mutant sequencing (**Table 1**), so it is a usefully functional confirmation strategy besides the genetic complementation and targeted mutagenesis.

3.4 Anther-specific expression analysis

The anther-specific expression analysis is another important method for functional confirmation of putative GMS gene. In general, the expression pattern of GMS gene could be analyzed by using the following approaches: semiquantitative reverse transcription (RT)-PCR, quantitative real-time RT-PCR (qRT-PCR), northern blotting, promoter-GUS or GMS-GFP transgenic plant analysis, RNA in situ hybridization, and immunoblotting (or western blotting). For instance, the spatiotemporal expression pattern of *Ms6021* was analyzed by qRT-PCR, RNA in situ hybridization, and western blotting, and the results indicated that *Ms6021* is mainly expressed in the tapetum and microspore in maize [23]. The anther- and tapetum-specific expression pattern of rice *PTC1* was analyzed by using RT-PCR, qRT-PCR, and $PTC1_{pro}$-*GUS* transgenic rice anther staining [35]. Spatiotemporal expression pattern of *TaMs2* was analyzed by using RT-PCR, RNA in situ hybridization, and *TaMs2*:GFP transgenic anther microscopy, indicating that *TaMs2* is an anther-specific expression and dominant GMS gene [50].

3.5 Phylogenetic analysis

In order to get more functional information of the putative GMS gene, phylogenetic analysis should be carried out for expounding the evolutionary relationship with other putative orthologs. The detailed method is as follows: protein sequences of the putative orthologs of the targeted GMS can be obtained from Gramene (http://www.gramene.org) or NCBI (https://www.ncbi.nlm.nih.gov/) and aligned using ClustalX program [98]. A phylogenetic tree can be generated using molecular evolutionary genetics analysis (MEGA6) program based on a Poisson model with the maximum likelihood method [99]. Support values are estimated by 1000 times of bootstrap replicates. For instance, by using phylogenetic analysis, maize Ms23 and its paralog bHLH122 fall in the same clade with two rice GMS proteins, TIP2 and EAT1. TIP2 is the rice ortholog of Ms23, whereas maize bHLH122 is the ortholog of rice EAT1. Maize bHLH51, rice TDR, and *Arabidopsis* AMS fall in the same clade, while maize Ms32, rice UDT1, and *Arabidopsis* DYT1 fall in the same clade [15]. These results not only confirm the function of Ms23 and Ms32 in regulating male sterility but also predict that their paralogs bHLH122 and bHLH51 may be involved in male sterility, and this needs to be confirmed by targeted mutagenesis analysis and/or other strategies.

3.6 Cytological observation

As to the forward genetic cloning of the GMS gene, cytological observation is one of the phenotypic analyses of the male-sterile mutant. When the candidate GMS gene is cloned by reverse genetic approaches, cytological observation is one of the most important strategies for functional confirmation of the putative GMS gene. Cytological observation methods include light microscopy of transverse sections, transmission electron microscopy (TEM), and scanning electron microscopy (SEM) of anther and pollen development. For instance, the functions of rice *OsTGA10* and *OsAGO2* in male sterility were confirmed by targeted mutagenesis of these genes with antisense and CRISPR-Cas9 systems and cytological characterization of mutants by transverse section observation and TEM analysis of anthers at different stages [84, 85]. The functions of wheat *TaMs26* in anther and pollen wall development in bread wheat were tested by targeted mutagenesis of all the three homologs and cytological analysis using SEM method [77]. Cytological observation is helpful to confirm the function mechanism of the putative GMS genes in the cellular level.

4. Application value evaluation of GMS genes and mutants in crop plants

Compared to CMS and environment-sensitive genic male sterility (EGMS), GMS has many advantages such as the high germplasm utilization efficiency, higher male-sterility stability under various environments, and lower linkage rate with adverse traits. As more and more GMS genes have been cloned in crops, the BMS systems by using GMS gene have been developed in several crop plants and come into commercial utilization, such as SPT and MCS systems [3]. However, before utilization in the BMS systems, many characteristics of GMS gene and its mutant should be assessed systemically, such as genetic stability analysis of male-sterility, heterosis comparison, and analysis of potential linkage with bad traits.

4.1 Genetic stability analysis of male-sterility

Firstly, the genetic stability of the male-sterile mutant should be appraised in different genetic backgrounds and various environments. The general procedure is as follows (**Figure 5A**; the recessive *ms* mutant is taken as an example): a homozygous *ms* mutant is used as female parent and crossed with hundreds of inbred lines with broad genetic backgrounds to get the heterozygous F_1 hybrids. Then one of the F_1 hybrids is self-pollinated to produce F_2 seeds. Thereafter 50–100 of the F_2 seeds from each cross are grown in various environments. The fertility segregation ratios

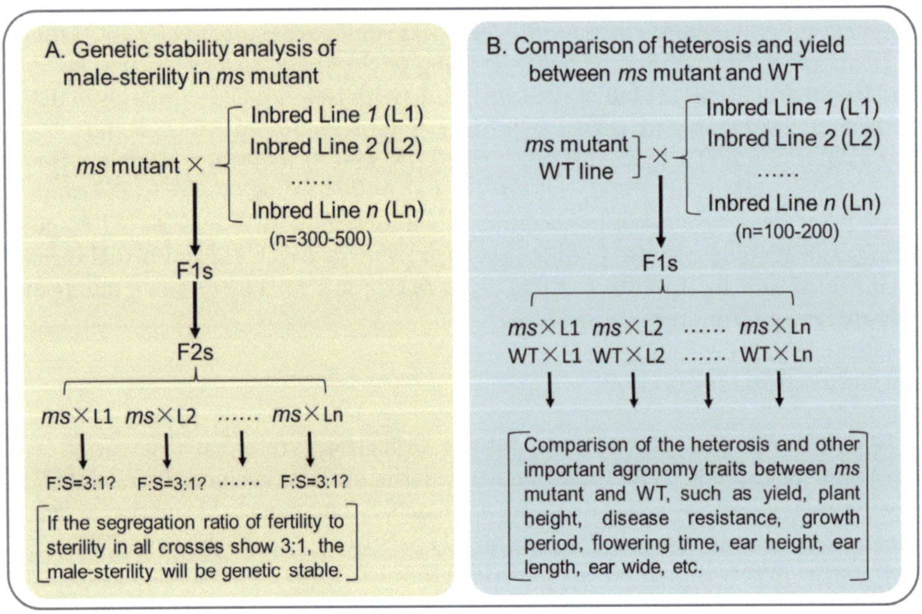

Figure 5.
The application value evaluation of GMS genes and mutants in crop plants.

of the F_2 populations are investigated, and anthers of three sterile individuals in each F_2 population are collected and stained with 1% I_2-KI solution to examine male-sterility status of pollen grains. If the segregation ratio of fertility to sterility in all crosses shows 3:1 as expected, we can say that the male sterility is genetically stable in different genetic backgrounds and various environments. Otherwise, if the ratio is not always 3:1 and confirmed by the molecular marker-assisted selection results, we can say that the male sterility is unstable in different genetic backgrounds and/or various environments. For instance, the male-sterility stability of maize *ms30-6028* mutant was analyzed by crossing with 329 maize inbred lines and observation of the segregation ratio of fertility to sterility in F_2 populations, suggesting that *ms30-6028* is a stable male-sterility mutant under diverse genetic backgrounds [18].

4.2 Heterosis comparison between *ms* mutant and wild type

Secondly, the effects of *ms* mutant on heterosis should be analyzed by comparing the yield and related agronomy traits between F_1 hybrid plants produced by using *ms* mutant and wild type (WT) as female parents and crossing with the same inbred line (**Figure 5B**). For instance, to test whether *ms30-6028* gene affects maize heterosis and grain yield, *ms30-6028* mutant and its homozygous WT line were used as female parents and crossed with 30 maize inbred lines, respectively. The harvested F_1 hybrids and their corresponding parental lines were grown according to the planting model of maize field production in two different locations. Eighteen agronomic traits such as plot yield, whole growth period, plant height, ear height, and hundred-kernel weight were investigated to compare the differences of heterosis and field production performance of 30 pairs of hybrid combinations using *ZmMs30* and *ms30-6028* homozygous plants as female parents, respectively. The results indicated that *ms30-6028* mutation has no obvious negative effects on maize heterosis and field production, suggesting that *ZmMs30* gene and its mutant *ms30-6028* are applicable for hybrid maize breeding and hybrid seed production [18].

4.3 Analysis of potential linkage with disadvantage genes and traits

Furthermore, other than the male-sterility stability analysis and heterosis comparison described above, the potential linkage with bad traits of *ms* locus should be analyzed. There are at least two ways to get this target: one is phenotypic observation of the hybrid plants that come from the homozygous *ms* mutant used as female parent, while those of the fertile sibling used as control. If the field production performances of the hybrid plants between *ms* mutant and WT are similar with each other, we can say that the *ms* mutation is not linked with disadvantage traits and thus can be applicable in hybrid seed breeding and production. For instance, maize *Ms44* hybrids showed no yield penalty in any of the tested environments, indicating that it is desirable for commercially viable products [22]. The other is sequencing of the putative genes near the *ms* locus and screening for the potential disadvantage genes based on bioinformatic analysis.

5. Application potential analyses of BMS systems by using GMS genes in crop plants

As described above, cloning and characterization of plant GMS genes have contributed significantly to our understanding of the molecular mechanisms of anther and pollen development in crop plants and have provided an important basis for developing BMS lines. Several attempts have been made to utilize GMS genes in combination with new technologies to achieve more feasible BMS systems in crop plants [3, 4, 6, 100]. Here, we introduce briefly the strategies, assessment, and applications of some typical BMS systems in crop plants (**Table 2**).

5.1 Development strategies of the BMS systems

The development strategies of BMS systems based on GMS genes and other new technologies have been reviewed thoroughly and systemically in our laboratory [3]. In general, there are two kinds of strategies to develop BMS systems that have an application potential in hybrid seed production: transgenic construct-driven non-transgenic seed systems and transgenic male-sterility systems. The former includes the SPT and MCS systems in maize, SPT-like systems in maize, rice, and wheat,

Strategy	BMS system	Crop	Application assessment	Application status	Ref.
Transgenic construct-driven non-transgenic product systems	MCS	Maize	1. Genetic stability and heterosis of *ms* line 2. Genetic stability analysis of MCS maintainer lines	Product test	[9, 18, 21]
	SPT	Maize	1. Genetic stability of SPT maintainer lines 2. SPT transgene transmission rate through pollen	Commercial application in maize	[62]
	SPT-like (based on dominant *ms44* gene)	Maize	1. *Ms44* plants increase kernel number 2. *Ms44* hybrids showed no yield penalty	Product test	[22]
	SPT-like (based on *OsNP1* gene)	Rice	The *osnp1* line was crossed with ~1200 rice germplasms, ~10% out-yielded the best local cultivars	Product test	[69]
	SPT-like (based on *TaMs1* gene)	Wheat	No data	No data	[49]
Transgenic male-sterility systems	RHS1: glyphosate-mediated male sterility	Maize	1. The consistency in performance across inbreds 2. The RHS inbreds showed no yield penalty	Commercial application in maize	[101]
	RHS2	Maize	1. The endogenous mts-siRNAs are present widely 2. The elite event was introgressed into 15 maize germplasms	Product test	[102]
	Barnase/Barstar system	Oilseed rape	1. It is feasible in some crop plants 2. Double female parent seeds needed	Commercial application in canola	[103, 104]

Table 2.
Strategy and application assessment of BMS systems in crop plants.

while the latter includes the RHS1 and RHS2 systems in maize and Barnase/Barstar system in oilseed rape (**Table 2**).

5.1.1 SPT- and SPT-like systems in crops

The SPT system is one of the representatives of transgenic construct-driven non-transgenic seed systems initially developed in maize by using a transgenic maintainer strategy [62]. The SPT transgenic maintainer line is created by transforming the plant of interest with an SPT construct consisting of three components: (i) a wild-type male-fertility gene (e.g., *Ms45*) to restore fertility, (ii) a pollen lethality gene (e.g., *ZmAA*) to disrupt normal pollen development, and (iii) a fluorescent seed color marker gene (e.g., *DsRed2*) for seed sorting. Of the pollen grains produced by the SPT maintainer line, all have the *ms45* genotype, 50% are non-transgenic, and 50% have the SPT transgenic elements. The latter grains are unable to germinate due to expression of the *ZmAA* gene. Thus, self-pollination of the SPT maintainer line produces both seeds with the same genotype of the SPT maintainer line (*ms45/ms45 + SPT-T-DNA*) and seeds with the male-sterile genotype (*ms45/ms45*). The two types of seeds can be efficiently separated by mechanical color sorting, since the 50% of seeds contain the SPT elements showing a red color under green excitation light. When the male-sterile line (*ms45/ms45*) is pollinated with the SPT maintainer line, almost 100% of the resulting seeds have the *ms45/ms45* genotype and can be used as male-sterile female lines for crossbreeding and hybrid seed production.

Since the maize SPT system was developed and applied successfully [62], several SPT-like systems have been developed in maize, rice, and wheat based on *ZmMs44*, *OsNP1*, and *TaMs1* genes, respectively [22, 49, 69]. Although there are potentially many advantages of the SPT system, the rate of transgene transmission through pollen was found to vary with the highest rate being 0.518% [62]. Therefore, there is an increased risk of transgenic pollen flow during the male-sterile line propagation phase, thus resulting in greatly limited application in the countries and regions with strict biotechnology regulatory oversight.

5.1.2 MCS System

To decrease the rate of transgene transmission through the pollen of SPT maintainer lines, our laboratory developed a MCS system by transforming a single MCS construct into the maize *ms7*, *ms30*, or *ms33* mutant [9, 105, 106]. The MCS construct contains five functional modules: (i) a male-fertility gene (e.g., *ZmMs7*, *ZmMs30* or *ZmMs33*) to restore fertility, (ii) two pollen disruption genes (e.g., *ZmAA* and *Dam*) to disrupt the production of transgenic pollen, (iii) a fluorescent color marker gene (e.g., *DsRed2* or *mCherry*) for seed color sorting, and (iv) an herbicide-resistant gene (e.g., *Bar*) to prevent sophistication of seeds because it is beneficial for the propagation of high-purity MCS transgenic maintainer line seeds through herbicide spraying during specific stages of production. As the MCS construct harbors two pollen disruption modules, both of which can inhibit transgenic pollen formation or function, the transgene transmission rate through pollen is greatly decreased. Furthermore, the *Bar* gene in the MCS construct is helpful for propagating highly pure seeds of the transgenic maintainer line. Compared with the SPT construct, the MCS construct, which harbors two additional functional modules, the *Bar* and *Dam* genes, can produce maintainer and male-sterile lines with higher purity and greatly decrease the transgene transmission rate as well as the risk of transgene flow in commercial maize hybrid seed production. To promote commercial application, a field test of the MCS system in China is currently underway.

As described above, although the final product of transgenic construct-driven male-sterility systems is non-transgenic, the use of these systems is often limited by the lack of GMS mutants and male-fertile genes in many crops. Consequently, many biotechnology strategies have been developed in the past 30 years to produce artificially dominant male-sterile plants independent of GMS mutants and male-fertility genes, such as the RHS systems in maize and Barnase/Barstar system in oilseed rape.

5.1.3 RHS system

The RHS system, which is based on glyphosate-mediated male sterility, is deployed for hybrid seed production by Monsanto [101]. The RHS system consists of RHS and RR transgene constructs. The RHS transgene cassette contains the CP4-EPSPS gene (encoding 5-enolpyruvyl-shikimate 3-phosphate synthase, which is insensitive or resistant to glyphosate) driven by the enhanced 35S promoter, which has been shown to be poorly expressed in tapetum cells and microspores, and thus the resulting RHS plant demonstrates male sterility following glyphosate application with little/no injury to the rest of the plant. The RR transgene construct comprises a double expression cassette providing high constitutive expression of CP4-EPSPS resulting in robust resistance to glyphosate. In hybrid seed production fields, rows of an RHS female line are interplanted with rows of an RR male line, and over-the-top sprays of glyphosate induce male sterility in RHS female plants, which are subsequently pollinated by RR male plants. By withholding glyphosate, the RHS plants remain fully fertile and are capable of self-pollination for propagation of female line without the need for a maintainer line.

The RHS system replaces mechanical detasseling with glyphosate spray and greatly simplifies the process of hybrid seed corn production. Recently, this system has been improved as RHS2 by using endogenous maize male tissue-specific small interfering RNAs to trigger cleavage of the CP4-EPSPS mRNA specifically in tassels, resulting in glyphosate-sensitive male cells [102].

5.1.4 Barnase/Barstar system

The Barnase/Barstar system was the first dominant BMS system developed in rapeseed and tobacco [103, 104] and then has been tested and tried in wheat and rice [107, 108]. The *barnase* and *barstar* genes are fused with the tapetum-specific TA29 promoter and then transformed individually into plants. The *TA29-barnase* transformed plants are completely male-sterile and are crossed with *TA29-barstar*-expressing fertile plants, which results in the co-expression of *barnase* and *barstar* genes in the anther tapetal cell layer. The inactivation of *barnase* by *barstar* leads to the restoration of fertility in the hybrid F1 plants [109].

5.2 Application assessment of the BMS systems

Although serval BMS systems had been developed during the past decades, only three of them were thoroughly assessed and applied in commercial hybrid seed production in some crops, such as SPT, RHS, and Barnase/Barstar systems.

In SPT system, the stability of transgenes in prospective SPT maintainer lines were examined based on Southern blot analyses of genomic DNA from T0 to T4 plants to assess the integration and structural fidelity of the transgenes. No changes in hybridization patterns with three different restriction enzyme digestions of the SPT transgenes indicated that the transgenes are stable over multiple generations. More importantly, the transgene transmission through pollen was tested by using the pollen of transgenic SPT maintainer to pollinate non-transgenic plants. Then ears were harvested from the non-transgenic female parent plants and examined under visible light for the presence of pink seeds expressing the DsRed2 protein. The transgene transmission rate through pollen varied from 0% to 0.518% with different constructs and transformants. As the transformant DP-32138-1 showed the lowest transgene transmission rate that was maintained across generations and in different inbred backgrounds, it was selected as the SPT maintainer line for use in maize male-sterile parent seed increase [62].

The RHS system was developed by minimizing the CP4-EPSPS expression in the tassel and maximizing glyphosate delivery to the tassel resulting in consistent male sterility for hybrid seed corn production [101]. Therefore, the glyphosate spray timing, dose, target, and mode should be examined firstly in different maize varieties. Subsequently, the consistency in performance of the RHS technology across a broad range of inbred varieties is essential and has been examined in field trials. The performance standard for RHS is 0.5% anther extrusion or >99.5% tassel sterility to insure high purity in hybrid seeds. The field data show that RHS has consistently surpassed the performance standard since 2007 when examined across an increasing number of inbred varieties. In fact, in 2011 and 2012, 100% sterility or zero anther extrusion was observed across 46 and 47 inbred varieties, respectively. The RHS inbreds have shown comparable yield to mechanical detasseling; furthermore, the F1 hybrid seeds produced by crossing RHS with RR showed full resistance to glyphosate and comparable performance to hybrid seeds produced by mechanical detasseling [101].

The Barnase/Barstar system was the first BMS system developed in tobacco and oilseed rape plants based on tapetal cell-specific expression of *TA29-barnase* and *TA29-barstar* genes [103, 104]. *TA29-barnase* transgene leads to dominant male sterility due to selective destruction of anther tapetal cells, while *TA29-barstar* transgene can suppress the expression of *TA29-barnase* transgene and restore the male fertility. The feasibility of this system was confirmed in many crop plants, such as oilseed rape, tobacco, lettuce, chicory, cauliflower, tomato, cotton, and maize. However, the dominant male-sterility line must maintained in heterozygous plants by crossing with a wild-type line in the same (isogenic) genetic background. The elimination of the fertile segregants by herbicide spray doubles the amount of female parent seed needed for hybrid seed production, which could limit the applicability of the system in crops with low multiplication factor and relatively low plant density [4].

5.3 Commercial application of the BMS systems

As shown in **Table 2**, there are only three BMS systems that have been applied in commercial hybrid seed production, including SPT, RHS, and Barnase/Barstar systems. The SPT system has been deregulated by USDA APHIS in 2011 and is thus available for commercial hybrid seed production in maize [110]. Unlike other BMS systems, the maize inbred parent lines produced using the SPT system do not inherit SPT transgene from the SPT maintainer line and thus are non-transgenic. Furthermore, both the commercial maize hybrid seed produced from the SPT system and the resulting commodity maize grain harvested from these hybrid plants are non-transgenic. Subsequently, acknowledgement of the non-transgenic status of progeny produced by the SPT system is also supported by regulatory agencies in Australia and Japan [111, 112]. Therefore, hybrid maize and commodity grain produced from the SPT system are non-genetically modified (non-GM) and subject only to those regulations applicable to conventional non-GM maize. The performance of RHS system has been evaluated by Monsanto manufacturing group which produces the hybrid seeds that are sold in the marketplace. A few modifications have been implemented to make the RHS system more practical and manageable in the field [101]. Most recently, the second-generation RHS (RHS2) technology combines the relative simplicity and convenience of a systemic herbicide spray methodology with targeted protein expression to create an inducible male sterility system for industrial production of maize hybrid seeds in an environmentally independent manner [102]. The Barnase/Barstar system has been used successfully for the commercial production of canola hybrids (*Brassica napus*) in Canada [4]. However, most of the BMS systems have not been used in commercial hybrid seed production, maybe because of lacking the cost-effective and environment-friendly BMS systems and/or the regulatory acceptance of using BMS systems among different countries.

6. Conclusions

In this chapter, we focus on the molecular cloning, functional confirmation, and application value assessment of GMS genes as well as their application in hybrid seed production via several BMS systems in cereal crops, such as rice, maize, and wheat. With the rapid development of the next-generation sequencing technology, more genome information of cereal crops are available, leading to plenty GMS genes cloned and characterized in crop plants. As shown in **Table 1**, there are more than 70 GMS genes cloned in cereal crops, and most of them (57/73) are identified by using forward genetic approach, including 38 genes isolated by map-based cloning, 15 genes identified by T-DNA/Transposon tagging and 4 genes isolated by MutMap method. Whereas the rest of GMS genes are identified *via* reverse genetic approach, including 7 genes isolated through homology-based cloning, 5 genes identified by anther-specific expression gene screening and 4 genes cloned by other reverse genetic methods. Among them, there are 49 GMS genes cloned in rice, 17 GMS genes in maize, 6 GMS genes in wheat, and 1 GMS gene in barley. From these data, we conclude that the forward genetic approaches, especially map-based cloning, are the most popular method for GMS gene cloning in crops; most GMS genes have been cloned in rice and maize, whereas only a few GMS genes are cloned in wheat and barley. Consider that the conserved role of GMS genes in different species and the sequence information of GMS genes in rice and maize can be used for cloning of the orthologs in wheat and barley through reverse genetic approaches. For example, the functions of *TaMs26* and *TaMs45*, the wheat homologs of maize *Ms26* and *Ms45*, were confirmed via a custom-designed homing endonuclease and CRISPR-Cas9-targeted mutagenesis in wheat, respectively [76, 77], while the role of *HvMs1*, the barley homolog of *Arabidopsis Ms1* and rice *PTC1*, was analyzed by using RNAi silencing in barley [93].

Although there are a lot of GMS genes identified in cereal crops up to now, less than 10 GMS genes are assessed for the value in heterosis utilization and hybrid seed production (**Table 1**). For example, *ZmMs7*, *ZmMs30*, and *ZmMs33* are tested in maize MCS system [9, 18, 21]; *ZmMs26*, *Zmms44*, and *ZmMs45* are tested in maize SPT (or SPT-like) system [16, 22, 62]; *OsNP1* is tested in rice SPT-like system [69]; and *TaMs1* is tested in wheat SPT-like system [49]. All these BMS systems belong to transgenic construct-driven non-transgenic product strategies, leading to potential application of these systems in commercial hybrid seed production, especially in the countries and/or regions with strict regulatory policy. These systems have many advantages, such as non-transgenic final products, environment-friendly without application of herbicide in hybrid seed production fields, and deregulated by the regulatory authority in some countries, whereas they are limited by using transgenic maintainer line based on completely male-sterile mutants and the male-fertility genes and requirement of fluorescent seed color-sorting machine. Therefore, the transgenic male-sterility systems, such as RHS system based on glyphosate-mediated male sterility, have also been developed and used in commercial hybrid seed production in maize [101, 102]. This system is independent of male-sterility mutants and male-fertility genes, no need for transgenic maintainer line and seed color sorting, and the herbicide-resistant male-sterility lines are helpful to highly efficient and mechanized hybrid seed production. However, this transgenic male-sterility system is limited by the "zero tolerance" regulatory policy preventing transgenic planting in many countries, need for application of herbicide in hybrid seed production fields, and potential risk of gene flow. In summary, both SPT and RHS systems have advantages and disadvantages compared with each other.

With the advance of molecular cloning methods including both forward and reverse genetic approaches, especially the next-generation sequencing technology and genome-editing technology (e.g., CRISPR-Cas9), more GMS genes in cereal crops with large and complex genome (e.g., wheat and barley) will be identified and characterized by using multiple strategies as described in this chapter. At the same time, the application value of the putative GMS genes should be assessed systemically in genetic stability of male sterility, effects on heterosis performance, and potential linkage with detrimental traits. This will not only boost our understanding in the molecular mechanism of anther and pollen development but also give great opportunity to develop novel BMS systems for commercial hybrid seed production in cereal crops.

Acknowledgements

The research in our lab was supported by the National Transgenic Major Program of China (2018ZX0800922B, 2018ZX0801006B), the National Natural Science Foundation of China (31771875, 31871702), the National Key Research and Development Program of China (2018YFD0100806, 2017YFD0102001, 2017YFD0101201), the Fundamental Research Funds for the Central Universities of China (06500060), and the "Ten Thousand Plan"—National High-Level Talents Special Support Plan (For Xiangyuan Wan).

Conflict of interest

The authors declared that they have no conflict of interest.

Abbreviations

BMS	biotechnology-based male sterility
BSA	bulked segregant analysis
CMS	cytoplasmic male sterility
CRISPR	clustered regularly interspersed short palindromic repeats
EGMS	environment-sensitive genic male sterility
EMS	methanesulfonate
EST	expressed sequence tag
GM	genetically modified
GMS	genic male sterility

MCS	multi-control sterility
MS	male sterility
MEGA	molecular evolutionary genetics analysis
qRT-PCR	quantitative real-time PCR
RHS	roundup hybridization systems
RT	reverse transcription
SEM	scanning electron microscopy
SPT	seed production technology
TAIL-PCR	thermal asymmetric interlaced-polymerase chain reaction
TEM	transmission electron microscopy
WT	wild type

Author details

Xiangyuan Wan[1,2*] and Suowei Wu[1,2*]

1 Biology and Agriculture Research Center, University of Science and Technology Beijing, Beijing, China

2 Beijing Engineering Laboratory of Main Crop Bio-Tech Breeding, Beijing International Science and Technology Cooperation Base of Bio-Tech Breeding, Beijing Solidwill Sci-Tech Co. Ltd., Beijing, China

*Address all correspondence to: wanxiangyuan@ustb.edu.cn; suoweiwu@ustb.edu.cn

References

[1] FAO U. How to Feed the World in 2050. Rome: Highlevel Expert Forum; 2009

[2] Miller JK, Herman EM, Jahn M, Bradford KJ. Strategic research, education and policy goals for seed science and crop improvement. Plant Science. 2010;**179**: 645-652. DOI: 10.1016/j.plantsci. 2010.08.006

[3] Wan X, Wu S, Li Z, Dong Z, An X, Ma B, et al. Maize genic male-sterility genes and their applications in hybrid breeding: Progress and perspectives. Molecular Plant. 2019;**12**:321-342. DOI: 10.1016/j.molp.2019.01.014

[4] Perez-Prat E, van Lookeren Campagne MM. Hybrid seed production and the challenge of propagating male-sterile plants. Trends in Plant Science. 2002;**7**:199-203

[5] Williams ME. Genetic engineering for pollination control. Trends in Biotechnology. 1995;**13**: 344-349

[6] Whitford R, Fleury D, Reif JC, Garcia M, Okada T, Korzun V, et al. Hybrid breeding in wheat: Technologies to improve hybrid wheat seed production. Journal of Experimental Botany. 2013;**64**:5411-5428. DOI: 10.1093/jxb/ ert333

[7] Jung KH, Han MJ, Lee YS, Kim YW, Hwang I, Kim MJ, et al. Rice undeveloped Tapetum1 is a major regulator of early tapetum development. The Plant Cell. 2005;**17**:2705-2722. DOI: 10.1105/tpc.105.034090

[8] Cigan AM, Unger E, Xu RJ, Kendall T, Fox TW. Phenotypic complementation of *ms45* maize requires tapetal expression of MS45. Sexual Plant Reproduction. 2001;**14**: 135-142

[9] Zhang D, Wu S, An X, Xie K, Dong Z, Zhou Y, et al. Construction of a multicontrol sterility system for a maize male-sterile line and hybrid seed production based on the ZmMs7 gene encoding a PHD-finger transcription factor. Plant Biotechnology Journal. 2018;**16**:459-471. DOI: 10.1111/pbi.12786

[10] Wang DX, Skibbe DS, Walbot V. Maize *Male sterile 8 (Ms8)*, a putative β-1,3-galactosyltransferase, modulates cell division, expansion, and differentiation during early maize anther development. Plant Reproduction. 2013;**26**:329-338. DOI: 10.1007/s00497-013-0230-y

[11] Albertsen M, Fox T, Leonard A, Li B, Loveland B, Trimnell M. Cloning and use of the *ms9* gene from maize. US patent US20160024520A1; 2016

[12] Somaratne Y, Tian Y, Zhang H, Wang M, Huo Y, Cao F, et al. ABNORMAL POLLEN VACUOLATION1 (APV1) is required for male fertility by contributing to anther cuticle and pollen exine formation in maize. The Plant Journal. 2017;**90**:96-110. DOI: 10.1111/tpj.13476

[13] Albertsen M, Fox T, Trimnell M, Wu Y, Lowe L, Li B, et al. *Msca1* nucleotide sequences impacting plant male fertility and method of using same. US patent US20090038027A1; 2009

[14] Chaubal R, Anderson JR, Trimnell MR, Fox TW, Albertsen MC, Bedinger P. The transformation of anthers in the msca1 mutant of maize. Planta. 2003; **216**:778-788. DOI: 10.1007/s00425-002-0929-8

[15] Nan GL, Zhai J, Arikit S, Morrow D, Fernandes J, Mai L, et al. MS23, a master basic helix-loop-helix factor, regulates the specification and development of the tapetum in maize. Development. 2017;**144**:163-172. DOI: 10.1242/ dev.140673

[16] Wu Y, Hershey H. Nucleotide sequences mediating plant male fertility and method of using same. USA patent US20110173725; 2011

[17] Djukanovic V, Smith J, Lowe K, Yang M, Gao H, Jones S, et al. Male-sterile maize plants produced by targeted mutagenesis of the cytochrome P450-like gene (MS26) using a re-designed I-CreI homing endonuclease. The Plant Journal. 2013;**76**:888-899. DOI: 10.1111/tpj.12335

[18] An X, Dong Z, Tian Y, Xie K, Wu S, Zhu T, et al. ZmMs30 encoding a novel GDSL lipase is essential for male fertility and valuable for hybrid breeding in maize. Molecular Plant. 2019;**12**: 343-359. DOI: 10.1016/j.molp.2019.01.011

[19] Moon J, Skibbe D, Timofejeva L, Wang CJ, Kelliher T, Kremling K, et al. Regulation of cell divisions and differentiation by MALE STERILITY32 is required for anther development in maize. The Plant Journal. 2013;**76**: 592-602. DOI: 10.1111/tpj.12318

[20] Xie K, Wu S, Li Z, Zhou Y, Zhang D, Dong Z, et al. Map-based cloning and characterization of Zea mays male sterility33 (ZmMs33) gene, encoding a glycerol-3-phosphate acyltransferase. Theoretical and Applied Genetics. 2018; **131**:1363-1378. DOI: 10.1007/s00122-018-3083-9

[21] Zhu T, Wu S, Zhang D, Li Z, Xie K, An X, et al. Genome-wide analysis of maize GPAT gene family and cytological characterization and breeding application of ZmMs33/ZmGPAT6 gene. Theoretical and Applied Genetics. 23 Apr 2019. DOI: 10.1007/s00122-019-03343-y. [Published online ahead of print]

[22] Fox T, DeBruin J, Haug Collet K, Trimnell M, Clapp J, Leonard A, et al. A single point mutation in Ms44 results in dominant male sterility and improves nitrogen use efficiency in maize. Plant Biotechnology Journal. 2017;**15**:942-952. DOI: 10.1111/pbi.12689

[23] Tian Y, Xiao S, Liu J, Somaratne Y, Zhang H, Wang M, et al. MALE STERILE6021 (MS6021) is required for the development of anther cuticle and pollen exine in maize. Scientific Reports. 2017;7:16736. DOI: 10.1038/s41598-017-16930-0

[24] Evans MM. The indeterminate gametophyte1 gene of maize encodes a LOB domain protein required for embryo Sac and leaf development. The Plant Cell. 2007;**19**:46-62. DOI: 10.1105/tpc.106.047506

[25] Wang CJ, Nan GL, Kelliher T, Timofejeva L, Vernoud V, Golubovskaya IN, et al. Maize multiple archesporial cells 1 (mac1), an ortholog of rice TDL1A, modulates cell proliferation and identity in early anther development. Development. 2012;**139**: 2594-2603. DOI: 10.1242/dev.077891

[26] Chen X, Zhang H, Sun H, Luo H, Zhao L, Dong Z, et al. IRREGULAR POLLEN EXINE1 is a novel factor in anther cuticle and pollen exine formation. Plant Physiology. 2017;**173**: 307-325. DOI: 10.1104/pp.16.00629

[27] Wang Y, Liu D, Tian Y, Wu S, An X, Dong Z, et al. Map-based cloning, phylogenetic, and microsynteny analyses of ZmMs20 gene regulating male fertility in maize. International Journal of Molecular Sciences. 2019;**20**: 1411. DOI: 10.3390/ijms20061411

[28] Hong L, Tang D, Zhu K, Wang K, Li M, Cheng Z. Somatic and reproductive cell development in rice anther is regulated by a putative glutaredoxin. The Plant Cell. 2012;**24**:577-588. DOI: 10.1105/tpc.111.093740

[29] Hong L, Tang D, Shen Y, Hu Q, Wang K, Li M, et al. MIL2 (MICROSPORELESS2) regulates early cell differentiation in the rice anther.

The New Phytologist. 2012;**196**:402-413. DOI: 10.1111/j.1469-8137.2012.04270.x

[30] Fu Z, Yu J, Cheng X, Zong X, Xu J, Chen M, et al. The rice basic helix-loop-helix transcription factor TDR INTERACTING PROTEIN2 is a central switch in early anther development. The Plant Cell. 2014;**26**:1512-1524. DOI: 10.1105/tpc.114.123745

[31] Ko SS, Li MJ, Sun-Ben Ku M, Ho YC, Lin YJ, Chuang MH, et al. The bHLH142 transcription factor coordinates with TDR1 to modulate the expression of EAT1 and regulate pollen development in rice. The Plant Cell. 2014;**26**: 2486-2504. DOI: 10.1105/tpc.114.126292

[32] Yang Z, Sun L, Zhang P, Zhang Y, Yu P, Liu L, et al. TDR INTERACTING PROTEIN 3 encoding a PHD-finger transcription factor regulates Ubisch bodies and pollen wall formation in rice. The Plant Journal. 25 Apr 2019. DOI: 10.1111/tpj.14365. [Published online ahead of print]

[33] Li H, Pinot F, Sauveplane V, Werck-Reichhart D, Diehl P, Schreiber L, et al. Cytochrome P450 family member CYP704B2 catalyzes the {omega}-hydroxylation of fatty acids and is required for anther cutin biosynthesis and pollen exine formation in rice. The Plant Cell. 2010;**22**:173-190. DOI: 10.1105/tpc.109.070326

[34] Yang X, Wu D, Shi J, He Y, Pinot F, Grausem B, et al. Rice CYP703A3, a cytochrome P450 hydroxylase, is essential for development of anther cuticle and pollen exine. Journal of Integrative Plant Biology. 2014;**56**: 979-994. DOI: 10.1111/jipb.12212

[35] Li H, Yuan Z, Vizcay-Barrena G, Yang C, Liang W, Zong J, et al. PERSISTENT TAPETAL CELL1 encodes a PHD-finger protein that is required for tapetal cell death and pollen development in rice. Plant Physiology. 2011;**156**:615-630. DOI: 10.1104/pp.111.175760

[36] Li N, Zhang DS, Liu HS, Yin CS, Li XX, Liang WQ, et al. The rice tapetum degeneration retardation gene is required for tapetum degradation and anther development. The Plant Cell. 2006;**18**:2999-3014. DOI: 10.1105/tpc.106.044107

[37] Liu Z, Lin S, Shi J, Yu J, Zhu L, Yang X, et al. Rice No Pollen 1 (NP1) is required for anther cuticle formation and pollen exine patterning. The Plant Journal. 2017;**91**:263-277. DOI: 10.1111/tpj.13561

[38] Men X, Shi J, Liang W, Zhang Q, Lian G, Quan S, et al. Glycerol-3-phosphate acyltransferase 3 (OsGPAT3) is required for anther development and male fertility in rice. Journal of Experimental Botany. 2017;**68**:513-526. DOI: 10.1093/jxb/erw445

[39] Shi J, Tan H, Yu XH, Liu Y, Liang W, Ranathunge K, et al. Defective pollen wall is required for anther and microspore development in rice and encodes a fatty acyl carrier protein reductase. The Plant Cell. 2011;**23**: 2225-2246. DOI: 10.1105/tpc.111.087528

[40] Xu D, Shi J, Rautengarten C, Yang L, Qian X, Uzair M, et al. Defective Pollen Wall 2 (DPW2) encodes an acyl transferase required for rice pollen development. Plant Physiology. 2017; **173**:240-255. DOI: 10.1104/pp.16.00095

[41] Yu J, Meng Z, Liang W, Behera S, Kudla J, Tucker MR, et al. A rice Ca^{2+} binding protein is required for tapetum function and pollen formation. Plant Physiology. 2016;**172**:1772-1786. DOI: 10.1104/pp.16.01261

[42] Zhang H, Liang W, Yang X, Luo X, Jiang N, Ma H, et al. Carbon starved anther encodes a MYB domain protein that regulates sugar partitioning required for rice pollen development. The Plant Cell. 2010;**22**:672-689. DOI: 10.1105/tpc.109.073668

[43] Zhao G, Shi J, Liang W, Xue F, Luo Q, Zhu L, et al. Two ATP binding cassette G transporters, rice ATP binding cassette G26 and ATP binding cassette G15, collaboratively regulate rice male reproduction. Plant Physiology. 2015;**169**:2064-2079. DOI: 10.1104/pp.15.00262

[44] Zhu X, Yu J, Shi J, Tohge T, Fernie AR, Meir S, et al. The polyketide synthase OsPKS2 is essential for pollen exine and Ubisch body patterning in rice. Journal of Integrative Plant Biology. 2017;**59**:612-628. DOI: 10.1111/jipb.12574

[45] Niu N, Liang W, Yang X, Jin W, Wilson ZA, Hu J, et al. EAT1 promotes tapetal cell death by regulating aspartic proteases during male reproductive development in rice. Nature Communications. 2013;**4**:1445. DOI: 10.1038/ncomms2396

[46] Zhu L, Shi J, Zhao G, Zhang D, Liang W. Post-meiotic deficient anther1 (PDA1) encodes an ABC transporter required for the development of anther cuticle and pollen exine in rice. Journal of Plant Biology. 2013; **56**:59-68. DOI: 10.1007/s12374-013-0902-z

[47] Tan H, Liang W, Hu J, Zhang D. MTR1 encodes a secretory fasciclin glycoprotein required for male reproductive development in rice. Developmental Cell. 2012;**22**:1127-1137. DOI: 10.1016/j.devcel.2012.04.011

[48] Yang X, Li G, Tian Y, Song Y, Liang W, Zhang D. A rice glutamyl-tRNA synthetase modulates early anther cell division and patterning. Plant Physiology. 2018;**177**:728-744. DOI: 10.1104/pp.18.00110

[49] Tucker EJ, Baumann U, Kouidri A, Suchecki R, Baes M, Garcia M, et al. Molecular identification of the wheat male fertility gene Ms1 and its prospects for hybrid breeding. Nature Communications. 2017;**8**:869. DOI: 10.1038/s41467-017-00945-2

[50] Ni F, Qi J, Hao Q, Lyu B, Luo MC, Wang Y, et al. Wheat Ms2 encodes for an orphan protein that confers male sterility in grass species. Nature Communications. 2017;**8**:15121. DOI: 10.1038/ncomms15121

[51] Xia C, Zhang L, Zou C, Gu Y, Duan J, Zhao G, et al. A TRIM insertion in the promoter of Ms2 causes male sterility in wheat. Nature Communications. 2017;**8**: 15407. DOI: 10.1038/ncomms15407

[52] Pallotta MA, Warner P, Kouidri A, Tucker EJ, Baes M, Suchecki R, et al. Wheat ms5 male-sterility is induced by recessive homoeologous A and D genome non-specific Lipid Transfer Proteins. The Plant Journal. 22 Apr 2019. DOI: 10.1111/tpj.14350. [Published online ahead of print]

[53] Li X, Gao X, Wei Y, Deng L, Ouyang Y, Chen G, et al. Rice APOPTOSIS INHIBITOR5 coupled with two DEAD-box adenosine 5′-triphosphate-dependent RNA helicases regulates tapetum degeneration. The Plant Cell. 2011;**23**:1416-1434. DOI: 10.1105/tpc.110.082636

[54] Moon S, Kim SR, Zhao G, Yi J, Yoo Y, Jin P, et al. Rice glycosyltransferase1 encodes a glycosyltransferase essential for pollen wall formation. Plant Physiology. 2013;**161**:663-675. DOI: 10.1104/pp.112.210948

[55] Han MJ, Jung KH, Yi G, Lee DY, An G. Rice Immature Pollen 1 (RIP1) is a regulator of late pollen development. Plant & Cell Physiology. 2006;**47**: 1457-1472. DOI: 10.1093/pcp/pcl013

[56] Jung KH, Han MJ, Lee DY, Lee YS, Schreiber L, Franke R, et al. Wax-deficient anther1 is involved in cuticle and wax production in rice anther walls and is required for pollen development. The Plant Cell. 2006;**18**:3015-3032. DOI: 10.1105/tpc.106.042044

[57] Lee S, Jung KH, An G, Chung YY. Isolation and characterization of a rice cysteine protease gene, OsCP1, using T-DNA gene-trap system. Plant Molecular Biology. 2004;**54**:755-765. DOI: 10.1023/B:PLAN.0000040904.15329.29

[58] Shi X, Sun X, Zhang Z, Feng D, Zhang Q, Han L, et al. GLUCAN SYNTHASE-LIKE 5 (GSL5) plays an essential role in male fertility by regulating callose metabolism during microsporogenesis in rice. Plant & Cell Physiology. 2015;**56**:497-509. DOI: 10.1093/pcp/pcu193

[59] Yi J, Kim SR, Lee DY, Moon S, Lee YS, Jung KH, et al. The rice gene DEFECTIVE TAPETUM AND MEIOCYTES 1 (DTM1) is required for early tapetum development and meiosis. The Plant Journal. 2012;**70**:256-270. DOI: 10.1111/j.1365-313X.2011.04864.x

[60] Yi J, Moon S, Lee YS, Zhu L, Liang W, Zhang D, et al. Defective tapetum cell death 1 (DTC1) regulates ROS levels by binding to metallothionein during tapetum degeneration. Plant Physiology. 2016;**170**:1611-1623. DOI: 10.1104/pp.15.01561

[61] Cigan AM, Unger-Wallace E, Haug-Collet K. Transcriptional gene silencing as a tool for uncovering gene function in maize. The Plant Journal. 2005;**43**: 929-940. DOI: 10.1111/j.1365-313X.2005.02492.x

[62] Wu Y, Fox TW, Trimnell MR, Wang L, Xu RJ, Cigan AM, et al. Development of a novel recessive genetic male sterility system for hybrid seed production in maize and other cross-pollinating crops. Plant Biotechnology Journal. 2016;**14**: 1046-1054. DOI: 10.1111/pbi.12477

[63] Vernoud V, Laigle G, Rozier F, Meeley RB, Perez P, Rogowsky PM. The HD-ZIP IV transcription factor OCL4 is necessary for trichome patterning and anther development in maize. The Plant Journal. 2009;**59**:883-894. DOI: 10.1111/j.1365-313X.2009.03916.x

[64] Kaneko M, Inukai Y, Ueguchi-Tanaka M, Itoh H, Izawa T, Kobayashi Y, et al. Loss-of-function mutations of the rice GAMYB gene impair alpha-amylase expression in aleurone and flower development. The Plant Cell. 2004;**16**:33-44. DOI: 10.1105/tpc.017327

[65] Nonomura KI, Miyoshi K, Eiguchi M, Suzuki T, Miyao A, Hirochika H, et al. The MSP1 gene is necessary to restrict the number of cells entering into male and female sporogenesis and to initiate anther wall formation in rice. Plant Cell. 2003;**15**:1728-1739. DOI: 10.1105/tpc.012401

[66] Ueda K, Yoshimura F, Miyao A, Hirochika H, Nonomura K, Wabiko H. Collapsed abnormal pollen1 gene encoding the Arabinokinase-like protein is involved in pollen development in rice. Plant Physiology. 2013;**162**:858-871. DOI: 10.1104/pp.113.216523

[67] Zou T, Xiao Q, Li W, Luo T, Yuan G, He Z, et al. OsLAP6/OsPKS1, an orthologue of Arabidopsis PKSA/LAP6, is critical for proper pollen exine formation. Rice (N Y). 2017;**10**:53. DOI: 10.1186/s12284-017-0191-0

[68] Chang Z, Chen Z, Yan W, Xie G, Lu J, Wang N, et al. An ABC transporter, OsABCG26, is required for anther cuticle and pollen exine formation and pollen-pistil interactions in rice. Plant Science. 2016;**253**:21-30. DOI: 10.1016/j.plantsci.2016.09.006

[69] Chang Z, Chen Z, Wang N, Xie G, Lu J, Yan W, et al. Construction of a male sterility system for hybrid rice breeding and seed production using a nuclear male sterility gene. Proceedings of the National Academy of Sciences. 2016;**113**:14145-14150. DOI: 10.1073/pnas.1613792113

[70] Wang Z, Li J, Chen S, Heng Y, Chen Z, Yang J, et al. Poaceae-specific MS1 encodes a phospholipid-binding protein for male fertility in bread wheat. Proceedings of the National Academy of Sciences of the United States of America. 2017;**114**:12614-12619. DOI: 10.1073/pnas.1715570114

[71] Cai C-F, Zhu J, Lou Y, Guo Z-L, Xiong S-X, Wang K, et al. The functional analysis of OsTDF1 reveals a conserved genetic pathway for tapetal development between rice and Arabidopsis. Science Bulletin. 2015;**60**:1073-1082. DOI: 10.1007/s11434-015-0810-3

[72] Li Y, Li D, Guo Z, Shi Q, Xiong S, Zhang C, et al. OsACOS12, an orthologue of Arabidopsis acyl-CoA synthetase5, plays an important role in pollen exine formation and anther development in rice. BMC Plant Biology. 2016;**16**:256. DOI: 10.1186/s12870-016-0943-9

[73] Zhang J, Tang W, Huang Y, Niu X, Zhao Y, Han Y, et al. Down-regulation of a LBD-like gene, OsIG1, leads to occurrence of unusual double ovules and developmental abnormalities of various floral organs and megagametophyte in rice. Journal of Experimental Botany. 2015;**66**:99-112. DOI: 10.1093/jxb/eru396

[74] Ni E, Zhou L, Li J, Jiang D, Wang Z, Zheng S, et al. OsCER1 plays a pivotal role in very-long-chain alkane biosynthesis and affects plastid development and programmed cell death of tapetum in rice (*Oryza sativa* L.). Frontiers in Plant Science. 2018; **9**:1217. DOI: 10.3389/fpls.2018.01217

[75] Wang A, Xia Q, Xie W, Datla R, Selvaraj G. The classical Ubisch bodies carry a sporophytically produced structural protein (RAFTIN) that is essential for pollen development. Proceedings of the National Academy of Sciences of the United States of America. 2003;**100**:14487-14492. DOI: 10.1073/pnas.2231254100

[76] Singh M, Kumar M, Albertsen MC, Young JK, Cigan AM. Concurrent modifications in the three homeologs of Ms45 gene with CRISPR-Cas9 lead to rapid generation of male sterile bread wheat (*Triticum aestivum* L.). Plant Molecular Biology. 2018;**97**:371-383. DOI: 10.1007/s11103-018-0749-2

[77] Singh M, Kumar M, Thilges K, Cho M-J, Cigan AM. MS26/CYP704B is required for anther and pollen wall development in bread wheat (*Triticum aestivum* L.) and combining mutations in all three homeologs causes male sterility. PLoS One. 2017;**12**:e0177632. DOI: 10.1371/journal.pone.0177632

[78] Zhang D, Liang W, Yin C, Zong J, Gu F, Zhang D. OsC6, encoding a lipid transfer protein, is required for postmeiotic anther development in rice. Plant Physiology. 2010;**154**:149-162. DOI: 10.1104/pp.110.158865

[79] Wan L, Zha W, Cheng X, Liu C, Lv L, Liu C, et al. A rice beta-1,3-glucanase gene Osg1 is required for callose degradation in pollen development. Planta. 2011;**233**:309-323. DOI: 10.1007/s00425-010-1301-z

[80] Li L, Li Y, Song S, Deng H, Li N, Fu X, et al. An anther development F-box (ADF) protein regulated by tapetum degeneration retardation (TDR) controls rice anther development. Planta. 2015;**241**:157-166. DOI: 10.1007/s00425-014-2160-9

[81] Sumiyoshi M, Inamura T, Nakamura A, Aohara T, Ishii T, Satoh S, et al. UDP-arabinopyranose mutase 3 is required for pollen wall morphogenesis in rice (*Oryza sativa*). Plant & Cell Physiology. 2015;**56**:232-241. DOI: 10.1093/pcp/pcu132

[82] Zou T, Li S, Liu M, Wang T, Xiao Q, Chen D, et al. An atypical strictosidine synthase, OsSTRL2, plays key roles in anther development and pollen wall formation in rice. Scientific Reports.

2017;7:6863. DOI: 10.1038/s41598-017-07064-4

[83] Song S, Chen Y, Liu L, See YHB, Mao C, Gan Y, et al. OsFTIP7 determines auxin-mediated anther dehiscence in rice. Nature Plants. 2018; **4**:495-504. DOI: 10.1038/s41477-018-0175-0

[84] Chen ZS, Liu XF, Wang DH, Chen R, Zhang XL, Xu ZH, et al. Transcription factor OsTGA10 is a target of the MADS protein OsMADS8 and is required for tapetum development. Plant Physiology. 2018; **176**:819-835. DOI: 10.1104/pp.17.01419

[85] Zheng S, Li J, Ma L, Wang H, Zhou H, Ni E, et al. OsAGO2 controls ROS production and the initiation of tapetal PCD by epigenetically regulating OsHXK1 expression in rice anthers. Proceedings of the National Academy of Sciences of the United States of America. 2019;**116**:7549-7558. DOI: 10.1073/pnas.1817675116

[86] Abe A, Kosugi S, Yoshida K, Natsume S, Takagi H, Kanzaki H, et al. Genome sequencing reveals agronomically important loci in rice using MutMap. Nature Biotechnology. 2012;**30**:174-178. DOI: 10.1038/nbt.2095

[87] Chen Z, Yan W, Wang N, Zhang W, Xie G, Lu J, et al. Cloning of a rice male sterility gene by a modified MutMap method. Hereditas (Beijing). 2014;**36**: 85-93

[88] Gomez JF, Talle B, Wilson ZA. Anther and pollen development: A conserved developmental pathway. Journal of Integrative Plant Biology. 2015;**57**:876-891. DOI: 10.1111/jipb.12425

[89] Ma H. Molecular genetic analyses of microsporogenesis and microgametogenesis in flowering plants. Annual Review of Plant Biology. 2005; **56**:393-434. DOI: 10.1146/annurev.arplant.55.031903.141717

[90] Shi J, Cui M, Yang L, Kim YJ, Zhang D. Genetic and biochemical mechanisms of pollen wall development. Trends in Plant Science. 2015;**20**:741-753. DOI: 10.1016/j.tplants.2015.07.010

[91] Wilson ZA, Zhang DB. From Arabidopsis to rice: Pathways in pollen development. Journal of Experimental Botany. 2009;**60**:1479-1492. DOI: 10.1093/jxb/erp095

[92] Zhang D, Luo X, Zhu L. Cytological analysis and genetic control of rice anther development. Journal of Genetics and Genomics. 2011;**38**:379-390. DOI: 10.1016/j.jgg.2011.08.001

[93] Fernández Gómez J, Wilson ZA. A barley PHD finger transcription factor that confers male sterility by affecting tapetal development. Plant Biotechnology Journal. 2014;**12**:765-777. DOI: 10.1111/pbi.12181

[94] Tsuchiya T, Toriyama K, Nasrallah ME, Ejiri S. Isolation of genes abundantly expressed in rice anthers at the microspore stage. Plant Molecular Biology. 1992;**20**:1189-1193

[95] Baulcombe D. RNA silencing in plants. Nature. 2004;**431**:356-363. DOI: 10.1038/nature02874

[96] Svitashev S, Schwartz C, Lenderts B, Young JK, Mark Cigan A. Genome editing in maize directed by CRISPR-Cas9 ribonucleoprotein complexes. Nature Communications. 2016;7:13274. DOI: 10.1038/ncomms13274

[97] Zhang L, Luo H, Zhao Y, Chen X, Huang Y, Yan S, et al. Maize male sterile 33 encodes a putative glycerol-3-phosphate acyltransferase that mediates anther cuticle formation and microspore development. BMC Plant Biology. 2018; **18**:318. DOI: 10.1186/s12870-018-1543-7

[98] Higgins DG, Thompson JD, Gibson TJ. Using CLUSTAL for multiple sequence alignments. Methods in Enzymology. 1996;**266**:383-402

[99] Tamura K, Stecher G, Peterson D, Filipski A, Kumar S. MEGA6: Molecular evolutionary genetics analysis version 6.0. Molecular Biology and Evolution. 2013;**30**:2725-2729. DOI: 10.1093/molbev/mst197

[100] Kim YJ, Zhang D. Molecular control of male fertility for crop hybrid breeding. Trends in Plant Science. 2018; **23**:53-65. DOI: 10.1016/j.tplants.2017.10.001

[101] Feng PC, Qi Y, Chiu T, Stoecker MA, Schuster CL, Johnson SC, et al. Improving hybrid seed production in corn with glyphosate-mediated male sterility. Pest Management Science. 2014;**70**:212-218. DOI: 10.1002/ps.3526

[102] Yang H, Qi Y, Goley ME, Huang J, Ivashuta S, Zhang Y, et al. Endogenous tassel-specific small RNAs-mediated RNA interference enables a novel glyphosate-inducible male sterility system for commercial production of hybrid seed in *Zea mays* L. PLoS One. 2018;**13**:e0202921. DOI: 10.1371/journal.pone.0202921

[103] Mariani C, De Beuckeleer M, Truettner J, Leemans J, Goldberg RB. Induction of male sterility in plants by a chimaeric ribonuclease gene. Nature. 1990;**347**:737-741

[104] Mariani C, Gossele V, Beuckeleer MD, Block MD, Goldberg RB, Greef WD, et al. A chimaeric ribonuclease-inhibitor gene restores fertility to male sterile plants. Nature. 1992;**357**:384-387

[105] Wan X, Xie K, Wu S, An X, Li J, Zhang D, et al. A strategy of maintaining and propagating male-sterile line based on Ms30 gene in maize. China Patent 201510300778.9; 2015

[106] Wan X, Xie K, Wu S, Li J, An X, Zhang D, et al. A method of maintaining and propagating male-sterile line by using a multi-control sterility construct based on Ms7 gene in maize. China Patent 201510301333.2; 2015

[107] De Block M, Debrouwer D, Moens T. The development of a nuclear male sterility system in wheat. Expression of the barnase gene under the control of tapetum specific promoters. Theoretical and Applied Genetics. 1997;**95**:125-131

[108] Abe K, Oshima M, Akasaka M, Konagaya KI, Nanasato Y, Okuzaki A, et al. Development and characterization of transgenic dominant male sterile rice toward an outcross-based breeding system. Breeding Science. 2018;**68**: 248-257. DOI: 10.1270/jsbbs.17090

[109] Shukla P, Singh NK, Gautam R, Ahmed I, Yadav D, Sharma A, et al. Molecular approaches for manipulating male sterility and strategies for fertility restoration in plants. Molecular Biotechnology. 2017;**59**:445-457. DOI: 10.1007/s12033-017-0027-6

[110] USDA-APHIS. Pioneer Hi-Bred International, Inc. Seed Production Technology (SPT) Process OECD Unique Identifier: DP-32138-1 Corn: Final Environmental Assessment. Riverdale, MD: United States Department of Agriculture Animal and Plant Health Inspection Service [Internet]. 2011. Available from: http://www.aphis.usda.gov/brs/aphisdocs/08_33801p_fea.pdf

[111] FSANZ. New Plant Breeding Techniques. Report of a Workshop hosted by Food Standards Australia New Zealand (FSANZ) [Internet]. 2012. Available from: http://www.foodstandards.gov.au/publications/Documents/New%20Plant%20Breeding%20Techniques%20Workshop%20Report.pdf

[112] MHLW J. The outcome of the discussion on F1 hybrid seeds produced with the DuPont's Seed Production Technology (SPT) using DP-32138-1. Japan Ministry of Health, Labor, and Welfare [Internet]. 2013. Available from: http://www.mhlw.go.jp/stf/shingi/2r9852000002tccm-att/2r9852000002tck7.pdf

Chapter 6

Silencing of Peroxiredoxin-4 in Anticancer Activity of Gamma-Tocotrienol

Afiah Nasuha Aznan and Zakiah Jubri

Abstract

Peroxiredoxin-4 (PRDX4) is known to have a role in protecting cells from oxidative stress. It has been previously reported to increase in HepG2 liver cancer cells treated with gamma-tocotrienol (GTT). As GTT treatment potentially kills the cancer cell by regulating multiple signaling pathways, this study aims to determine the involvement of PRDX4 in GTT anticancer activity by silencing the *PRDX4* gene. The efficiency of PRDX4 silencing is achieved by optimizing HepG2 cell density, effect of serum presence in transduction media, incubation time of the cells with lentivirus, polybrene concentration, puromycin dose, functional titer, and multiplicity of infection (MOI) of the lentivirus. Silenced HepG2-PRDX4 cells (HepG2-shRNA-PRDX4) were treated with 70 μM of GTT for 18 h. GTT treatment significantly decreased the HepG2-shRNA-PRDX4 cell viability, increased apoptosis rate, and reduced free radical production compared to untreated HepG2-shRNA-PRDX4 cells. These findings are further supported by proteomic analysis, which showed that pro-apoptotic and DNA damage proteins were upregulated, and proteins involved in cell cycle arrest, carcinogenesis, and anti apoptotic signaling pathways were downregulated in HepG2-shRNA-PRDX4 cells treated with GTT compared to control. In conclusion, PRDX4 plays a role in GTT anticancer activity by increasing free radical production and oxidative damage to induce apoptosis in HepG2 cell.

Keywords: silencing, peroxiredoxin-4, anticancer, gamma-tocotrienol, antioxidant

1. Introduction

Peroxiredoxin-4 (PRDX4) is one of the unique isomers of peroxiredoxin (PRDX) and is located in the endoplasmic reticulum. It has a peroxidase site to oxidize hydrogen peroxide (H_2O_2) and thus functions as an antioxidant, increases cell proliferation, and is involved in regulating multiple signaling transduction pathways [1, 2]. Double cysteine residues at the peroxidase site of PRDX4 oxidize H_2O_2 and form water molecule. Oxidation is one of the processes that control H_2O_2 homeostasis in the cells and thus indirectly reduces the risk of high level of oxidative stress [3]. The increase in reactive oxygen species (ROS) production in the tumor cells has been linked to increased PRDX4 expression, which makes the cell susceptible toward apoptosis [4]. Besides that, PRDX4 is a potential tumor biomarker [5] because of its high expression in most of the tumor tissues as it plays a role in tumor growth and progression. The pattern of *PRDX4* gene expression is different among cancer cells and depends on its role. *PRDX4* gene may be involved in increasing the immune system of a normal cell to kill the cancer cells or reducing the level of oxidative stress to make the cancer cell more insusceptible toward the anticancer activity. *PRDX4* gene expression is high in hepatocellular, pancreas, colon, and prostate cancer cells, whereas its expression is low in the lung, kidney, and thymus cancer cells [6]. Recent findings have shown that *PRDX4* gene is highly expressed in HepG2 liver cancer cells treated with gamma-tocotrienol (GTT) [7] and reduces the HepG2 viability [8]. However, currently, there are no studies yet that focus on the role of PRDX4 in GTT treatment.

GTT is one of the tocotrienol isomers of vitamin E. It has an unsaturated and short phenyl chain and is differentiated based on the methyl group located on the chromanol ring [9]. This structure enables GTT to pass through the saturated lipid bilayer membrane and to be absorbed by the cells efficiently. GTT and other tocotrienol isomers are renowned as antioxidants [10]. Besides that, GTT has also been proven to have the capability as a signaling molecule to induce anticancer mechanism through activation of multiple pathways [11]. Previous studies have shown that GTT has an effective antitumor activity compared to other tocotrienol isomers [12]. GTT as an anticancer agent is selective on malignant cells, is capable of targeting multiple signaling pathways simultaneously, and has a synergistic effect with chemotherapy [13, 14]. Hence, various studies have been done to identify GTT capabilities and its mechanism in anticancer activities.

To determine the role of PRDX4 in anticancer activity of GTT, *PRDX4* gene in HepG2 cells was silenced using lentivirus particles that carry the RNA sequence of *PRDX4* gene (shRNA-PRDX4). The shRNA-PRDX4 is complementary with the *PRDX4* gene sequence in the HepG2 cell. The *PRDX4* gene and protein expression was reduced and indirectly caused the genotypic and phenotypic changes in the cell [15]. The silenced HepG2 cells were resistant toward puromycin and also encoded green fluorescent protein (GFP). Puromycin resistance enabled the culture of only silenced cell in the media. The presence of GFP as a reporter gene that exhibits bright green fluorescence when exposed to ultraviolet light was used as a visual tag for the expression of other genes. To silence the gene using lentivirus, there are several critical factors to be considered to avoid false positive and to increase silencing efficiency [16]. In this study, the silenced HepG2 cells were treated with GTT for 48 h. Then, cell viability, apoptosis rate, and ROS production were determined. Protein profiling was done to further confirm the proteins involved in the pathways.

2. Gene silencing

Gene silencing is used to study the role of specific genes by introducing antisense RNA to block the translation of messenger RNA (mRNA) and inhibit gene expression or translation. This biological process is known as RNA interference (RNAi). RNA plays a role as a mediator in regulating gene expression. In relation to this, synthetic RNAi is developed to mimic the targeted gene and reduce its expression [17]. The silencing possibly occurs during the transcription or translation phase. When the targeted gene is silenced, its expression is reduced to 70% without eliminating the whole expression [18]. This technique offers one step forward for the therapeutic strategy of specialized medication for patients to undergo treatment for cancer or infectious diseases [19].

There are three types of RNAi which are small interference RNA (siRNA), microRNA (miRNA), and small hairpin RNA (shRNA). siRNA is a double-stranded RNA comprising 20–25 nucleotides. siRNA sequences are coupled with a polymer and liposome carrier to enter the cell by using exogenous mechanism to silence the gene [20]. This process is known as transfection. shRNA is encoded specific RNA transcription which comprises 19–29 nucleotides. These nucleotides form a bridge for small hairpin of nine nucleotides [21]. shRNA silencing mechanism is known as transduction. The delivery of shRNA to the cell is through vectors such as plasmid, adenovirus, lentivirus, or retrovirus with a U6 promoter to regulate shRNA expression [22]. The vector will ensure that shRNA is expressed to silence the targeted gene. The silenced gene is inherited by the daughter cells [23]. miRNA is single-stranded RNA (ssRNA) which comprises 21–23 nucleotides. This type of RNAi is complementary with mRNA molecule and can be used to silence the gene [24].

In vivo studies have shown that RNAi silences the targeted gene without affecting other cellular activities such as interferon action which may inhibit protein synthesis [25]. siRNA can only be used in actively dividing cells and the silencing effect is temporary. This is because siRNA concentration decreases when the silenced cell divides. siRNA is also limited to cells with low susceptibility toward a foreign molecule [26]. In relation to this, the improvement of transfection method is required by introducing shRNA, which is able to silence the targeted gene in a more specific and effective way. In comparison to siRNA, shRNA and its lentivirus vector have the ability to stably integrate into the host genome. The silencing effect is passed to the daughter cell, resulting in permanent gene silencing. It increases the potential of the targeted gene to be silenced in nondividing cells, and the silencing effect can be delivered to cells that have low susceptibility toward lipid penetration. Thus, it can be applied in cell and animal model [27].

Both siRNA and shRNA have the same silencing mechanism; however, the choice of RNAi method to be used depends on the cell type, the time required to silence the gene, and the duration to silence the gene whether temporarily or permanently. The lentivirus plasmid used in this study has a GFP sequence, which functions as reporter gene, puromycin-resistance sequence for silenced cell selection, and a shRNA sequence that is antisense to the *PRDX4* sequence. Thus, the percentage of transduced cells can be determined by viewing the cells under a fluorescent microscope and culturing the cells with an optimal dose of puromycin in the culture media to select for the silenced cells.

3. Mechanism of gene silencing

The purpose of gene silencing is to regulate gene expression by degrading the targeted gene's product or reducing its mRNA translation through the delivery of RNAi agents into the cytoplasm [28]. Gene silencing mechanism involves both exogenous and endogenous pathways. The silencing mechanism of synthetic RNAi agents such as siRNA, shRNA, and miRNA is through the exogenous pathway, whereas the silencing mechanism for miRNA that exists naturally in the cell is through the endogenous pathway [29]. The mechanism of these three synthetic RNAi agents depends on the RNA-induced silencing complex (RISC) to cleave or degrade the mRNA of the targeted gene.

Further process of siRNA silencing occurs in the cytoplasm, whereas for shRNA and pre-miRNA, DNA integration occurs in the nucleus prior to the changes of pri-miRNA/pri-shRNA to the pre-miRNA/pre-shRNA [30]. The siRNA pathway is activated when dsRNA, together with the carrier complex, penetrates the cell membrane. Then, an endogenous dicer enzyme identifies the dsRNA sequence and splits it into small fragments of siRNA. The RISC complex binds to the siRNA fragments and causes RNA splitting for gene silencing to occur [31]. Plasmid carried by the lentiviral vector encodes the shRNA sequence of the targeted gene and also shRNA transcripts on the promoter of RNA pol III or pol II. When the lentivirus infects the cells, lentiviral plasmids are transferred to the cytoplasm. An endogenous dicer enzyme identifies the plasmid and splits the shRNA into small fragments of pri-shRNA [32]. The small fragments of pri-shRNA enter the nucleus, are multiplied by reverse transcription, and integrate into the host cell's genome. The integrated genome will enter the shRNA silencing pathway to silence the gene.

Pre-shRNA and microRNA primers (pri-miRNA) are transcribed in the nucleus using a complex of Drosha microprocessors and DGCR8 as intermediators to produce the precursor microRNA (pre-miRNA)/pre-shRNA. Pre-miRNA/pre-shRNA is then exported to the cytoplasm by exportin-5 and splits by a dicer enzyme to dsRNA [33]. The dsRNA is combined with RISC and is resolved by a helicase. The disassembled dsRNA activates the mRNA thread guide to recognize the target gene and Argonaute protein (Ago) in RISC [34]. The RISC complex helps to locate the mRNA thread guide which is complementary to the mRNA molecules of the targeted gene. The targeted gene's mRNA is then degraded by the endonuclease and inactivated [35].

3.1 Critical factors of gene silencing

Each cell has a different level of susceptibility toward lentivirus infection, and this is the biggest challenge to overcome in order to achieve optimal conditions for successful transduction [36]. The efficiency of shRNA silencing on the targeted gene is measured manually by experiment. Therefore, several critical factors must be considered to achieve specificity and efficiency of cell transduction. The factors are cell density, polybrene concentration, serum presence in the transduction media, incubation time, and lentivirus and puromycin dosage [37]. Furthermore, the functional titer and the multiplicity of infection (MOI) should be determined so that the minimum amount of lentivirus needed to transduce the cell is used. The ideal shRNA structure and experimental design should also be taken into account [38].

3.2 Basic conditions of gene silencing

One of the basic conditions that needs to be optimized for successful gene silencing is the cell density. The recommended cell density for transduction is 40–50% of cell confluence [16]. However, it depends on the size and growth rate of the cell. This confluence is to ensure that the cells have enough space to divide during transduction, which takes about 96 h. A previous study showed that cell confluence of more than 50% limits the interaction of lentivirus, cells, and DNA complex [39]. On the other hand, cell confluence of less than 30% will slow down cell growth [40]. Besides that, the cells used for transduction process must be active. This is because active cells take up foreign molecules more efficiently compared to quiescent cells.

The lentivirus membrane and cell wall are negatively charged. This causes difficulty for the lentivirus to infect the cell. Polybrene is a cation polymer that facilitates the lentivirus's infiltration into the cells [41]. Higher concentration of polybrene results in a more effective lentiviral infection. However, if the concentration of polybrene is too high and it is incubated with the cells for a long duration, it may cause toxic effects to the cells [42]. Therefore, a polybrene concentration that does not affect cell viability in long culture periods was chosen as the optimum condition. Studies have reported that the absence of serum in the culture media increases the efficiency of lentivirus DNA uptake by the cell [43]. However, the absence of serum may affect cell growth. Therefore, the presence of serum in the media during the transduction process has to be determined for efficient transduction.

Stable silenced cells are selected through puromycin resistance. Non-transduced cells will die as puromycin inhibits protein synthesis [44]. Cells are cultured in media containing different concentrations of puromycin for 7 days. Then, a kill curve is constructed. The optimal dosage of puromycin to be used is the lowest dosage of puromycin that kills the cell significantly from the third to the seventh day. Cell viability is calculated starting from the third day because the cells only respond to the antibiotic exposure after 48 h.

Each cell type has different susceptibilities to lentivirus infection. Therefore, the functional titer needs to be determined in order to know the minimum lentivirus concentration required to infect the cell. Functional titer is the smallest transducing unit required for lentivirus to infect the cell. The transducing unit needs to be parallel to the ratio between the lentivirus and cell in culture, which is known as MOI. Functional titer and MOI are important to ensure optimum condition for shRNA expression for transduction to occur. Technically, only a small concentration of functional titer is required to transduce cells at a consistent MOI ratio [45]. MOI is the ratio of lentivirus that can infect the cell at one time. As the MOI increases, the lentivirus volume required in a fixed amount of functional titer also increases. The minimum MOI should be determined so that the optimum concentration of shRNA that is sufficient to infect the cells at the recommended confluence is used [46].

3.3 Small hairpin RNA (shRNA) design

The design of shRNA vector is important to control the optimum expression of shRNA. The optimum expression of shRNA is determined by the lentiviral vector, promoters, and shRNA structures [47]. A study reported that human cytomegalovirus (hCMV) promoter is able to infect 95% of HepG2 cells and stably integrate into the host cell genome [48]. Lentivirus infection has low toxicity and does not affect the phenotype of the cell [49]. An efficient combination of promoter and vector will have an influence on the functional titer. Thus, shRNA can be expressed optimally to specifically silence a target gene.

3.4 Experimental design

A good experimental design is essential in gene silencing so that the silencing effect can be validated as specific silencing without any false positive. The recommended experimental design for transduction method comprises a positive control, a negative control, and unsilenced cell [50]. The positive control is a sequence of normalized genes that are highly expressed in cells to identify whether the silencing have effects on the cell cycle or any pathways that may affect the growth of the silenced cells [51]. The presence of nontargeted lentivirus negative control (NTC) is to validate whether the plasmid of the lentivirus itself has an effect on the targeted gene expression. NTC is consists of shRNA sequence that is not complementary to any mammalian gene by having three or less nucleotide equivalents. It also contains GFP and also puromycin-resistance sequences. This control is important to avoid any false positive.

The NTC control should have no effect on the targeted gene and the transduced cell [52]. The non-transduced cell controls are standardized to be compared with NTC controls. If the NTC and non-transduced cell controls show no difference in mRNA and protein expression of targeted proteins, this proves that the plasmid carried by the lentivirus has no effect on the cell. Although shRNA functions are at the mRNA level, only changes in protein expression may contribute to phenotypic changes. Therefore, validation of the mRNA and protein expression of the targeted proteins should be carried out to ensure that the gene expression is suppressed [53]. In addition, it is essential to validate the silencing effect by using more than two sequences of targeted gene shRNA. Every segment of gene sequence has a different effect in silencing the gene. The best sequence is selected based on the higher silencing rates shown through reduction of mRNA and protein expression of targeted gene.

4. Peroxiredoxin-4

4.1 Peroxiredoxin-4 and its function

H_2O_2 is produced during the disulfide bond formation in protein synthesis and from a side effect of cell biology mechanism located in the ER lumen and extracellular matrix [54]. PRDX4 is localized in the endoplasmic reticulum and highly expressed in the pancreas, liver, and heart but is low in blood and brain leukocytes [5]. PRDX4 plays a role as an antioxidant by scavenging H_2O_2 and is a chaperone molecule to activate ER stress pathway [55]. PRDX4 is important for cell protection by reducing H_2O_2 to water in order to reduce oxidative stress.

In addition, PRDX4 has a role in regulating the activation of NF-κB transcription factor and TNF-related apoptosis-inducing ligand (TRAIL) [56]. TRAIL is a transmembrane protein involved in apoptosis extrinsic pathway by binding to receptors DR4 or DR5. A reduction in PRDX4 expression leads to TRAIL activation and apoptosis induction, whereas an increase in PRDX4 expression inhibits the TRAIL activation and leads to cell survival [57]. The expression of PRDX4 in the cytosol increases NF-κB activity through phosphorylation of IκB-α [58]. Meanwhile, the expression of PRDX4 in the endoplasmic reticulum reduces NF-κB activity. NF-κB plays a role in cell proliferation and survival. A study has shown that PRDX4 is bound to the endothelium and is secreted when there is a redox change in the extracellular matrix [59]. This study is supported with the presence of high PRDX4 in the serum that indicates membrane leakage due to tissue destruction and cell apoptosis [60].

4.2 Mechanism of peroxiredoxin-4 as an antioxidant

PRDX4 triggers H_2O_2 signaling and protects cells from oxidative stress by oxidizing thioredoxin (Trx) proteins. Trx is a group of co-factor proteins with chaperone activity to control cell homeostasis and inhibit H_2O_2 signaling pathway [61]. PRDX4 requires Trx peroxidase activity as an electron donor. The oxidized Trx is recycled by Trx reductase and NADPH as the primary electron donor. The main target of H_2O_2 molecules is two cysteine residues on PRDX4 to form catalytic peroxide mechanisms [62]. PRDX4 has two cysteine residues known as peroxidatic cysteine residue (CysP-) and resolution cysteine residue (CysR-). These two cysteine subunits have peroxidatic properties to oxidize H_2O_2.

When the oxidative stress level is high, CysP- acts on peroxide to form sulfenic acid (CysP-SOH). CysP- is one of the cysteine units located near the N-terminal of PRXD4. CysP-SOH then reacts with another systemic subunit known as CysR- to form a stable disulfide bond, and water molecule is produced. Trx enzyme reduces the disulfide bond and completes the PRDX4 catalytic cycle by detoxifying the peroxide and producing an active thiol. If the oxidative stress keeps increasing, –SOH is oxidized to $-SO_2H$ [63]. PRDX4 in $-SO_2H$ is reduced and re-oxidized by sulfiredoxin (Srx) through the reduction of ATP to ADP. This process is reversible [1]. However, in high oxidation state, $-SO_2H$ is continuously oxidized to $-SO_3H$, and PRDX4 will undergo hyperoxidation. This will cause inhibition of oxidation, and PRDX4 will activate other pathways to counteract the oxidation state. In conclusion, PRDX4 antioxidant activity is inhibited in high oxidation state and indirectly activates the ER-pressure pathway [64].

Studies have shown that the ER produces higher level of H_2O_2 than the mitochondria [65]. The main source of H_2O_2 in the ER lumen is the reaction of oxidase-1 in the ER (Ero1) with disulfide isomerase protein (PDI) for disulfide bond formations during protein synthesis. The disulfide bonds are important to prevent the protein from degrading after it is excreted from the ER lumen. Disulfide bonds formation involves high oxidative processes, and the unfolded bonds on damaged proteins may cause unfolded protein response (UPR). Unfolded proteins are degraded by dissolution of disulfide bonds before the protein is bound to the cytosol membrane [66]. UPR is the action of cells to balance the increasing oxidative stress and repair the function of or degrade the unfolded protein. The UPR will activate chaperone proteins of multiple pathways to balance the oxidative stress [67]. High oxidative stress in the ER will induce UPR and activate Ero1 to oxidize PDI catalytic enzymes by using oxygen molecules as the electron receiver [68]. The UPR action will form three intermediate sensors which are ATF6, IRE1α, and PERK and at the same time increase Ero1 and PRDX4 expressions as homeostatic chaperones [69].

5. The effect of viability, apoptosis rate, and reactive oxygen species production in HepG2 cell silenced with peroxiredoxin-4 and treated with GTT

Gamma-tocotrienol has been shown to have high antitumor activity [12] that exhibits cell cycle arrest and apoptosis in alveolar adenocarcinoma epithelial cells, A549 [70], and colorectal cancer cell HT-29 [71]. Its action is specific and causes the cancer cells to be more susceptible and sensitive to treatment [72]. A previous study by Sazli et al. [7] reported that PRDX4 was upregulated when HepG2 cells were treated with GTT. In this study, we silenced *PRDX4* gene and treated with 70 μM of GTT to determine the role of PRDX4 in anticancer activity of GTT. Finding has shown that GTT treatment reduces HepG2-shRNA-PRDX4 cell viability significantly ($p < 0.01$) compared to its control (HepG2-shRNA-PRDX4) and also compared to HepG2 treated with GTT ($p < 0.05$) (**Table 1**). This viability assay is the first line of observation to show that GTT treatment does have an effect toward the silenced *PRDX4* gene.

To investigate further the cause of reduction in cell viability, an apoptosis assay was done. The findings showed that the apoptosis rate was significantly increased ($p < 0.05$) in HepG2 treated with GTT compared to HepG2 control. Besides that, apoptosis rate increased in HepG2-shRNA-PRDX4-GTT ($p < 0.05$) compared to HepG2-shRNA-PRDX4 and HepG2-GTT ($p < 0.05$). GTT is capable to induce intrinsic and extrinsic apoptotic pathways in cancer cells such are breast cancer cell line, MCF-7, and MDA-MB-231 by increasing biomarker stress in the endoplasmic reticulum [73]. It is suggested that the main reason for the apoptosis in GTT-treated group is high level of ROS production. GTT has triggered ROS production through PRDX4 activity. Studies reported that one of the anticancer activities of GTT is apoptosis induction through increases of ROS production [74]. We have postulated that GTT might trigger the ROS production through PRDX4 activity.

Cell groups	Cell viability (%)	Apoptosis rate (%)	Free radical production (arbitrary unit)
HepG2	100 ± 0.08	13.26 ± 1.97	1.00 ± 0.01
HepG2-shRNA-PRDX4	98 ± 12.33	18.91 ± 2.90	3.59 ± 0.33[a]
HepG2 with 70 μM GTT	90 ± 8.98	76.09 ± 4.89[a]	2.32 ± 0.09[a]
HepG2-shRNA-PRDX4 with 70 μM GTT	63 ± 10.38[b,c]	92.65 ± 6.58[b,c]	1.61 ± 0.01[b]

The data is presented as the mean ± standard deviation. Each group consists of technical triplicate and three biological replicates. GTT, gamma-tocotrienol; PRDX4, peroxiredoxin-4; HepG2-shRNA-PRDX4, HepG2 cell with PRDX4 gene silenced.
[a]A significant difference compared to HepG2 group ($p < 0.05$).
[b]A significant difference compared to HepG2-shRNA-PRDX4 group ($p < 0.01$).
[c]A significant difference compared to HepG2 GTT-treated group ($p < 0.05$).

Table 1.
The effect of GTT treatment on HepG2 and HepG2-shRNA-PRDX4 cell viability, apoptosis rate, and free radical production.

Hence, the level of ROS in each group was measured. The result showed that GTT increased ROS production ($p < 0.05$) in HepG2 group compared to the control but reduced ROS production in HepG2-shRNA-PRDX4 group. In HepG2-shRNA-PRDX4, ROS production was even higher compared to other groups but causes no effect on the cell viability. This proves that the function of PRDX4 is to reduce ROS level and oxidative stress. GTT either increases ROS production [75] to stimulate apoptosis pathway in HepG2 group or directly activate the apoptosis pathway in HepG2-shRNA-PRDX4.

To investigate further, protein profiling was done using LCMS machine to detect proteins expressed in HepG2-shRNA-PRDX4 group treated with GTT compare with HepG2-shRNA-PRDX4 as its control group. Protein profiling has shown a total of 3413 proteins expressed in HepG2-shRNA-PRDX4 and 3659 proteins expressed in HepG2-shRNA-PRDX4 treated with GTT. There are 2121 similar proteins expressed in both HepG2-shRNA-PRDX4 control group and HepG2-shRNA-PRDX4 treated with GTT. Statistical analysis has been done to differentiate protein which significantly expressed HepG2-shRNA-PRDX4 treated with GTT compared to HepG2-shRNA-PRDX4 control group using Fisher Exact test. The proteins are significantly expressed if the p value is less than 0.00398. Then, the significantly expressed protein is filtered and selected based on their functional processes that are involved in anticancer activity using UniProt and Reactome database.

There are 6 upregulated protein expressions that are CLU, NDRG1, NUDT2, PRDX5, RALB, and SLC25A6 (**Table 2**) and 14 downregulated proteins expression (**Table 3**) in HepG2-shRNA-PRDX4 group treated with GTT compared to HepG2-shRNA-PRDX4 control group. The downregulated protein expressions are EEF1A1, DHX9, PRDX1, RPS27, HIST2H2AA3, UBA52, UTP20, GSTP1, HSPB1 NPM1, PRDX2, PRDX6, PRKDC, and TXN—the significant different expressed proteins involved in multiple anticancer mechanism targeted pathway. Most of the upregulated proteins are involved in apoptotic pathway and DNA damage, whereas for the 14 downregulated proteins are involved in carcinogenesis pathway, anti-apoptotic, and cell cycle arrest. NDRG1, NUDT2, and PRDX5 expressions resulted from cellular response on ROS production causes on the downstream action. Those proteins trigger cell cycle arrest due to DNA damage and apoptosis [76]. This situation worsens the cell conditions; thus, GTT has increased pro-apoptotic proteins to induce apoptosis. The apoptotic pathway is regulated by the expression of RALB, SLC25A6, and CLU which mediate the releases of cytochrome c from mitochondria [77].

Functional cluster/ protein name	Accession name (Swiss Prot)	*P*-value	Fold change	Functional process	Mechanism
Clusterin	CLU	0.0013	1.0	Release of cytochrome c from mitochondria	Pro-apoptosis
Protein NDRG1	NDRG1	0.0001	3.4	DNA damage response, signal transduction by p53 class mediator, cellular response to hypoxia	DNA damage
Bis(5′-nucleosil)-tetraphosphatase	NUDT2	0.00056	8.5	Apoptotic process, cellular response to oxidative stress	Pro-apoptosis
Peroxiredoxin-5, mitochondrial	PRDX5	0.0023	1.6	Apoptotic process, cell redox homeostasis, cellular response to reactive oxygen species	Pro-apoptosis
Ras-related protein Ral-B	RALB	0.0020	4.8	Apoptotic process, cell cycle	Pro-apoptosis
ADP/ATP translocase 3	SLC25A6	0.0003	1.4	Apoptotic process	Pro-apoptosis

Table 2.
List of upregulated protein expression in HepG2-shRNA-PRDX4 treated with GTT compared to HepG2-shRNA-PRDX4 control group.

The treatment of GTT on HepG2-shRNA-PRDX4 causes downregulated protein expression that is involved in cell cycle arrest, carcinogenesis pathway, proteins resulted in the ER stress, and anti-apoptotic. The level of ROS production was reduced in HepG2-shRNA-PRDX4 group treated with GTT, while the apoptosis activity was induced. EEF1A1, PRDX 1, PRDX2, PRDX6, and TXN are the proteins that function to reduce ROS level and thus become negative regulator for cell apoptosis [78]. Thus, GTT has shown to reduce the ROS accumulation in HepG2-shRNA-PRDX4. GTT also suppressed the HIST2H2AA3, UBA52, and UTP20 protein expressions that are involved in cell cycle arrest. The reduction of ROS level promotes cell proliferation [79], and this justifies the downregulation of protein expression for cell cycle arrest. The expression of DHX9 is downregulated, and it plays a role in regulating DNA repair. GTT in silenced cells reduces the ROS level and stimulates an apoptotic pathway to cause cell death.

GTT also suppressed PRDX1 and RPS27 expression that are involved in carcinogenesis. PRDX1 is a positive regulator of stress-activated MAPK cascade, whereas protein RPS27 is involved in JNK cascade and Wnt signaling pathway. The activation of ER stress response leads to the expression of protein that involves the MAPK pathway through the activation of JNK as mediator [80]. Most of the downregulated proteins are involved in direct negative regulator of apoptosis or negative regulator of oxidative stress-induced proteins. The proteins are GSTP1, HSPB1, NPM1, PRDX2, PRDX6, PRKDC, TXN, and UBA52. Protein profiling of HepG2-shRNA-PRDX4 showed that GTT induces apoptosis by reducing oxidative stress in the endoplasmic reticulum and upregulated pro-apoptotic protein expression.

Functional cluster/protein name	Accession name (Swiss Prot)	*P*-value	Fold change	Functional process	Mechanism
ATP-dependent RNA helicase A	DHX9	0.0015	0.80	Positive regulation of DNA repair	Carcinogenesis
Cluster of elongation factor 1-alpha 1	EEF1A1	0.0001	0.80	Response to endoplasmic reticulum stress	ER stress
Glutathione S-transferase P	GSTP1	0.0001	0.60	Negative regulation of extrinsic apoptotic signaling pathway	Anti-apoptosis
Cluster of histone H2A type 2-A	HIST2H2AA3	0.0001	0.70	Negative regulation of cell proliferation	Cell cycle arrest
Heat shock protein beta-1	HSPB1	0.0001	0.70	Negative regulation of oxidative stress-induced intrinsic apoptotic signaling pathway	Anti-apoptosis
Nucleophosmin	NPM1	0.0018	0.80	Negative regulation of apoptotic process	Anti-apoptosis
Peroxiredoxin-1	PRDX1	0.0001	0.60	Regulation of stress-activated MAPK cascade, response to oxidative stress	Carcinogenesis
Peroxiredoxin-2	PRDX2	0.0001	0.70	Negative regulation of apoptotic process, response to oxidative stress	Anti-apoptosis
Peroxiredoxin-6	PRDX6	0.0001	0.60	Negative apoptosis regulation by regulating reactive oxygen species	Anti-apoptosis
DNA-dependent protein kinase catalytic subunit	PRKDC	0.0001	0.80	Negative regulation of apoptotic process	Anti-apoptosis
Cluster of 40S ribosomal protein S27	RPS27	0.0025	0.30	JNK cascade, Wnt signaling pathway	Carcinogenesis

Functional cluster/protein name	Accession name (Swiss Prot)	*P*-value	Fold change	Functional process	Mechanism
Thioredoxin	TXN	0.0001	0.01	Negative regulation of hydrogen peroxide-induced cell death	Anti-apoptosis
Ubiquitin-60S ribosomal protein L40	UBA52	0.0011	0.70	Signal transduction by p53 class mediator resulting in cell cycle arrest, negative regulation of apoptotic process	Cell cycle arrest and Anti-apoptosis
Small subunit processome component 20 homolog	UTP20	0.00010	0.20	Negative regulation of cell proliferation	Cell cycle arrest

Table 3.
List of downregulated protein expression in HepG2-shRNA-PRDX4 treated with GTT compared to HepG2-shRNA-PRDX4 control group.

6. Conclusion

Gene silencing is a technique to prevent the expression of certain genes. This technique is very useful to study biochemical pathway or produce therapeutics to treat cancer and diseases. Optimizing on the basic criteria for gene silencing is very important to achieve efficient silencing. GTT treatment reduces cell viability and causes apoptosis in both silenced HepG2-shRNA-PRDX4 and non-silenced HepG2 groups, but ROS production was increased non-silenced cells. The silencing of *PRDX4* gene in HepG2 cells caused ROS accumulation but did not cause cell death. Proteomic technique showed that GTT caused HepG2 cell death through activation of multiple pathways. It either triggers the apoptosis pathway directly in silenced cell or increases ROS production through PRDX4 activity, thus increasing pro-apoptotic and reducing anti-apoptotic protein expressions.

Acknowledgements

The authors would like to express gratitude to all researchers and staff of the Biochemistry Department, Faculty of Medicine, the National University of Malaysia. This study was funded by the National University of Malaysia Medical Centre grant (FF-2016-063) and the Ministry of Higher Education under the Fundamental Research Grant Scheme (FRGS/1/2013/SKK01/UKM/02/2).

Conflict of interest

The authors declare no conflict of interest.

Author details

Afiah Nasuha Aznan and Zakiah Jubri*
Department of Biochemistry, Faculty of Medicine Medical Centre,
Universiti Kebangsaan Malaysia, Kuala Lumpur, Malaysia

*Address all correspondence to: zakiah.jubri@ppukm.ukm.edu.my

References

[1] Fujii J, Ikeda Y. Advances in our understanding of peroxiredoxin, a multifunctional, mammalian redox protein. Redox Report. 2002;**7**(3):123-130. DOI: 10.1179/135100002125000352

[2] Sato Y, Kojima R, Okumura M, Hagiwara M, Masui S, Maegawa K-I, et al. Synergistic cooperation of PDI family members in peroxiredoxin 4-driven oxidative protein folding. Scientific Reports. 2013;**3**:1-13. DOI: 10.1038/srep02456

[3] Zhu L, Yang K, Wang X, Wang C-C. A novel reaction of peroxiredoxin 4 towards substrates in oxidative protein folding. PLoS One. 2014;**9**(8):e105529. DOI: 10.1371/journal.pone.0105529

[4] Hwang K-E, Park D-S, Kim Y-S, Kim B-R, Park S-N, Lee M-K, et al. Prx1 modulates the chemosensitivity of lung cancer to docetaxel through suppression of FOXO1-induced apoptosis. International Journal of Oncology. 2013;**43**(1):72-78. DOI: 10.3892/ijo.2013.1918

[5] Schulte J. Peroxiredoxin 4: A multifunctional biomarker worthy of further exploration. BMC Medicine. 2011;**9**(1):137. DOI: 10.1186/1741-7015-9-137

[6] Yi NAN, Xiao MB, Ni WK, Jiang F, Lu CH, Ni R-Z. High expression of peroxiredoxin 4 affects the survival time of colorectal cancer patients, but is not an independent unfavorable prognostic factor. Molecular and Clinical Oncology. 2014;**2**(5):767-772. DOI: 10.3892/mco.2014.317

[7] Sazli FAR, Jubri Z, Rahman MA, Karsani SA, Top AGM, Ngah WZW. Gamma-tocotrienol treatment increased peroxiredoxin-4 expression in HepG2 liver cancer cell line. BMC Complementary and Alternative Medicine. 2015;**15**(1):1. DOI: 10.1186/s12906-015-0590-y

[8] Zakiah J, WZ WN. The antiproliferative effect of palm oil gamma-tocotrienol on isoprenoid pathway of hepatoma cell line. European Journal of Scientific Research. 2005;**18**(4):576-583

[9] Wada S, Satomi Y, Murakoshi M, Noguchi N, Yoshikawa T, Nishino H. Tumor suppressive effects of tocotrienol in vivo and in vitro. Cancer Letters. 2005;**229**(2):181-191. DOI: 10.1016/j.canlet.2005.06.036

[10] Sen CK, Khanna S, Roy S. Tocotrienols in health and disease: The other half of the natural vitamin E family. Molecular Aspects of Medicine. 2007;**28**(5):692-728. DOI: 10.1016/j.mam.2007.03.001

[11] Ahsan H, Ahad A, Iqbal J, Siddiqui WA. Pharmacological potential of tocotrienols: A review. Nutrition and Metabolism. 2014;**11**(1):52. DOI: 10.1186/1743-7075-11-52

[12] Aggarwal B, Nesaretnam K. Vitamin E tocotrienols: Life beyond tocopherols. Genes and Nutrition. 2012;**7**(1):1. DOI: 10.1007/s12263-011-0234-x

[13] Abubakar IB, Lim K-H, Kam T-S, Loh H-S. Enhancement of apoptotic activities on brain cancer cells via the combination of γ-tocotrienol and jerantinine A. Phytomedicine. 2017;**30**:74-84. DOI: 10.1016/j.phymed.2017.03.004

[14] Bachawal SV, Wali VB, Sylvester PW. Combined γ-tocotrienol and erlotinib/gefitinib treatment suppresses Stat and Akt signaling in murine mammary tumor cells. Anticancer Research. 2010;**30**(2):429-437

[15] Nash KL, Jamil B, Maguire AJ, Alexander GJ, Lever AM. Hepatocyte-specific gene expression from integrated lentiviral vectors. The Journal of Gene Medicine. 2004;**6**(9):974-983. DOI: 10.1002/jgm.591

[16] Aznan AN, Abdul Karim N, Wan Ngah WZ, Jubri Z. Critical factors for lentivirus-mediated PRDX4 gene transfer in the HepG2 cell line. Oncology Letters. 2018;**16**(1):73-82. DOI: 10.3892/ol.2018.8650

[17] Mocellin S, Provenzano M. RNA interference: Learning gene knock-down from cell physiology. Journal of Translational Medicine. 2004;**2**(1):39. DOI: 10.1186/1479-5876-2-39

[18] Hood E. RNAi: What's all the noise about gene silencing? Environmental Health Perspectives. 2004;**112**(4):A224. DOI: 10.1289/ehp.112-a224

[19] Castanotto D, Rossi JJ. The promises and pitfalls of RNA-interference-based therapeutics. Nature. 2009;**457**(7228):426. DOI: 10.1038/nature07758

[20] Meister G, Tuschl T. Mechanisms of gene silencing by double-stranded RNA. Nature. 2004;**431**(7006):343-349. DOI: 10.1038/nature02873

[21] Lingor P. Regulation of cell death and survival by RNA interference—The roles of miRNA and siRNA. In: Cecconi F, D'amelio M, editors. Apoptosome: An Up-and-Coming Therapeutical tool. Dordrecht, The Netherlands: Springer; 2010. pp. 95-117

[22] Xia XG, Zhou H, Ding H, Affar EB, Shi Y, Xu Z. An enhanced U6 promoter for synthesis of short hairpin RNA. Nucleic Acids Research. 2003;**31**(17):e100-e100. DOI: 10.1093/nar/gng098

[23] Fellmann C, Lowe SW. Stable RNA interference rules for silencing. Nature Cell Biology. 2013;**16**:10

[24] Dalmay T. Mechanism of miRNA-mediated repression of mRNA translation. Essays in Biochemistry. 2013;**54**:29-38. DOI: 10.1042/bse0540029

[25] Agrawal N, Dasaradhi PVN, Mohmmed A, Malhotra P, Bhatnagar RK, Mukherjee SK. RNA interference: Biology, mechanism, and applications. Microbiology and Molecular Biology Reviews. 2003;**67**(4):657-685

[26] Takasaki S, Kotani SF, Konagaya A, Konagaya A. An effective method for selecting siRNA target sequences in mammalian cells. Cell Cycle. 2004;**3**(6):1551-4005

[27] Rao DD, Vorhies JS, Senzer N, Nemunaitis J. siRNA vs. shRNA: Similarities and differences. Advanced Drug Delivery Reviews. 2009;**61**(9):746-759. DOI: 10.1016/j.addr.2009.04.004

[28] Zamore PD, Tuschl T, Sharp PA, RNAi BDP. Double-stranded RNA directs the ATP-dependent cleavage of miRNA at 21 to 23 nucleotide intervals. Cell. 2000;**101**(1):25-33. DOI: 10.1016/S0092-8674(00)80620-0

[29] Donzé O, Picard D. RNA interference in mammalian cells using siRNAs synthesized with T7 RNA polymerase. Nucleic Acids Research. 2002;**30**(10):e46-e46. DOI: 10.1093/nar/30.10.e46

[30] Khatri N, Rathi MN, Baradia D, Trehan S, Misra A. In vivo delivery aspects of miRNA, shRNA and siRNA. Critical Reviews™ in Therapeutic Drug Carrier Systems. 2012;**29**(6):487-527. DOI: 10.1615/CritRevTherDrugCarrierSyst.v29.i6.20

[31] Pratt AJ, Macrae IJ. The RNA-induced silencing complex: A versatile gene-silencing machine. The Journal of Biological Chemistry. 2009;**284**(27):17897-17901. DOI: 10.1074/jbc.R900012200

[32] Taxman DJ, Moore CB, Guthrie EH, Huang MTH. Short hairpin RNA (shRNA): Design, delivery, and assessment of gene knockdown. RNA Therapeutics: Function, Design, and Delivery. 2010:139-156. DOI: 10.1007/978-1-60761-657-3_10

[33] Kim VN, Han J, Siomi MC. Biogenesis of small RNAs in animals. Nature Reviews Molecular Cell Biology. 2009;**10**(2):126-139. DOI: 10.1038/nrm2632

[34] Bartel DP. microRNAs: Target recognition and regulatory functions. Cell. 2009;**136**(2):215-233. DOI: 10.1016/j.cell.2009.01.002

[35] Maniataki E, Mourelatos Z. A human, ATP-independent, risk assembly machine fueled by pre-miRNA. Genes & Development. 2005;**19**(24):2979-2990

[36] Yang L, Bailey L, Baltimore D, Wang P. Targeting lentiviral vectors to specific cell types in vivo. Proceedings of the National Academy of Sciences. 2006;**103**(31):11479-11484. DOI: 10.1073/pnas.0604993103

[37] Andreadis S, Lavery T, Davis HE, Le Doux JM, Yarmush ML, Morgan JR. Toward a more accurate quantitation of the activity of recombinant retroviruses: Alternatives to titer and multiplicity of infection. Journal of Virology. 2000;**74**(3):1258-1266

[38] Zhang B, Metharom PF, Jullie H, Jullie HF, Ellem KAO, Ellem KF, et al. The significance of controlled conditions in lentiviral vector titration and in the use of multiplicity of infection (MOI) for predicting gene transfer events. Genetic Vaccines and Therapy. 2004;**2**(6):1479-0556. DOI: 10.1186/1479-0556-2-6

[39] Parr-Brownlie LC, Bosch-Bouju C, Schoderboeck L, Sizemore RJ, Abraham WC, Hughes SM. Lentiviral vectors as tools to understand central nervous system biology in mammalian model organisms. Frontiers in Molecular Neuroscience. 2015;**8**:14. DOI: 10.3389/fnmol.2015.00014

[40] Prijic S, Sersa G. Magnetic nanoparticles as targeted delivery systems in oncology. Radiology and Oncology. 2011;**45**(1):1-16. DOI: 10.2478/v10019-011-0001-z

[41] Le Bihan O, Chèvre R, Mornet S, Garnier B, Pitard B, Lambert O. Probing the in vitro mechanism of action of cationic lipid/DNA lipoplexes at a nanometric scale. Nucleic Acids Research. 2011;**39**(4):1595-1609. DOI: 10.1093/nar/gkq921

[42] Denning W, Das S, Guo S, Xu J, Kappes JC, Hel Z. Optimization of the transductional efficiency of lentiviral vectors: Effect of sera and polycations. Molecular Biotechnology. 2013;**53**(3):308-314. DOI: 10.1007/s12033-012-9528-5

[43] Davis HE, Rosinski M, Morgan JR, Yarmush ML. Charged polymers modulate retrovirus transduction via membrane charge neutralization and virus aggregation. Biophysical Journal. 2004;**86**(2):1234-1242. DOI: 10.1016/S0006-3495(04)74197-1

[44] Watanabe S, Iwamoto M, Suzuki SI, Fuchimoto D, Honma D, Nagai T, et al. A novel method for the production of transgenic cloned pigs: Electroporation-mediated gene transfers to non-cultured cells and subsequent selection with puromycin. Biology of Reproduction. 2005;**72**(2):309-315. DOI: 10.1095/biolreprod.104.031591

[45] Wotherspoon S, Dolnikov A, Symonds G, Nordon R. Susceptibility of cell populations to transduction by retroviral vectors. Journal of Virology. 2004;**78**(10):5097-5102. DOI: 10.1128/JVI.78.10.5097-5102.2004

[46] Logan AC, Nightingale SJ, Haas DL, Cho GJ, Pepper KA, Kohn DB. Factors influencing the titer and infectivity of lentiviral vectors. Human Gene Therapy. 2004;**15**(10):976-988. DOI: 10.1089/hum.2004.15.976

[47] Matveeva O, Nechipurenko Y, Rossi L, Moore B, Sætrom P, Ogurtsov AY, et al. Comparison of approaches for rational siRNA design leading to a new efficient and transparent method. Nucleic Acids Research. 2007;**35**(8):e63. DOI: 10.1093/nar/gkm088

[48] Nasri M, Karimi A, Farsani MA. Production, purification and titration of a lentivirus-based vector for gene delivery purposes. Cytotechnology. 2014;**66**(6):1031-1038. DOI: 10.1007/s10616-013-9652-5

[49] Zamule SM, Strom SC, Omiecinski CJ. Preservation of hepatic phenotype in lentiviral-transduced primary human hepatocytes. Chemico-Biological Interactions. 2008;**173**(3):179-186. DOI: 10.1016/j.cbi.2008.03.015

[50] Shearer RF, Saunders DN. Experimental design for stable genetic manipulation in mammalian cell lines: Lentivirus and alternatives. Genes to Cells. 2015;**20**(1):1-10. DOI: 10.1111/gtc.12183

[51] Feng Y, Nie L, Thakur MD, Su Q, Chi Z, Zhao Y, et al. A multifunctional lentiviral-based gene knockdown with concurrent rescue that controls for off-target effects of RNAi. Genomics, Proteomics & Bioinformatics. 2010;**8**(4):238-245. DOI: 10.1016/S1672-0229(10)60025-3

[52] Svoboda P. Off-targeting and other non-specific effects of RNAi experiments in mammalian cells. Current Opinion in Molecular Therapeutics. 2007;**9**(3):248

[53] Valinezhad OA, Safaralizadeh R, Kazemzadeh-Bavili M. Mechanisms of miRNA-mediated gene regulation from common downregulation to miRNA-specific upregulation. International Journal of Genomics. 2014;**2014**:1-15. DOI: 10.1155/2014/970607

[54] Bulleid NJ. Disulfide bond formation in the mammalian endoplasmic reticulum. Cold Spring Harbor Perspectives in Biology. 2012;**4**(11):a013219. DOI: 10.1101/cshperspect.a013219

[55] Schieber M, Chandel NS. ROS function in redox signaling and oxidative stress. Current Biology. 2014;**24**(10):R453-RR62. DOI: 10.1016/j.cub.2014.03.034

[56] Knoops B, Argyropoulou V, Becker S, Ferté L, Kuznetsova O. Multiple roles of peroxiredoxins in inflammation. Molecules and Cells. 2016;**39**(1):60-64. DOI: 10.14348/molcells.2016.2341

[57] Wang HQ, Du ZF, Liu B-Q, Liu BF, Gao Y-Y, Gao YF, et al. TNF-related apoptosis-inducing ligand suppresses PRDX4 expression. FEBS Letters. 2009;**583**:1511-1515. DOI: 10.1016/j.febslet.2009.04.009

[58] Christian F, Smith EL, Carmody RJ. The regulation of NF-kB subunits by phosphorylation. Cell. 2016;**5**(1):12. DOI: 10.3390/cells5010012

[59] Okado-Matsumoto A, Matsumoto A, Fujii J, Taniguchi N. Peroxiredoxin IV is a secretable protein with heparin-binding properties under reduced conditions. The Journal of Biochemistry. 2000;**127**(3):493-501

[60] Ito R, Takahashi M, Ihara H, TsukamotoH, FujiiJ, IkedaY. Measurement of peroxiredoxin-4 serum levels in rat tissue and its use as a potential marker for hepatic disease. Molecular Medicine Reports. 2012;**6**(2):379-384. DOI: 10.3892/mmr.2012.935

[61] Brown JD, Day AM, Taylor SR, Tomalin LE, Morgan BA, Veal EA. A

peroxiredoxin promotes H_2O_2 signalling and oxidative stress resistance by oxidizing a thioredoxin family protein. Cell Reports. 2013;**5**(5):1425-1435. DOI: 10.1016/j.celrep.2013.10.036

[62] Rhee SG, Woo HA, Kil IS, Bae SH. Peroxiredoxin functions as a peroxidase and a regulator and sensor of local peroxides. Journal of Biological Chemistry. 2012;**287**(7):4403-4410. DOI: 10.1074/jbc.R111.283432

[63] Perkins A, Nelson KJ, Parsonage D, Poole LB, Karplus PA. Peroxiredoxins: Guardians against oxidative stress and modulators of peroxide signalling. Trends in Biochemical Sciences. 2015;**40**(8):435-445. DOI: 10.1016/j.tibs.2015.05.001

[64] Martin RE, Cao Z, Bulleid NJ. Regulating the level of intracellular hydrogen peroxide: The role of peroxiredoxin IV. Biochemical Society Transactions. 2014;**42**(1):1470-8752. DOI: 10.1042/BST20130168

[65] Enyedi B, Várnai P, Geiszt M. Redox state of the endoplasmic reticulum is controlled by ERO 1l-Alpha and intraluminal calcium. Antioxidants & Redox Signaling. 2010;**13**(6):721-729. DOI: 10.1089/ars.2009.2880

[66] Ushioda R, Hoseki JF, Araki K, Araki KF, Jansen G, Jansen GF, et al. Erdj5 is required as a disulfide reductase for degradation of misfolded proteins in the ER. Science. 2008;**321**:1095-9203. DOI: 10.1126/science.1159293

[67] Hetz C. The unfolded protein response: Controlling cell fate decisions under ER stress and beyond. National Review of Molecular Cell Biology. 2012;**13**(2):89-102. DOI: 10.1038/nrm3270

[68] Kakihana T, Araki K, Vavassori S, Iemura SI, Cortini M, Fagioli C, et al. Dynamic regulation of Ero1α and peroxiredoxin 4 localization in the secretory pathway. Journal of Biological Chemistry. 2013;**288**(41):29586-29594. DOI: 10.1074/jbc.M113.467845

[69] Tavender T, Sheppard A, Bulleid N. Peroxiredoxin IV is an Endoplasmic reticulum-localized enzyme forming oligomeric complexes in human cells. Biochemistry Journal. 2008;**411**:191-199. DOI: 10.1042/BJ20071428

[70] Phutthaphadoong S, Yodkeeree S, Chaiyasut C, Limtrakul P. Anti-cancer activities of α-and γ-tocotrienol against the human lung cancer. African Journal of Pharmacy and Pharmacology. 2012;**6**(9):620-629. DOI: 10.5897/AJPP11.806

[71] Xu W-L, Liu J-R, Liu H-K, Qi G-Y, Sun X-R, Sun W-G, et al. Inhibition of proliferation and induction of apoptosis by γ-tocotrienol in human colon carcinoma HT-29 cells. Nutrition. 2009;**25**(5):555-566. DOI: 10.1016/j.nut.2008.10.019

[72] Yap W, Chang P, Han H-Y, Lee D, Ling M, Wong YC, et al. γ-Tocotrienol suppresses prostate cancer cell proliferation and invasion through multiple-signalling pathways. British Journal of Cancer. 2008;**99**(11):1832-1841. DOI: 10.1038/sj.bjc.6604763

[73] Chang PN, Yap WN, Wing Lee DT, Ling M, Wong YC, Yap YL. Evidence of γ-tocotrienol as an apoptosis-inducing, invasion-suppressing, and chemotherapy drug-sensitizing agent in human melanoma cells. Nutrition and Cancer. 2009;**61**(3):357-366. DOI: 10.1080/01635580802567166

[74] Zhao K, Zhao GF, Wu D, Wu DF, Soong Y, Soong YF, et al. Cell-permeable peptide antioxidants targeted to inner mitochondrial membrane inhibit mitochondrial swelling, oxidative cell death, and reperfusion injury. The Journal of Biological Chemistry 2004;**279**(33):34682-34690. DOI: 10.1074/jbc.M402999200

[75] Birringer M, Lington D, Vertuani S, Manfredini S, Scharlau D, Glei M, et al. Proapoptotic effects of long-chain vitamin E metabolites in HepG2 cells are mediated by oxidative stress. Free Radical Biology & Medicine. 2010;**49**:1315-1322. DOI: 10.1016/j.freeradbiomed.2010.07.024

[76] Yedjou CG, Tchounwou HM, Tchounwou PB. DNA Damage, Cell Cycle Arrest, and Apoptosis Induction Caused by Lead in Human Leukemia Cells. International Journal Environmental Research Public Health. 2015;**22**(13):1660-1672. DOI: 10.3390/ijerph13010056

[77] Argüelles S, Camandola S, Cutler RG, Ayala A, Mattson MP. Elongation factor 2-diphthamide is critical for translation of two IRES-dependent protein targets, XIAP and FGF2, under oxidative stress conditions. Free Radical Biology & Medicine. 2014;**67**:131-138. DOI: 10.1016/j.freeradbiomed.2013.10.015

[78] Kupsco A, Schlenk D. Oxidative stress, unfolded protein response, and apoptosis in developmental toxicity. International Review of Cell and Molecular Biology. 2015;**317**:1-66. DOI: 10.1016/bs.ircmb.2015.02.002

[79] Kumari S, Badana AK, G MM, G S, Malla R. Reactive oxygen species: A key constituent in cancer survival. Biomarker Insights. 2018;**13**:35-42. DOI: 10.1177/1177271918755391

[80] Son Y, Cheong Y-K, Kim N-H, Chung H-T, Kang DG, Pae H-O. Mitogen-activated protein kinases and reactive oxygen species: How can ROS activate MAPK pathways? Journal of Signal Transduction. 2011;**2011**:6. DOI: 10.1155/2011/792639

Chapter 7

A Noninvasive, Orally Stable, Mucosa-Penetrating Polyvalent Vaccine Platform Based on Hepatitis E Virus Nanoparticle

Shizuo G. Kamita, Mo A. Baikoghli, Luis M. de la Maza and R. Holland Cheng

Abstract

Hepatitis E virus nanoparticle (HEVNP) is an orally stable, mucosa-penetrating delivery platform for noninvasive, targeted delivery of therapeutic and diagnostic agents. HEVNP does not carry HEV genomic RNA and is incapable of replication. The key characteristics that make HEVNP an ideal and unique vehicle for diagnostic and therapeutic delivery include surface plasticity, resistance to the harsh environment of the gastrointestinal (GI) tract, significant payload capacity, platform sustainability, and safety. Furthermore, HEVNP is easily produced using currently available expression/purification technologies; can be easily formulated as a liquid, powder, or solid; and can be distributed (and stored) without the need for a temperature-controlled supply chain.

Keywords: hepatitis E virus, HEV, nanoparticle, HEVNP, noninvasive vaccine, mucosal delivery, cryo-EM

1. Introduction

1.1 Noninvasive vaccine delivery by nanocarriers

Currently, most vaccines, drugs, and diagnostic/therapeutic agents are administered through invasive routes such as injection. There has been vast interest in the development of noninvasive, targeted, stable, and convenient drug delivery platforms that obviate the drawbacks of invasive delivery methods (reviewed in [1–6]). Systemic drug delivery through noninvasive routes requires that the delivery platform protects the drug compound while it traverses physiological barriers. Noninvasive delivery platforms, as in the case of traditional delivery platforms, should also distribute the drug effectively and selectively so that only the targeted cells receive the therapeutic agent. The rapid evolution of nanotechnology has shed light on the huge potential of nanocarrier platforms for targeting and drug delivery. Recent developments in the optimization of drug nanocarriers in terms of packaging, delivery, and targeting have the potential to revolutionize noninvasive administration and delivery of therapeutics and diagnostics through the mucosa. Several nanocarrier systems have been developed that take advantage of these

IntechOpen

developments and additionally show diminished toxicity in nontargeted cells and tissues. Despite these early successes, instability under physiological conditions, inefficient targeting, toxicity, and lack of bioavailability impose serious limitations for the development of an effective mucosal delivery platform.

While there are several routes of mucosal drug delivery, the oral and nasal routes are among the most safe and preferred by patients. The inherent characteristics of a nanocarrier such as structural composition, size, and natural stability play major roles in the potential success of a drug delivery system (reviewed in [1–4, 7–9]). For many nanocarrier platforms, problems with enzymatic degradation, limited penetration of the thick mucosal layer, and subsequently transportation of drugs through transcellular or paracellular routes are major shortcomings. The majority of currently available nanocarriers consist of simple structures that are on the nanometer to micrometer scale. Theranostic delivery vehicles that are currently used or considered for use fall into a handful of categories including polymers, lipids, solid-lipid carriers, gold carriers, nanotubes, immunostimulant complexes, magnetic carriers, and virus-like particles (VLPs) [3, 8, 9]. The size and exact composition of these nanocarriers are commonly altered and optimized based on their intended application. The key factors required for entry and distribution of theranostics include high degrees of bioavailability, the ability to withstand physiological conditions without degradation or premature exposure of the drug, and efficient distribution by overcoming the physical and enzymatic barriers through noninvasive routes.

1.2 Nanocarrier platform based on viral capsids

Evolutionarily, viruses adapt and coevolve with their host. Genetic engineering techniques and elucidation of viral structures have enabled virologist to generate empty capsids, called VLPs, which retain the physical characteristics of the capsid structure but lack the viral genome. VLPs thus exhibit the structural characteristics of the authentic virus but are incapable of replicating. In addition to being noninfectious, VLPs are generally nontoxic, biodegradable, and highly biocompatible. Structurally, the symmetrical configuration of VLPs allows them to be developed as nanocarrier systems that can entrap not only foreign nucleic acids but also peptides and imaging agents within their internal cavity. The exterior surface of VLPs, in some cases, can be tagged with targeting ligands without disruption of the VLP structure. The VLP assembles spontaneously and forms highly ordered structures following recombinant expression of the capsid protein (CP) in prokaryotic, eukaryotic, and cell-free protein expression systems. Currently, there are numerous ongoing VLP-based clinical trials worldwide [10–13]. From these clinical trials, a handful of VLP-based vaccines have been approved by the US FDA and other governmental regulatory agencies. For example, VLPs of hepatitis B virus (HBV), human papillomavirus (HPV), influenza virus, human parvovirus, and Norwalk virus have shown success in clinical trials or have been commercially developed as vaccines. The effectiveness of the delivery of therapeutic and/or diagnostic payloads using VLPs, as well as VLP surface modulation by attachment of ligands and tracking molecules, has been recently reviewed [10, 11, 14]. Here, a description of the key advantages and application of hepatitis E virus nanoparticles for use in vaccine development will be discussed.

2. Structure of hepatitis E virus capsid and HEVNP

Significant effort has been invested in characterizing the structure of the capsid of HEV by biochemical methods, imaging (X-ray crystallography and cryogenic electron microscopy (cryo-EM)), and molecular biological techniques [15–22]. These studies have revealed the underlying architecture and biochemical composition of HEV (reviewed in [1, 2, 23, 24]). The authentic HEV is composed of 180 monomers of capsid protein (CP) that are assembled into an icosahedral cage in an RNA-dependent manner with a triangulation number of 3 (T = 3). Native HEV has a virion diameter of approximately 45 nm. When the native CP is truncated (leaving amino acid (aa) residues 112–608), this truncated CP forms a smaller particle with a diameter of approximately 27 nm. This structure, known as the HEV nanoparticle (HEVNP), is composed of 60 monomers (i.e., 30 CP dimers) of the truncated CP and forms a T = 1 icosahedral conformation. The CP is comprised of three domains: S (shell domain, aa 118–317), M (middle domain, aa 318–451), and P (protrusion domain, aa 452–606) (**Figure 1**). The S domain is the most conserved region among HEV genotypes and, along with the M domain, is responsible for the formation of the HEV capsid base [17, 19, 25]. The P domain, as the name suggests, protrudes from the capsid surface and plays a role in CP dimerization [18, 26], HEV capsid antigenicity [19, 27, 28], and recognition by the host cell receptor [29]. The M domain interacts strongly with the P domain through a long proline-rich hinge; however, the biological roles of the S, M, and P domains are independent [19, 22, 25]. This modular functionality allows the P domain to be genetically modified while (i) causing no or minimal effects on capsid formation and (ii) retaining capsid stability and resistance to acidic and proteolytic conditions found in the mammalian GI tract. Additionally, genetic modification of the P domain results in invisibility of the capsid to host immune surveillance as will be discussed below. Since the P domain of HEVNP is repeated

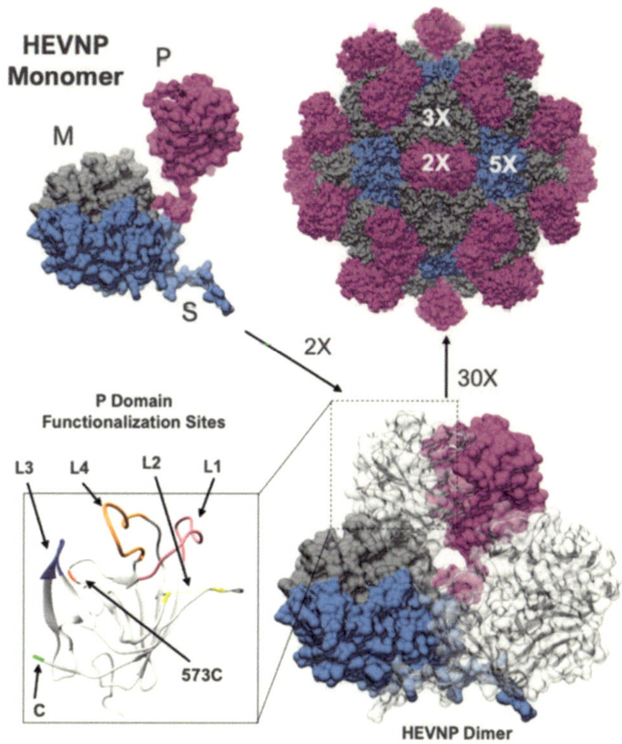

Figure 1.
Modular composition of HEVNP. HEVNP is formed by 30 homodimers of the HEVNP monomer. The dimer is the building block of HEVNP. The HEVNP monomer is composed of three domains: Shell (S), middle (M), and protrusion (P). The P domain has four surface-exposed loops (L1–L4) and a C-terminus that can be genetically or chemically (e.G., at N573C) modified in order to functionalize the HEVNP surface.

60 times on the surface of the capsid, it provides high accessibility for surface modulations that may include targeting ligands, imaging molecules, tracking molecules, and immunogenic peptides.

3. Advantages of waterborne HEVNP for vaccine development

As mentioned above, 30 dimers of the truncated CP of HEV will spontaneously self-assemble into HEVNP following heterologous expression in insect cells or bacteria. Unlike HEV, HEVNP does not encapsulate genomic RNA and is, thus, incapable of replication. HEVNP is, however, capable of encapsulating foreign RNA or DNA. As a vaccine delivery vehicle, HEVNP possesses a combination of advantageous characteristics including surface plasticity, stability within the harsh conditions of the GI tract, significant payload capacity, and platform sustainability.

3.1 Surface plasticity

The utility of the HEVNP as a mucosa-penetrating vaccine delivery platform was successful demonstrated by the development of an orally administered HEVNP-based HIV vaccine [21]. In this groundbreaking study, a 15-amino-acid-long peptide from the V3 loop of HIV-1 gp120 (called P18) was genetically inserted on the surface of HEVNP, generating the HEVNP-P18 construct (also known as 18-VLP). This insertion was successfully made after residue Y485 of the truncated CP, a location that is within the antibody-binding site of HEVNP. Cryo-EM studies revealed that the HEVNP capsid maintained its icosahedral shape and was not disrupted by the P18 insertion. The successful insertion after Y485 resulted in fully formed, stable HEVNP. In contrast, attempts of insertion after aa residues A179, R366, A507, and R542 all failed to achieve the quaternary assembly of HEVNP. Clearly, surface modification of HEVNP via modulation at Y485 by peptide insertion does not interfere with capsid stability or the formation of $T = 1$ icosahedral organization.

Following the successful insertion of P18 after Y485, four additional aa residues (T489, S533, N573, and T586) have been identified as targets for modulating the surface of HEVNP [30]. These sites are found within four surface-accessible loops (L1, aa 483–491; L2, aa 530–535; L3, aa 554–561; and L4, aa 582–593) that are found on the P domain (**Figure 1**). These sites (as well as Y485) were identified based on (i) their three-dimensional localization on the surface of HEVNP and (ii) the likelihood that mutation would result in minimal or no distortion of the HEVNP structure. In order to test the hypotheses generated by the structural analyses regarding these sites, site-directed mutagenesis was performed in order to replace these residues with a cysteine residue. All of the cysteine mutation constructs successfully assembled into stable icosahedral capsids and were subjected to surface modulation through covalent chemical conjugation. The conjugations were performed via a cysteine acylation reaction with maleimide-linked biotin, and the conjugation efficiency at each site was determined using labeled streptavidin. Of the mutations that were generated (HEVNP-485C, HEVNP-489C, HEVNP-533C, HEVNP-573C, and HEVNP-586C), the HEVNP-573C construct showed the greatest streptavidin signal. This indicated that the N573C mutation of HEVNP-573C is the most surface-visible site for modulation. More recent structural analysis has identified additional aa residues that are found on the P domain (aa residues 510–514 and 520–525) as well as the M domain (residues 342–344 and 402–408) that may be utilized as conjugation sites in a future study.

In order to demonstrate the functionality of the HEVNP-573C construct, a breast cancer cell-targeting ligand LXY30 [31] was chemically conjugated to HEVNP-573C in order to generate HEVNP-573C-LXY30 [30]. The HEVNP-573C-LXY30 construct

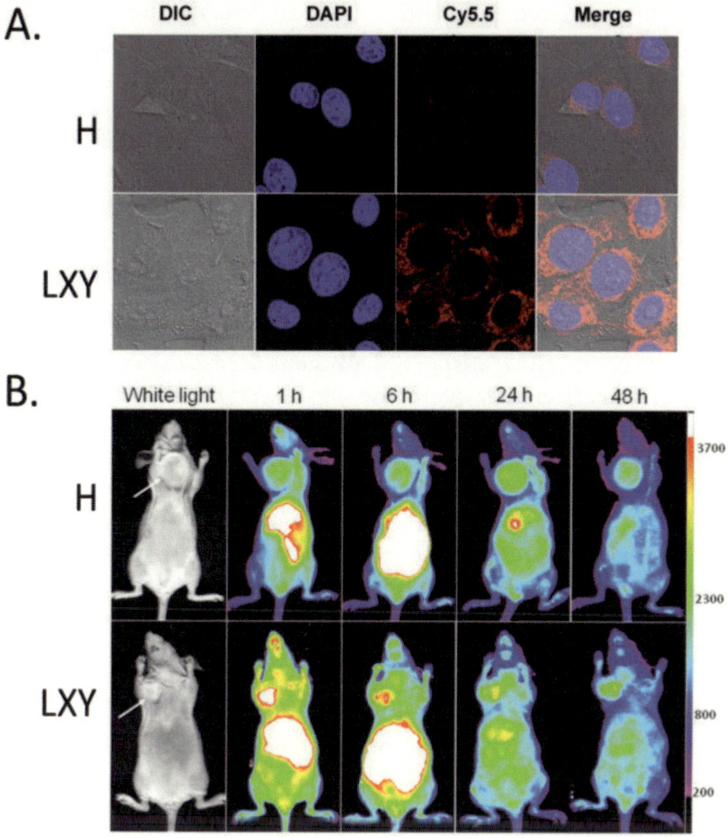

Figure 2.
Selective binding and internalization of LXY30-tagged HEVNP. Breast cancer cells (MDA-MB-231) were inoculated with Cy5.5-labeled HEVNP (row H) or Cy5.5-labeled HEVNP tagged with LXY30 (row LXY). At 1 h post inoculation, the cells were visualized for nuclear dsDNA (DAPI) or Cy5.5. Cy5.5 staining is significantly higher in the cytoplasm of cells inoculated with HEVNP tagged with LXY30 (A). Female SPF BALB/c mice were injected with MDA-MB-231 cells (5 x 10^5). Following the formation of tumors (white arrows), 0.1 nmoles of Cy5.5-labeled HEVNP (row H) or Cy5.5-labeled HEVNP tagged with LXY30 (row LXY) was injected into the tail vein. Optical imaging of live mice at 1, 6, 24, and 48 h post injection (p.i.) showed that LXY30-tagged HEVNP selectively binds to the tumor at 1 h p.i. Staining was also seen in the abdominal regions at 1 and 6 h p.i., likely due to the accumulation of HEVNPs in the liver or other organs prior to degradation (B). Modified from Chen et al., 2016.

selectively binds to cells in the breast cancer cell line MDA-MB-231 (**Figure 2A**). Furthermore, in vivo fluorescence microscopy demonstrates that HEVNP-573C-LYX30, unlike HEVNP-573C, is selectively delivered to breast cancer tumors (formed following the subcutaneous injection of MDA-MB-231 cells in female SPF BLAB/c mice) (**Figure 2B**). These findings demonstrate that HEVNP can be engineered for surface modulation by covalent attachment of a small molecule while maintaining the integrity of the capsid structure. HEVNP thus presents a unique platform for surface functionalization.

3.2 Gastrointestinal tract stability

The human GI tract is divided into the upper tract and lower tract with the upper tract consisting of the mouth, pharynx, esophagus, stomach, and first part of the small intestine (i.e., the duodenum) and the lower tract consisting of the remainder of the small intestine (i.e., jejunum and ileum) and large intestine [32]. Although the duodenum is the shortest portion of the small intestine, it is connected to and/

or associated with the liver, gallbladder, and pancreas through various ducts, veins, and arteries. Following ingestion of HEV, the virus capsid will be exposed to extreme conditions including highly acidic and then alkaline pH, a wide range of digestive enzymes, bile, bacteria and other microorganisms, thick mucosal layers, and mucosal flow throughout the 5-plus-meter length of the human digestive tract. At the cellular level, the inner surface of the intestines is lined with a layer of several types of simple columnar cells including villi and goblet cells that face the lumen. The villi and goblet cells are primarily involved in the absorption of digested nutrients and secretion of a thick (ca. 200 μm) layer of mucosa composed primarily of mucin, respectively. Microfold cells (M cells) are also found in the intestines which play important roles in the initiation of mucosal immunity and the transport of antigens across the epithelial cell layer. HEV has evolved to efficiently overcome these barriers (chemical, enzymatic, mechanical, physical, immunological, etc.) and to eventually initiate a productive infection of cells of the liver and other tissues. Although HEVNP is unable to replicate, it retains the inherent ability of HEV to efficiently target and deliver therapeutic agents through the GI tract with little or no toxicity [1, 2]. This ability of HEVNP to deliver, through oral dosing, a therapeutic payload in a targeted manner using a modular format is currently unavailable through other nanocarrier platforms. Additionally, HEVNP is highly stable to long-term storage at room temperature. Thus, the need for a temperature-controlled supply chain for storage and distribution of HEVNP is minimized or eliminated. This makes the storage and distribution of HEVNP significantly less difficult especially in less developed regions. In addition to being stable at room temperature, HEVNP is water soluble and can be formulated as a liquid (as well as a cream, powder, or solid) which allows HEVNP to be administered noninvasively as a drink or droplet.

3.3 Significant payload capacity

HEVNP functions as an epitope nanocarrier through display of the epitope on its surface. HEVNP also has a large hollow core with a width that ranges from approximately 10 to 12 nm (**Figure 3A**) that can be loaded with a payload such as a nucleic acid chain, peptide, or small molecule. This large hollow core results from the space within HEVNP that in HEV encapsulates genomic RNA. A payload can be encapsulated within the hollow core of HEVNP using a simple process that reversibly disassembles HEVNP and then reassembles it in the presence of the payload molecules. This reversible process occurs through chemical reduction, chelation of Ca^{2+}, and the subsequent return of Ca^{2+} (**Figure 3B**). Specifically, HEVNP disassembles in the presence of DTT and EGTA and reassembles by the slow addition of Ca^{2+}. If peptide molecules such as insulin or inorganic molecules such as ferrite are present during the reassembly process, these molecules are encapsulated within the reassembled HEVNP. Similarly, in the presence of DNA or RNA, the reassembled HEVNP will incorporate the nucleic acid molecule, and HEVNP can function as an orally deliverable DNA vaccine nanocarrier (reviewed in [2]). For example, plasmid DNA-encoding HIV envelope gp120 has been encapsulated by HEV VLP, and this construct has been used to orally deliver the plasmid to the spleen, Peyer's patches, and mesenteric lymph nodes of mice [33]. Cell-mediated immune (specific cytotoxic T-lymphocyte (CTL) response) and specific humoral responses are generated locally and systemically. A payload is not essential for HEVNP capsid formation or capsid stability, but having this capacity offers a way to further increase the epitope signal beyond the 60 epitope copies that can be placed through chemical conjugation or genetic insertion on the HEVNP surface via the P domains.

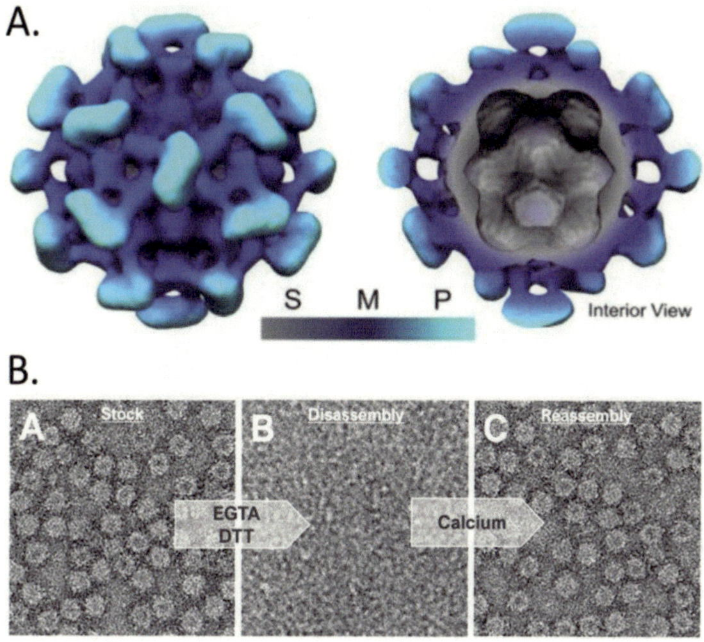

Figure 3.
Structure and disassembly/reassembly of HEVNP. The HEVNP monomer is composed of three domains: Shell (S), middle (M), and protrusion (P). The surface and interior localization of these domains is indicated by the color map (A). A large hollow core is found in the interior of HEVNP (right image in A). The hollow core can encapsulate various payloads such as nucleic acids, peptides, small proteins, or small molecules. Electron microscopic images of the process of HEVNP disassembly (following the addition of EGTA and DTT) and reassembly following the addition of calcium (B).

3.4 Platform sustainability by prevention of self-immunity

While HEVNP exhibits natural tolerance against the harsh enzymatic environment associated with the digestive tract, its repeated use as a drug delivery vehicle will quickly result in self-immunity if a mechanism is not in place to avoid this common problem. As discussed above, insertion of the HIV-1 P18 peptide onto the surface P domain maintains the icosahedral arrangement of P18-HEVNP and indicates that intermolecular forces between the truncated CP of the recombinant nucleocapsid are not disrupted by the insertion of P18. Additionally, since the antigenicity of HEVNP lies specifically within the P domain, the insertion of the P18 peptide significantly lowers immune detection of the HEVNP vehicle [21] (**Figure 4A**). The immune reactivity of P18-HEVNP has been tested by two antibodies, 447-52D and HEP224. Antibody 447-52D specifically targets the V3 loop of HIV-1 gp120, and monoclonal antibody HEP224 targets the conformational epitope (i.e., the three loops around Y485) of the P domain of HEV CP. Based on ELISA experiments, antibody 447-52D shows preferential binding of P18-HEVNP. On the other hand, the binding of antibody HEP224 to the conformational epitope of the P domain of HEV CP is disrupted by the insertion of HIV P18 without altering the structural characteristic of HEVNP. Thus, insertion of specific peptides into the exposed P domain serves as a practical strategy to escape antibody recognition by the immune system (i.e., issues with self-immunity) while triggering the desired humoral and cellular responses against the attached/inserted antigen. Similarly, an HEV-specific monoclonal antibody, Fab230, fails to recognize HEVNP after maleimide-biotin conjugation at position N573C of HEVNP [30] (**Figure 4B**). Additionally, the geometrical constraints provided by the M domain provide a

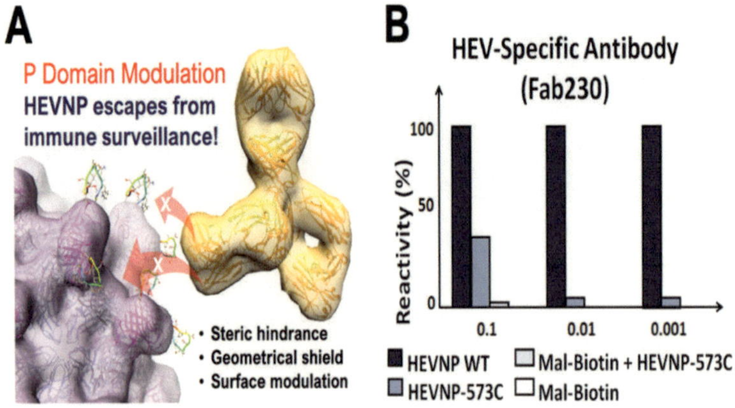

Figure 4.
3-D modeling of HEVNP surface modulation. Surface modulation through chemical conjugation or genetic modification promotes the escape of HEVNP from immune surveillance (A). Surface modulation of HEVNP with maleimide-biotin or mutation of the P domain at residue N573 dramatically reduces cross reactivity with the HEV-specific monoclonal antibody fab230 by ELISA (B).

physical barrier for antibody binding which helps HEVNP avoid immune system surveillance by HEV-specific antibodies. These findings show the sustainability of the HEVNP nanocarrier platform.

3.5 Safety of HEVNP

HEV annually causes acute and self-limiting infection in about 20 million people worldwide [34–36]. The majority of people infected with HEV show clinical symptoms that are relatively mild, and death rates from hepatitis E are low. The disease, however, is more severe in pregnant women, and chronic infection may occur in immunocompromised individuals. Although the exact mechanism of the increased severity of the disease during pregnancy is unknown, there is some evidence that increased viral replication in placental tissues plays a role [34, 35]. Thus, in a large proportion of the population, HEV is naturally a low-virulence pathogen. The low virulence of HEV and the inability of HEVNP to replicate (because it does not carry HEV genomic RNA) suggest that an HEVNP-based nanocarrier will not induce undue virulence in patients.

3.6 Established production and engineering technology

A common eukaryotic cell-based technology for vaccine production utilizes recombinant baculoviruses and insect cells. Baculoviruses are arthropod-specific viruses that are commonly used to produce recombinant proteins for basic research and commercial applications. Baculoviruses have been successfully used to produce human therapeutics and diagnostics since the late 1990s [12]. A recent example of a baculovirus-based vaccine is Flublok (released in 2013 by Protein Sciences Corporation), a vaccine against human influenza virus. The baculovirus expression vector system is also used to express the major capsid protein L1 of human papilloma virus. The recombinant L1 capsid protein forms a VLP-based vaccine (Cervarix™) that protects against cervical cancer [12, 37]. The commercial GMP technology that is currently used to express and purify these vaccines and others can be easily adapted for the production of recombinant truncated CP and the engineering of HEVNP-based vaccine delivery nanocarriers.

4. Single epitope modification of HEVNP: HIV-1 GP120 P18 example

As discussed earlier, insertion of the P18 peptide from the GP120 protein of HIV-1 results in a stable HEVNP that displays P18 on its surface (in the P domain after residue Y485). Additionally, the P18 insertion significantly lowers the immune system response against HEVNP. When the P18-HEVNP construct is orally inoculated into mice, it induces strong and specific cell-mediated and humoral responses in comparison to immunization with HEVNP [21]. After three rounds of oral immunization, the cell-mediated response includes the lysis of cytotoxic T lymphocytes (CTLs) in three immune system-associated organs. Similarly, humoral responses (IgG, IgA, and IgM induction) in the sera and intestinal fluids are detected by ELISA. These responses were generated by P18-HEVNP without the need for an external adjuvant coadministration.

5. Multiple epitope modifications of HEVNP: MOMP example

Over 120 million people are annually infected with *Chlamydia trachomatis*. Because the initial stages of chlamydia are generally asymptomatic, many individuals are unaware that they are infected and do not seek antibiotic treatment. As the infection spreads, chronic abdominal pain, pelvic inflammatory disease, ectopic pregnancy, and infertility can result. The major outer membrane protein (MOMP) of *Chlamydia*, in its native trimeric form (nMOMP), has been demonstrated to impart significant protection against chlamydial infection and disease in a mouse model. MOMP is a structurally rigid, 40 kDa trimer-forming protein that makes up about 60% of the total mass of the outer membrane of *Chlamydia* [38, 39]. MOMP itself is characterized by five constant domains (CDs) and four variable domains (VDs) which help to define the immunogenicity of various serovars of *Chlamydia* [40, 41].

MOMP is the immunodominant antigen of *Chlamydia* and has multiple epitopes for T-cell and B-cell activation; thus, it induces both cell-mediated and humoral immunity [42–46]. Mice that are vaccinated with the nMOMP with Freund's adjuvant are significantly protected from the effects of *Chlamydia* in terms of a shedding assay and infertility [47]. In contrast, denatured MOMP does not offer this protection. The denatured MOMP, however, induces a greater humoral response than nMOMP. Robust protective activity following vaccination with nMOMP and other adjuvants has also been reported [45, 48]; this activity was similar to that of mice that were immunized intranasally with live *Chlamydia* elementary bodies (EBs). These and other studies [47, 49–52] using various readouts (i.e., body weight, lung weight, number of inclusions forming units recovered, length of shedding, etc.) demonstrate the important role of MOMP in inducing protection against *Chlamydia*.

Formulating a vaccine with a properly folded membrane protein such as MOMP remains a genetic engineering challenge. The use of membrane proteins for vaccine applications requires a platform that can be engineered to enable proper folding of the membrane protein, potentially allow for adjuvant incorporation, and be amenable to the display of multiple epitopes employing multiple display strategies. In the past 10 years, incorporating membrane proteins into nanolipoprotein particles for both solubility and stabilization has become increasingly common with varied success.

In our laboratory, HEVNP has been used as a platform to display two MOMP VD epitope sequences (VD1 and VD4). With this construct, HEVNP-VD1/HEVNP-VD4, the VD1 and VD4 peptide sequences were genetically incorporated at S533 and T485, respectively, of the truncated capsid protein, a region corresponding

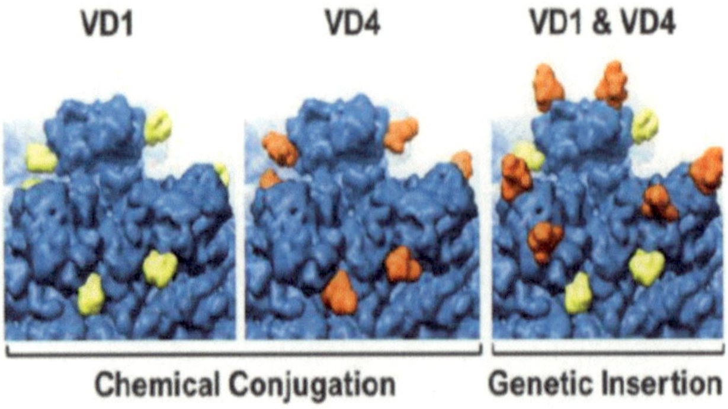

Figure 5.
Chlamydial vaccine design. Peptide sequences from variable domain 1 (VD1, yellow epitopes) and/or VD4 (orange epitopes) from the major outer membrane protein of Chlamydia *were chemically conjugated to amino acid residue N573C (left and center panels) or genetically inserted (after amino acid residues S533 and T485, respectively, right panel) to the P domain of HEVNP.*

to surface-exposed loops L2 and L1, respectively. Analysis of the visibility of these epitopes by structural modeling (**Figure 5**) and by ELISA using VD1- or VD4-specific antibodies (data not shown) indicates that all three of these constructs are highly immunogenic, suggesting that the epitopes are authentically displayed on the surface of HEVNP. Furthermore, in preliminary animal experiments, anti-MOMP IgG levels in the serum of mice that are immunized by HEVNP-VD1/HEVNP-VD4 (prime and two boosts) are like those found following immunization with a whole *Chlamydia* cell vaccine. These findings are highly exciting; and we are currently investigating whether there is also a cell-mediated immune response induced by HEVNP-VD1/HEVNP-VD4 and, if there is, how this response compares with that induced by a whole cell vaccine.

6. Conclusions

As a nanocarrier, HEVNP is a structure that can display multiple epitopes on its surface; and simultaneously it can deliver a payload, for example, an epitope encoding nucleotide sequence, peptide, or small molecule. Unlike nanoparticles generated from polymers, lipids, nanotubes, or other carriers, HEVNP delivers epitopes and payload through the mucosa of the GI tract without the need for any, potentially deleterious, exogenous enhancers such as a mucosal breakdown enzyme, pH regulator, or uptake cofactor. The key characteristics that make HEVNP an ideal and unique vehicle for vaccine delivery include: (i) *Surface plasticity*. Sites on the P domain can be engineered for site-specific attachment or insertion of the epitope(s). Even when the surface of HEVNP is genetically or chemically modified, the core structure of HEVNP remains intact. (ii) *GI tract stability*. Even when surface modified, HEVNP is stable to the harsh conditions of low pH and proteolytic enzymes that are found in the GI tract. This allows HEVNP to deliver epitopes orally. HEVNP has the capability to penetrate the mucosal lining of the entire GI tract and other mucosa-lined cavities or organs and directly target cells of the basement membrane. (iii) *Significant payload capacity*. The large hollow core of HEVNP can package and protect large biological molecules including DNA and RNA. (iv) *Platform sustainability*. Immune recognition of the carrier platform is negated with HEVNP. The surface P domain carries the primary antigenic sites of HEV (and HEVNP). Thus, modification of the P domain by chemical conjugation or genetic insertion of a vaccine epitope completely neutralizes endogenous immunogenicity

DOI: http://dx.doi.org/10.5772/intechopen.86830

against HEVNP carrier platform. In addition, the HEVNP nanocarrier platform can overcome many of the drawbacks of other nanocarrier platforms including issues with (1) formulation, (2) production, (3) safety, (4) cold chain distribution, (5) target selectivity, and (6) signal amplification.

Acknowledgements

This work was partially supported by grant from the National Institutes of Health (AI095382, EB21230, and CA198880) and National Institute of Food and Agriculture. RHC is a Finland distinguished professor.

Conflict of interest

None.

Author details

Shizuo G. Kamita[1], Mo A. Baikoghli[1], Luis M. de la Maza[2] and R. Holland Cheng[1]*

1 Department of Molecular and Cellular Biology, University of California, Davis, California, USA

2 Department of Pathology and Laboratory Medicine, University of California, Irvine, California, USA

*Address all correspondence to: rhch@ucdavis.edu

References

[1] Baikoghli MA, Chen C-C, Cheng RH. Hepatitis E nanoparticle: A capsid-based platform for non-invasive vaccine delivery and imaging-guided cancer treatment. Advanced Research in Gastroenterology Hepatology. 2018;**9**: 1-5. DOI: 10.19080/argh.2018.09.555752

[2] Holla P, Baikoghli MA, Soonsawad P, Cheng RH. Toward mucosal DNA delivery: Structural modularity in vaccine platform design. In: Skwarczynski M, Toth I, editors. Micro- and Nanotechnology in Vaccine Development. Amsterdam: Elsevier Inc; 2016. pp. 303-326. DOI: 10.1016/B978-0-323-39981-4.00016-6

[3] Agrahari V, Vivek Agrahari AKM. Nanocarrier fabrication and macromolecule drug delivery: Challenges and opportunities. Therapeutic Delivery. 2016;7:257-278

[4] Marasini N, Skwarczynski M, Toth I. Oral delivery of nanoparticle-based vaccines. Expert Review of Vaccines. 2014;**13**:1361-1376. DOI: 10.1586/14760584.2014.936852

[5] Jitendra, Sharma PK, Bansal S, Banik A. Noninvasive routes of proteins and peptides drug delivery. Indian Journal of Pharmaceutical Sciences. 2011;**73**:367-375. DOI: 10.4103/0250-474X.95608

[6] Allen TM, Cullis PR. Drug delivery systems: Entering the mainstream. Science. 2004;**303**:1818-1822. DOI: 10.1126/science.1095833

[7] Danhier F. To exploit the tumor microenvironment: Since the EPR effect fails in the clinic, what is the future of nanomedicine? Journal of Controlled Release. 2016;**244**:Part A:108-121. DOI: 10.1016/j.jconrel.2016.11.015

[8] Danhier F, Ansorena E, Silva JM, Coco R, Le Breton A, Préat V. PLGA-based nanoparticles: An overview of biomedical applications. Journal of Controlled Release. 2012;**161**:505-522. DOI: 10.1016/j.jconrel.2012.01.043

[9] Cho K, Wang X, Nie S, Chen Z, Shin DM. Therapeutic nanoparticles for drug delivery in cancer. Clinical Cancer Research. 2008;**14**:1310-1316. DOI: 10.1158/1078-0432.CCR-07-1441

[10] Deng F. Advances and challenges in enveloped virus-like particle (VLP)-based vaccines. Journal of Immunology Science. 2018;**2**:36-41. DOI: 10.29245/2578-3009/2018/2.1118

[11] Hill BD, Zak A, Khera E, Wen F. Engineering virus-like particles for antigen and drug delivery. Current Protein & Peptide Science. 2017;**19**:112-127. DOI: 10.2174/1389203718666161122113041

[12] Van Oers MM, Pijlman GP, Vlak JM. Thirty years of baculovirus-insect cell protein expression: From dark horse to mainstream technology. The Journal of General Virology. 2015;**96**:6-23. DOI: 10.1099/vir.0.067108-0

[13] Herbst-Kralovetz M, Mason HS, Chen Q. Norwalk virus-like particles as vaccines. Expert Review of Vaccines. 2010;**9**:299-307. DOI: 10.1586/erv.09.163

[14] Neek M, Il KT, Wang SW. Protein-based nanoparticles in cancer vaccine development. Nanomedicine: Nanotechnology, Biology and Medicine. 2019;**15**:164-174. DOI: 10.1016/j.nano.2018.09.004

[15] Li TC, Yamakawa Y, Suzuki K, Tatsumi M, Razak MA, Uchida T, et al. Expression and self-assembly of empty virus-like particles of hepatitis E virus. Journal of Virology. 1997;**71**:7207-7213

[16] Xing L, Kato K, Li T, Takeda N, Miyamura T, Hammar L, et al. Recombinant hepatitis E capsid protein

self-assembles into a dual-domain T = 1 particle presenting native virus epitopes. Virology. 1999;**265**:35-45. DOI: 10.1006/viro.1999.0005

[17] Wang CY, Miyazaki N, Yamashita T, Higashiura A, Nakagawa A, Li TC, et al. Crystallization and preliminary X-ray diffraction analysis of recombinant hepatitis e virus-like particle. Acta Crystallographica. Section F, Structural Biology and Crystallization Communications. 2008;**64**:318-322. DOI: 10.1107/S1744309108007197

[18] Li S, Tang X, Seetharaman J, Yang C, Gu Y, Zhang J, et al. Dimerization of hepatitis E virus capsid protein E2s domain is essential for virus-host interaction. PLoS Pathogens. 2009;**5**:e1000537. DOI: 10.1371/journal.ppat.1000537

[19] Xing L, Li TC, Mayazaki N, Simon MN, Wall JS, Moore M, et al. Structure of hepatitis E virion-sized particle reveals an RNA-dependent viral assembly pathway. The Journal of Biological Chemistry. 2010;**285**:33175-33183. DOI: 10.1074/jbc.M110.106336

[20] Mori Y, Matsuura Y. Structure of hepatitis E viral particle. Virus Research. 2011;**161**:59-64. DOI: 10.1016/j.viruses.2011.03.015

[21] Jariyapong P, Xing L, van Houten NE, Li TC, Weerachatyanukul W, Hsieh B, et al. Chimeric hepatitis E virus-like particle as a carrier for oral-delivery. Vaccine. 2013;**31**:417-424. DOI: 10.1016/j.vaccine.2012.10.073

[22] Yamashita T, Mori Y, Miyazaki N, Cheng RH, Yoshimura M, Unno H, et al. Biological and immunological characteristics of hepatitis E virus-like particles based on the crystal structure. Proceedings of the National Academy of Sciences. 2009;**106**:12986-12991. DOI: 10.1073/pnas.0903699106

[23] Cao D, Meng XJ. Molecular biology and replication of hepatitis E virus. Emerging Microbes & Infections. 2012;**1**:e17. DOI: 10.1038/emi.2012.7

[24] Purdy MA, Harrison TJ, Jameel S, Meng XJ, Okamoto H, Van Der Poel WHM, et al. ICTV virus taxonomy profile: Hepeviridae. The Journal of General Virology. 2017;**98**:2645-2646. DOI: 10.1099/jgv.0.000940

[25] Guu TSY, Liu Z, Ye Q, Mata DA, Li K, Yin C, et al. Structure of the hepatitis E virus-like particle suggests mechanisms for virus assembly and receptor binding. Proceedings of the National Academy of Sciences. 2009;**106**:15148-15153. DOI: 10.1073/pnas.0904848106

[26] Xiaofang L, Zafrullah M, Ahmad F, Jameel S. A C-terminal hydrophobic region is required for homo-oligomerization of the hepatitis E virus capsid (ORF2) protein. Journal of Biomedicine & Biotechnology. 2001;**1**:122-128. DOI: 10.1155/S1110724301000262

[27] Schofield DJ, Purcell RH, Nguyen HT, Emerson SU. Monoclonal antibodies that neutralize HEV recognize an antigenic site at the carboxyterminus of an ORF2 protein vaccine. Vaccine. 2003;**22**:257-267. DOI: 10.1016/j.vaccine.2003.07.008

[28] Zhang J, Gu Y, Ge SX, Li SW, He ZQ, Huang GY, et al. Analysis of hepatitis E virus neutralization sites using monoclonal antibodies directed against a virus capsid protein. Vaccine. 2005;**22**:2881-2892. DOI: 10.1016/j.vaccine.2004.11.065

[29] Yu H, Li S, Yang C, Wei M, Song C, Zheng Z, et al. Homology model and potential virus-capsid binding site of a putative HEV receptor Grp78. Journal of Molecular Modeling. 2011;**17**:987-995. DOI: 10.1007/s00894-010-0794-5

[30] Chen CC, Xing L, Stark M, Ou T, Holla P, Xiao K, et al. Chemically activatable viral capsid functionalized for cancer targeting. Nanomedicine. 2016;**11**:377-390. DOI: 10.2217/nnm.15.207

[31] Xiao W, Li T, Bononi FC, Lac D, Kekessie IA, Liu Y, et al. Discovery and characterization of a high-affinity and high-specificity peptide ligand LXY30 for in vivo targeting of α3 integrin-expressing human tumors. EJNMMI Research. 2016;**6**:1-12. DOI: 10.1186/s13550-016-0165-z

[32] Reed KK, Wickham R. Review of the gastrointestinal tract: From macro to micro. Seminars in Oncology Nursing. 2009;**25**:3-14. DOI: 10.1016/j.soncn.2008.10.002

[33] Takamura S, Niikura M, Li TC, Takeda N, Kusagawa S, Takebe Y, et al. DNA vaccine-encapsulated virus-like particles derived from an orally transmissible virus stimulate mucosal and systemic immune responses by oral administration. Gene Therapy. 2004;**11**:628-635. DOI: 10.1038/sj.gt.3302193

[34] Kamar N, Dalton HR, Abravanel F, Izopet J. Hepatitis E virus infection. Clinical Microbiology Reviews. 2014;**27**:116-138. DOI: 10.1128/CMR.00057-13

[35] Wedemeyer H, Pischke S, Manns MP. Pathogenesis and treatment of hepatitis E virus infection. Gastroenterology. 2012;**142**:1388-1397. DOI: 10.1053/j.gastro.2012.02.014

[36] Takahashi H, Zeniya M, Hepatitis E. In: Gershwin ME, Vierling JM, Manns MP, editors. Liver Immunology: Principles and Practice. New York: Springer; 2014. pp. 243-252. DOI: 10.1007/978-3-319-02096-9_17

[37] Harper DM. Impact of vaccination with Cervarix™ on subsequent HPV-16/18 infection and cervical disease in women 15-25 years of age. Gynecologic Oncology. 2008;**110**:10-17. DOI: 10.1016/j.ygyno.2008.06.029

[38] Caldwell HD, Kromhout J, Schachter J. Purification and partial characterization of the major outer membrane protein of *Chlamydia trachomatis*. Infection and Immunity. 1981;**31**:1161-1176

[39] Hatch TP, Vance DW, Al-Hossainy E. Identification of a major envelope protein in *Chlamydia* spp. Journal of Bacteriology. 1981;**146**:426-429

[40] Stephens RS, Kalman S, Lammel C, Fan J, Marathe R, Aravind L, et al. Genome sequence of an obligate intracellular pathogen of humans: *Chlamydia trachomatis*. Science. 1998;**282**:754-759. DOI: 10.1126/science.282.5389.754

[41] Stephens RS, Sanchez-Pescador R, Wagar EA, Inouye C, Urdea MS. Diversity of *Chlamydia trachomatis* major outer membrane protein genes. Journal of Bacteriology. 1987;**169**:3879-3885. DOI: 10.1128/jb.169.9.3879-3885.1987

[42] Caldwell HD, Perry LJ. Neutralization of *Chlamydia trachomatis* infectivity with antibodies to the major outer membrane protein. Infection and Immunity. 1982;**38**:745-754

[43] Baehr W, Zhang YX, Joseph T, Su H, Nano FE, Everett KD, et al. Mapping antigenic domains expressed by *Chlamydia trachomatis* major outer membrane protein genes. Proceedings of the National Academy of Sciences of the United States of America. 1988;**85**:4000-4004. DOI: 10.1073/pnas.85.11.4000

[44] Ortiz L, Demick KP, Petersen JW, Polka M, Rudersdorf RA, Van der Pol B, et al. *Chlamydia trachomatis* major outer membrane protein (MOMP) epitopes

that activate HLA class II-restricted T cells from infected humans. Journal of Immunology. 1996;**157**:4554-4567

[45] Pal S, Peterson EM, De La Maza LM. Vaccination with the *Chlamydia trachomatis* major outer membrane protein can elicit an immune response as protective as that resulting from inoculation with live bacteria. Infection and Immunity. 2005;**73**:8153-8160. DOI: 10.1128/IAI.73.12.8153-8160.2005

[46] Stephens RS. High-resolution mapping of serovar-specific and common antigenic determinants of the major outer membrane protein of *Chlamydia trachomatis*. The Journal of Experimental Medicine. 2004;**167**: 817-831. DOI: 10.1084/jem.167.3.817

[47] Pal S, Theodor I, Peterson EM, De la Maza LM. Immunization with the *Chlamydia trachomatis* mouse pneumonitis major outer membrane protein can elicit a protective immune response against a genital challenge. Infection and Immunity. 2001;**69**:6240-6247. DOI: 10.1128/IAI.69.10.6240-6247.2001

[48] Pal S, Tatarenkova OV, de la Maza LM. A vaccine formulated with the major outer membrane protein can protect C3H/HeN, a highly susceptible strain of mice, from a *Chlamydia muridarum* genital challenge. Immunology. 2015;**146**:432-443. DOI: 10.1111/imm.12520

[49] Farris CM, Morrison SG, Morrison RP. CD4+ T cells and antibody are required for optimal major outer membrane protein vaccine-induced immunity to *Chlamydia muridarum* genital infection. Infection and Immunity. 2010;**78**:4374-4383. DOI: 10.1128/IAI.00622-10

[50] Sun G, Pal S, Weiland J, Peterson EM, de la Maza LM. Protection against an intranasal challenge by vaccines formulated with native and recombinant preparations of the *Chlamydia trachomatis* major outer membrane protein. Vaccine. 2009;**27**:5020-5025. DOI: 10.1016/j.vaccine.2009.05.008

[51] Tifrea DF, Sun G, Pal S, Zardeneta G, Cocco MJ, Popot JL, et al. Amphipols stabilize the *Chlamydia* major outer membrane protein and enhance its protective ability as a vaccine. Vaccine. 2011;**29**:4623-4631. DOI: 10.1016/j.vaccine.2011.04.065

[52] Carmichael JR, Pal S, Tifrea D, De la Maza LM. Induction of protection against vaginal shedding and infertility by a recombinant *Chlamydia* vaccine. Vaccine. 2011;**29**:5276-5283. DOI: 10.1016/j.vaccine.2011.05.013

Chapter 8

PCR and Infectious Diseases

Danielle Alves Gomes Zauli

Abstract

Since the 1950s, the medical community has been faced with infectious diseases, which have brought significant public health and financial challenges. Currently, routine testing for the laboratory diagnosis for infectious agents is based on cell culture, serological, and molecular methods. However, cell culture-based methods are used mainly in research laboratories and are less sensitive methods when compared with serological and molecular methods. The diagnosis of infectious diseases has been revolutionized by the development of molecular techniques, mainly with the applications of polymerase chain reaction (PCR). The high sensitivity, specificity, and ease with which the PCR can be used to detect genetic sequences known have led to your wide application in science. A great number of qualitative and quantitative molecular assays are mostly based on what have been described such as real-time PCR, multiplex PCR, LAMP-PCR, and digital PCR. These assays could identify active infection by detecting infectious agents and nucleic acid in various clinical conditions including arboviruses, sexually transmitted infections, and bacterial infections. Further advancement of molecular technology is needed to improve the capacity to detect infectious agents in order to control the spread of infectious diseases and lead to appropriate actions which help to benefit patients and health-care workers themselves.

Keywords: infectious disease, PCR, molecular techniques, diagnosis

1. Introduction

Infectious diseases (ID) are caused by pathogenic microorganisms, such as bacteria, viruses, parasites, or fungi, and the diseases can be spread, directly or indirectly, from one person to another. Scientific advances in the biomedical area since the first half of last century, represented by the development of therapeutic drugs, vaccines, and advanced sanitation technologies, were carried as result of the control or prevention of infectious diseases. These diseases are considered, at the global level, as some of the most common public health problems. The relevance of these pathologies is evidenced by the number of individuals reached, the lack of knowledge about the infectious agents, their socioeconomic impact, the deepening of the molecular studies involving a precise and fast diagnosis, and appeals public health agency studies aimed at the development of diagnostic techniques for the early detection of symptomatic carriers as well as the asymptomatic carriers of these infections.

Changes in society, technology, and the microorganisms themselves are contributing to the emergence of new diseases, the reemergence of diseases once controlled, and to the development of antimicrobial resistance. According to the World Health Organization (WHO), the IDs constitute a significant proportion of all human diseases known, and at least 25% of about 60 million deaths that occur worldwide each year are estimated to be due to infectious diseases [1, 2].

Scientific studies of infectious agents and diseases provide a knowledge for the development of diagnostic tests for such diseases, drugs to treat, and vaccines for prevention. Earlier, specific and effective diagnosis is one of the most appropriate forms and strategies for managing. According to [3], in American hospitals, about 5 million cases of infectious disease are reported annually. Besides that, most of the cases are unreported, resulting in substantial morbidity and mortality [3]. In the last 20 years, analysis methods based on the detection and sequencing of 16S rDNA have been widely used in place of conventional culture methods.

Unfortunately, despite in clinical laboratories, the diagnosis of infectious diseases is directly associated with time of pathogen identification by conventional culture methods as these tests suffer from long turnaround times, from hours to days. A technical difficulty encountered in these methods performed before the advent of the molecular techniques was that not all pathogens are cultivable, and culture conditions ordinarily are not known. Other limitations of the traditional diagnostic include requirements for additional testing and wait times for characterizing detected pathogens (i.e., discernment of species, virulence factors, and antimicrobial resistance) [3, 4].

Nucleic acid amplification is one of the most valuable tools in virtually all life science fields, including application-oriented fields such as clinical medicine, for diagnosis of infectious diseases.

The serological methods are limited by the cross-reactions between the types of agents and by the fact that some infectious agents have no clearly identified epitopes that are sufficiently specific, requiring them as a stringent clinic diagnostic. In addition, the specific IgM antibodies are detected only in acute phase of infection, and for detecting infections, the serological tests are inaccurate, labor-intensive, and unreliable. In the last 20 years, analysis methods based on the nucleic acid amplification have been widely used in all life science fields as a new way for the diagnosis of human pathogens like virus, bacteria, and parasites.

The use of amplification techniques such as Polymerase Chain Reaction (PCR) has long been used to detection, genotyping, and quantification of virus and bacteria in various clinical specimens, such as serum, plasma, urine, semen, and liquid cerebrospinal fluid (CSF).

PCR-based diagnostics have been effectively developed for a wide range of microorganisms. Due to its incredible sensitivity, specificity, reproducibility, broad dynamic range, and speed of amplification, PCR has been championed by infectious disease experts for identifying organisms that cannot be grown in vitro, or in instances where existing culture techniques are insensitive and/or need prolonged incubation times [5].

Advances in development of molecular technology and diagnostics have enhanced understanding IDs' etiology, pathogenesis, and molecular epidemiology, which provide basis for appropriate detection, quantification, prevention, and control measures as well as rational design of vaccine, by which some diseases have been successfully eliminated.

Since 1985, many PCR amplification-based techniques have been designed for detection and identification, including: multiplex PCR (M-PCR), LAMP-PCR, digital PCR (dPCR), and real-time PCR.

2. PCR techniques and clinical applications in diagnostic of infectious disease

2.1 Multiplex PCR

In diagnostic laboratories, the use of PCR is often limited by its cost and sometimes by the availability of adequate sample volume. To overcome these issues and also to increase the diagnostic capacity of PCR, there is a type termed multiplex PCR (mPCR). The mPCR refers to the use of different pairs of primers to simultaneously amplify multiple regions of the nucleic acid of the sample with visualization of the amplified products by gel electrophoresis. The use of multiple primer pairs in mPCRs is an innovation that offers significant benefits in cost, time, and exact diagnosis. The main advantage of this technology is to minimize the number of separate reactions, for example, to detect several pathogens at the same time in a single specimen such as sexually transmitted pathogens [6–8]. This technique makes it possible to diagnose several diseases with a single diagnostic test, with sensitivity, specificity, and speed, indispensable values in diagnostic tests.

This technique has become a mainstay of research and clinical diagnostic applications, such as sexually transmitted infections (STIs). Considering a major public health problem, the STIs are common everywhere from developed countries and developing countries. It is estimated that each year more than 340 million new cases of bacterial STI arise, including gonorrhea, chlamydia, and syphilis, and the incidence is increased worldwide in adults of 15–49 years of age [9]. The susceptibility to sexually transmitted infections, including the human immunodeficiency virus (HIV), and the high cost of treatment have led to the need for fast and reliable laboratory techniques for the identification of pathogens. Procedures for nucleic acid amplification to detect sexually transmitted pathogens have been developed, especially mPCR methods [10].

The multiplex PCR has the potential to analyze many samples in a single reaction, and it is useful for diagnostic of multipathogenic infection. However, it has some limitations such as the nonspecific products generated through primer-primer interactions that may interfere with the amplification of targets, decreasing sensitivity, and selectivity of reactions.

2.2 Loop-mediated isothermal amplification

Nucleic acid amplification is commonly used in the field of life science research. With the development of molecular biology, many new molecular diagnostic technologies have been developed subsequently [11].

The loop-mediated isothermal amplification (LAMP-PCR) was first developed over 15 years ago, and it has emerged as powerful method to concurrently detect multiple pathogens [12, 13]. The method employs a DNA polymerase with strand displacement activity and a set of four inner and outer primers that recognize a total of six distinct sequences of the target DNA. Moreover, the method involves two successive steps of amplification, with the first step comprising mPCR and the second step LAMP. Amplicons of the first step serve as templates in the second step. The amplification protocol requires only a single temperature for the reaction, and the amplification is diagnosed without the need for electrophoretic techniques, using in situ detection process with colorimetric dye or with a fluorescent dye. The final products are the accumulation of 10^9 copies of target DNA in less than an hour. The LAMP-PCR has been regarded as an innovative technology and emerged as an alternative to PCR-based methodologies in clinical laboratory with significant increase of detection limits, efficiency, selectivity, and specificity over single-stage.

With more and more scientists focusing their attention on the application of LAMP technology, the range of its use is not limited to the bacteria detection and identification any more [14]. The LAMP-PCR was developed and employed to detect species that cause chorioamnionitis and premature labor, *Ureaplasma parvum*, and *Ureaplasma urealyticum* [15].

It was also applied to the parasite and virus detection [16–18]. Recently, Kurosaki et al. in their study [19] in 2017 developed a LAMP-PCR assay for the detection of

Zika virus plasma, serum, and urine samples collected from 120 suspected cases of arbovirus infection in Brazil.

2.3 Real-time PCR

According to [20], clinical diagnostic approaches rely on quantitative PCR (qPCR) as a method to detect and quantify infectious agents. Fluorescence chemistry-based methods have revolutionized molecular diagnostics and become the gold standard for viral load quantification and detection of bacterial and viral pathogens. During qPCR, the nucleic acid is amplified until it produces a certain level of signal which is supplied through a DNA intercalating dye or sequence-specific fluorescent probe. The cycle threshold (Cq), defined as the number of amplification cycles required to reach that signal level, is used to calculate the number of target molecules originally present based on a standard curve [20]. In qPCR, the targets are detected in real time from the sealed PCR plate, and there is no post-PCR processing required; therefore, the risk of false-positive results due to amplicon carryover is substantially decreased compared to conventional [21].

During the past decade, advantages on PCR have become gold standard procedure in the diagnosis of infectious diseases, particularly the diagnosis of viral diseases, such as arboviruses. Arboviruses are causing an unprecedented health calamity in world, especially in Latin American countries, with rising statistics on a daily basis. The diagnosis of these diseases is difficult to establish only by clinical features. A substantial proportion of these infections are asymptomatic, but some patients may also present clinical symptoms similar to the arboviruses such as those caused by the Dengue, Zika, and Chikungunya virus. The qPCR technique is more sensitive and specific than serological tests. Besides that, in serum samples, it is only possible to perform the diagnosis in the acute phase of the disease that lasts up to 4–7 days after the onset of symptoms. In relation to the detection of Zika virus (ZIKV), for example, recent data from the literature indicate that in human urine, viral RNA was found longer compared to serum, up to 20 days after the onset of the first symptoms. In semen, studies show that the genetic material of ZIKV was found for weeks and even months after infection [22]. However, the determination of viral load presents some particular challenges when using qPCR methodology. This is because reliable absolute concentration results of qPCR are dependent on assay efficiency, instrument calibration metrics, and comparison with a known reference sample to convert the Cq measurements to a sample unknown.

2.4 Digital PCR

In contrast to qPCR, the digital PCR (dPCR) uses an alternative method that is not dependent upon the determination of the amplification cycle that the reporter dye signal exceeds a threshold. Instead, prior to amplification, the samples to be subjected to dPCR are divided into thousands of independent PCR reactions and are scored as either positive or negative for amplification of the viral sequence of interest. The positive wells are counted and converted to a target concentration in the original sample. This binary assignment of each reaction greatly minimizes the dependence of measurement on parameters such as the efficiency of the assay and the calibration of the instrument. Therefore, dPCR is the absolute quantification methodology with the greatest potential for quantification of low-load viral nucleic acids.

In the diagnostic routine, it is very common to obtain positive qPCR results obtained at the detection limit of this methodology, which may generate uncertainty of the result. dPCR is a complementary methodology that works beyond

	qPCR	dPCR
Results	Cq, ΔCq, or ΔΔCq	Copies/mL
Quantification	Relative quantification	Absolut quantification, without standard curve
Factors affecting the signal	Standard curve	Results are not affected by any parameter
	Instrument	
	Primers and probes	

Table 1.
Comparative analysis between RT-qPCR and dPCR.

the limit of detection of qPCR, since it is based on the Poisson distribution. Consequently, this methodology has a significant impact on research as well as on diagnostic applications [23–25].

Some benefits of digital PCR in virology can be cited [25]:

- Quantification of viral genomes in samples without the need to use a standard curve;
- Detection of viruses that have a very low viral load;
- Use of low concentration of samples;
- Reduction of the impact of inhibitors present on complex samples.

Table 1 shows a comparison between the two methodologies: qPCR and dPCR.

A great number of studies use dPCR to diagnose infectious disease-related viruses, including hepatitis B virus (HBV), cytomegalovirus, human influenza, and HIV [26–28]; bacterial infections (*Mycobacterium tuberculosis*, *Chlamydia trachomatis*, and *Staphylococcus aureus*) [29–31]; and parasitic infectious such as detection of *Plasmodium falciparum* and *Plasmodium vivax* [32].

3. Conclusions

The ability to concurrently detect multiple pathogens infecting a host is crucial for accurate diagnosis of infectious diseases, identification of coinfections, and assessment of disease state for an effective patient management. PCR technology has been widely used to detect and quantify pathogenic microorganisms that cause various infectious diseases including some arboviruses, STIs, and bacterial infection. This methodology is revolutionizing the area of molecular diagnostics because of its high sensitivity of detection and specificity for the determination of infectious agents. In addition, there is a reduction in run time and cost over traditional cultivation methods, for example, to determine the amount of a particular pathogen in a clinical specimen. The main advantages of PCR are its higher sensitivity and specificity compared with other diagnostic methods such as serological assays and culture methods, as well as its rapidity, utility, and versatility in clinical laboratory.

Although the conventional PCR is the most widely used molecular technique, other methodologies have been developed including real-time PCR, multiplex PCR, LAMP-PCR, and digital PCR. The biochemical mechanisms of these techniques are based on enzyme-mediated processes, target, signal or probe amplification, and isothermal conditions.

Considering the clinical importance of these diseases, the number of infected individuals worldwide and the serious health consequences for population is extremely relevant to the precise, rapid, and sensitive diagnosis of these diseases in laboratories. Regardless, there is still the need for advances in basic science research and development of molecular technologies, which provide basis for the precise diagnostic and molecular epidemiology of infectious diseases as well as control measures, prevention, and design of vaccines and monitoring of infections face-to-face the treatment applied in clinical practice.

Acknowledgements

This chapter was supported by grants from the Financiadora de Inovação e Pesquisa (FINEP).

Conflict of interest

The author declares that he has no conflict of interest.

Author details

Danielle Alves Gomes Zauli
Instituto Hermes Pardini, Belo Horizonte, Brazil

*Address all correspondence to: danielle.zauli@hermespardini.com.br

References

[1] Nii-Trebi NI. Emerging and neglected infectious diseases: Insights, advances, and challenges. BioMed Research International. 2017;**2017**:1-15. DOI: 10.1155/2017/5245021

[2] Cohen ML. Changing patterns of infectious disease. Nature. 2000;**406**:762-767

[3] Yang S, Rothman RE. PCR-based diagnostics for infectious diseases: Uses, limitations, and future applications in acute-care settings. The Lancet Infectious Diseases. 2004;**4**:337-348. DOI: 10.1016/S1473-3099(04)01044-8

[4] Vouga M, Greub G. Emerging bacterial pathogens: The past and beyond. Clinical Microbiology and Infection. 2016;**22**:12-21. DOI: 10.1016/j.cmi.2015.10.010

[5] Louie M, Louie L, Simor A. The role of DNA amplification technology in the diagnosis of infectious disease. CMAJ. 2000;**163**:301-309

[6] Elnifro EM, Ashshi AM, Cooper RJ, Klapper PE. Multiplex PCR: Optimization and application in diagnostic virology. Clinical Microbiology Reviews. 2000;**13**:559-570

[7] McIver CJ, Jacques CFH, Chow SSW, Munro SC, Scott GM, Roberts JA, et al. Development of multiplex PCRs for detection of common viral pathogens and agents of congenital infections. Journal of Clinical Microbiology. 2005;**43**:5102-5110. DOI: 10.1128/JCM.43.10.5102-5110.2005

[8] Ratcliff RM, Chang G, Kok T, Sloots TP. Molecular diagnosis of medical viruses. Current Issues in Molecular Biology. 2007;**9**:87-102

[9] Tucker JD, Bien CH, Peeling RW. Point-of-care testing for sexually transmitted infections: Recent advances and implications for disease control. Current Opinion in Infectious Diseases. 2013;**26**:73-79. DOI: 10.1097/QCO.0b013e32835c21b0

[10] Zauli DAG, Lima LM, Fradico JRB, Menezes CLP, Diniz CG, Silva VL, et al. In house real time PCR assays for detection of sexually transmitted pathogens: *Neisseria gonorrhoeae, Chlamydia trachomatis, Ureaplasma urealyticum, Mycoplasma hominis and Mycoplasma genitalium*. International Journal of Recent Advances in Multidisciplinary Research. 2017;**4**:2561-2565

[11] Yanmei L, Penghui F, Shishui Z, Li Z. Loop-mediated isothermal amplification (LAMP): A novel rapid detection platform for pathogens. Microbial Pathogenesis. 2017;**107**:54-61. DOI: 10.1016/j.micpath.2017.03.016

[12] Iwamoto T, Sonobe T, Hayashi K. Loop-mediated isothermal amplification for direct detection of complex, and in sputum samples. Journal of Clinical Microbiology. 2003;**41**:2616-2622

[13] Notomi T, Okayama H, Masubuchi H, Yonekawa T, Watanabe K, Amino N, et al. Loop mediated isothermal amplification of DNA. Nucleic Acids Research. 2000;**28**:e63

[14] Maruyama F, Kenzaka T, Yamaguchi N. Detection of bacteria carrying the stx2 gene by in situ loop-mediated isothermal amplification. Applied and Environmental Microbiology. 2003;**69**:5023-5028. DOI: 10.1128/AEM.69.8.5023-5028.2003

[15] Fuwa K, Seki M, Hirata Y, Yanagihara I, Nakura Y, Takano C, et al. Rapid and simple detection of Ureaplasma species from vaginal swab samples using a loop- mediated isothermal amplification method.

American Journal of Reproductive Immunology. 2017;**79**:1-8. DOI: 10.1111/aji.12771

[16] Kaneko H, Iida T, Aoki K. Sensitive and rapid detection of herpes simplex virus and varicella-zoster virus DNA by loop-mediated isothermal amplification. Journal of Clinical Microbiology. 2005;**43**:3290-3296. DOI: 10.1128/JCM.43.7.3290-3296.2005

[17] Enomoto Y, Yoshikawa T, Ihira M. Rapid diagnosis of herpes simplex virus infection by a loop-mediated isothermal amplification method. Journal of Clinical Microbiology. 2005;**43**:951-955. DOI: 10.1128/JCM.43.2.951-955.2005

[18] Varlet-Marie E, Sterkers Y, Perrotte M, Bastien P. A new LAMP-based assay for the molecular diagnosis of toxoplasmosis: Comparison with a proficient PCR assay. International Journal for Parasitology. 2018;**48**:457-462. DOI: 10.1016/j.ijpara.2017.11.005. Epub 2018 Feb 22

[19] Kurosaki Y, Martins DBG, Kimura M, Catena AS, Borba MACSM, Mattos SS, et al. Development and evaluation of a rapid molecular diagnostic test for Zika virus infection by reverse transcription loop-mediated isothermal amplifcation. Nature. 2017;7:13503-13513. DOI: 10.1038/s41598-017-13836-9

[20] Bustin SA, Benes V, Garson JA, Hellemans J, Huggett J, Kubista M, et al. The MIQE guidelines: Minimum information for publication of quantitative real-time PCR experiments. Clinical Chemistry. 2009;**55**:611-622. DOI: 10.1373/clinchem.2008.112797

[21] Sibley CD, Peirano G, Church DL. Molecular methods for pathogen and microbial community detection and characterization: Current and potential application in diagnostic microbiology. Infection, Genetics and Evolution. 2012;**12**:505-521. DOI: 10.1016/j.meegid.2012.01.011. Epub 2012 Feb 9

[22] Wahid B, Ali A, Rafique S, Idrees M. Zika: As an emergent epidemic. Asian Pacific Journal of Tropical Medicine. 2016;**9**:723-729. DOI: 10.1016/j.apjtm.2016.06.019

[23] Huggett JF, Foy CA, Benes V, Emslie K, Garson JA, Haynes R, et al. The digital MIQE guidelines: Minimum information for publication of quantitative digital PCR experiments. Clinical Chemistry. 2013;**59**:892-902. DOI: 10.1373/clinchem.2013.206375

[24] Huggett JF, Cowen S, Foy CA. Considerations for digital PCR as an accurate molecular diagnostic tool. Clinical Chemistry. 2015;**61**:79-88. DOI: 10.1373/clinchem.2014.221366

[25] Sedlak RH, Jerome KR. Viral diagnostics in the era of digital polymerase chain reaction. Diagnostic Microbiology and Infectious Disease. 2013;**75**:1-4. DOI: 10.1016/j.diagmicrobio.2012.10.009

[26] Whale AS, Bushell CA, Grant PR, Cowen S, Gutierrez-Aguirre I, O'Sullivan DM. Detection of rare drug resistance mutations by digital PCR in a human influenza a virus model system and clinical samples. Journal of Clinical Microbiology. 2016;**54**:392-400. DOI: 10.1128/JCM.02611-15

[27] Huang JT, Liu YJ, Wang J, Xu ZG, Yang Y, Shen F. Next generation digital PCR measurement of hepatitis b virus copy number in formalin-fixed paraffin-embedded hepatocellular carcinoma tissue. Clinical Chemistry. 2015;**61**:290-296. DOI: 10.1373/clinchem.2014.230227

[28] Sedlak RH, Cook L, Cheng A, Magaret A, Jerome KR. Clinical utility of droplet digital PCR for human cytomegalovirus. Journal of Clinical

Microbiology. 2014;**52**:2844-2848. DOI: 10.1128/JCM.00803-14

[29] Yang J, Han X, Liu A, Bai X, Xu C, Bao F, et al. Use of digital droplet PCR to detect *Mycobacterium tuberculosis* DNA in whole blood-derived DNA samples from patients with pulmonary and extrapulmonary tuberculosis. Frontiers in Cellular and Infection Microbiology. 2017;**11**:7-369. DOI: 10.3389/fcimb.2017.00369

[30] Roberts CH, Last A, Molina-Gonzalez S, Cassama E, Butcher R, Nabicassa M, et al. Development and evaluation of a next-generation digital PCR diagnostic assay for ocular *Chlamydia trachomatis* infections. Journal of Clinical Microbiology. 2013;**51**:2195-2203. DOI: 10.1128/JCM.00622-13

[31] Luo J, Li J, Yang H, Yu J, Wei H. Accurate detection of methicillin-resistant *Staphylococcus aureus* in mixtures by use of single-bacterium duplex droplet digital PCR. Journal of Clinical Microbiology. 2017;**55**: 2946-2955. DOI: 10.1128/JCM.00716-17

[32] Koepfli C, Nguitragool W, Hofmann NE, Robinson LJ, Ome-Kaius M, Sattabongkot J. Sensitive and accurate quantification of human malaria parasites using droplet digital PCR (ddPCR). Scientific Reports. 2016;**6**:39183. DOI: 10.1038/srep39183

Chapter 9

Polymerase Chain Reaction (PCR): Principle and Applications

Karim Kadri

Abstract

The characterization of the diversity of species living within ecosystems is of major scientific interest to understand the functioning of these ecosystems. It is also becoming a societal issue since it is necessary to implement the conservation or even the restoration of biodiversity. Historically, species have been described and characterized on the basis of morphological criteria, which are closely linked by environmental conditions or which find their limits especially in groups where they are difficult to access, as is the case for many species of microorganisms. The need to understand the molecular mechanisms in species has made the PCR an indispensable tool for understanding the functioning of these biological systems. A number of markers are now available to detect nuclear DNA polymorphisms. In genetic diversity studies, the most frequently used markers are microsatellites. The study of biological complexity is a new frontier that requires high-throughput molecular technology, high speed computer memory, new approaches to data analysis, and the integration of interdisciplinary skills.

Keywords: PCR, molecular markers, genetic diversity

1. Introduction

Polymerase chain reaction (PCR) was invented by Mullis in 1983 and patented in 1985. Its principle is based on the use of DNA polymerase which is an in vitro replication of specific DNA sequences. This method can generate tens of billions of copies of a particular DNA fragment (the sequence of interest, DNA of interest, or target DNA) from a DNA extract (DNA template). Indeed, if the sequence of interest is present in the DNA extract, it is possible to selectively replicate it (we speak of amplification) in very large numbers. The power of PCR is based on the fact that the amount of matrix DNA is not, in theory, a limiting factor. We can therefore amplify nucleotide sequences from infinitesimal amounts of DNA extract. PCR is therefore a technique of purification or cloning. DNA extracted from an organism or sample containing DNAs of various origins is not directly analyzable. It contains many mass of nucleotide sequences. It is therefore necessary to isolate and purify the sequence or sequences that are of interest, whether it is the sequence of a gene or noncoding sequences (introns, transposons, mini or microsatellites). From such a mass of sequences that constitutes the matrix DNA, the PCR can therefore select one or more sequences and amplify them by replication to tens of billions of copies. Once the reaction is complete, the amount of matrix DNA that is not in the area of interest will not have varied. In contrast, the amount of the amplified sequence(s) (the DNA of interest) will be very big. PCR makes it possible to amplify a signal from a background noise, so it is a molecular cloning method, and clone comes back to purity.

There are many applications of PCR. It is a technique now essential in cellular and molecular biology. It permits, especially in a few hours, the "acellular cloning" of a DNA fragment through an automated system, which usually takes several days with standard techniques of molecular cloning. On the other hand, PCR is widely used for diagnostic purposes to detect the presence of a specific DNA sequence of this or that organism in a biological fluid. It is also used to make genetic fingerprints, whether it is the genetic identification of a person in the context of a judicial inquiry, or the identification of animal varieties, plant, or microbial for food quality testing, diagnostics, or varietal selection. PCR is still essential for performing sequencing or site-directed mutagenesis. Finally, there are variants of PCR such as real-time PCR, competitive PCR, PCR in situ, RT-PCR, etc.

At present, the revolutionary evolutions of the molecular biological research are based on the PCR technique which provides the suitable and specific products especially in the field of the characterization and the conservation of the genetic diversity. Several applications are possible in downstream of the PCR technique: (1) the establishment of a complete sequence of the genome of the most important livestock breeds; (2) development of a technology measuring scattered polymorphisms at loci throughout the genome (e.g., SNP detection methods); and (3) the development of a microarray technology to measure gene transcription on a large scale. The study of biological complexity is a new frontier that requires high throughput molecular technology, high speed and computer memory, new approaches to data analysis, and the integration of interdisciplinary skills.

2. Principle of the PCR

PCR makes it possible to obtain, by in vitro replication, multiple copies of a DNA fragment from an extract. Matrix DNA can be genomic DNA as well as complementary DNA obtained by RT-PCR from a messenger RNA extract (poly-A RNA), or even mitochondrial DNA. It is a technique for obtaining large amounts of a specific DNA sequence from a DNA sample. This amplification is based on the replication of a double-stranded DNA template. It is broken down into three phases: a denaturation phase, a hybridization phase with primers, and an elongation phase. The products of each synthesis step serve as a template for the following steps, thus exponential amplification is achieved [1].

The polymerase chain reaction is carried out in a reaction mixture which comprises the DNA extract (template DNA), Taq polymerase, the primers, and the four deoxyribonucleoside triphosphates (dNTPs) in excess in a buffer solution. The tubes containing the mixture reaction are subjected to repetitive temperature cycles several tens of times in the heating block of a thermal cycler (apparatus which has an enclosure where the sample tubes are deposited and in which the temperature can vary, very quickly and precisely, from 0 to 100°C by Peltier effect) [1, 2]. The apparatus allows the programming of the duration and the succession of the cycles of temperature steps. Each cycle includes three periods of a few tens of seconds. The process of the PCR is subdivided into three stages as follows:

2.1 The denaturation

It is the separation of the two strands of DNA, obtained by raising the temperature. The first period is carried out at a temperature of 94°C, called the denaturation

DOI: http://dx.doi.org/10.5772/intechopen.86491

temperature. At this temperature, the matrix DNA, which serves as matrix during the replication, is denatured: the hydrogen bonds cannot be maintained at a temperature higher than 80°C and the double-stranded DNA is denatured into single-stranded DNA (single-stranded DNA).

2.2 Hybridization

The second step is hybridization. It is carried out at a temperature generally between 40 and 70°C, called primer hybridization temperature. Decreasing the temperature allows the hydrogen bonds to reform and thus the complementary strands to hybridize. The primers, short single-strand sequences complementary to regions that flank the DNA to be amplified, hybridize more easily than long strand matrix DNA. The higher the hybridization temperature, the more selective the hybridization, the more specific it is.

2.3 Elongation

The third period is carried out at a temperature of 72°C, called elongation temperature. It is the synthesis of the complementary strand. At 72°C, Taq polymerase binds to primed single-stranded DNAs and catalyzes replication using the deoxyribonucleoside triphosphates present in the reaction mixture. The regions of the template DNA downstream of the primers are thus selectively synthesized. In the next cycle, the fragments synthesized in the previous cycle are in turn matrix and after a few cycles, the predominant species corresponds to the DNA sequence between the regions where the primers hybridize. It takes 20–40 cycles to synthesize an analyzable amount of DNA (about 0.1 μg). Each cycle theoretically doubles the amount of DNA present in the previous cycle. It is recommended to add a final cycle of elongation at 72°C, especially when the sequence of interest is large (greater than 1 kilobase), at a rate of 2 minutes per kilobase [1–3]. PCR makes it possible to amplify sequences whose size is less than 6 kilobases. The PCR reaction is extremely rapid, it lasts only a few hours (2–3 hours for a PCR of 30 cycles).

2.4 Primers

To achieve selective amplification of nucleotide sequences from a DNA extract by PCR, it is essential to have least one pair of oligonucleotides. These oligonucleotides, which will serve as primers for replication, are synthesized chemically and must be the best possible complementarity with both ends of the sequence of interest that one wishes to amplify. One of the primers is designed to recognize complementarily a sequence located upstream of the fragment 5′–3′ strand DNA of interest; the other to recognize, always by complementarity, a sequence located upstream complementary strand (3′–5′) of the same fragment DNA. Primers are single-stranded DNAs whose hybridization on sequences flanking the sequence of interest will allow its replication so selective. The size of the primers is usually between 10 and 30 nucleotides in order to guarantee a sufficiently specific hybridization on the sequences of interest of the matrix DNA [1–5].

2.5 Taq polymerase

DNA polymerase allows replication. We use a DNA polymerase purified or cloned from of an extremophilic bacterium, *Thermus aquaticus*, which lives in hot springs and resists temperatures above 100°C. This polymerase (Taq polymerase) has the characteristic remarkable to withstand temperatures of around 100°C, which are usually sufficient to denature most proteins. *Thermus aquaticus* finds its temperature of comfort at 72°C, optimum temperature for the activity of its polymerase [4].

3. The reaction conditions

The volumes of reaction medium vary between 10 and 100 μl. There are a multitude of reaction medium formulas. However, it is possible to define a standard formula that is suitable for most polymerization reactions. This formula has been chosen by most manufacturers and suppliers, who, moreover, deliver a ready-to-use buffer solution with Taq polymerase. Concentrated 10 times, its formula is approximately the following: 100 mM Tris-HCl, pH 9.0; 15 mM $MgCl_2$, 500 mM KCl [2, 4].

It is possible to add detergents (Tween 20, Triton X-100) or glycerol in order to increase the conditions of stringency that make it harder and therefore more selective hybridization of the primers. This approach is generally used to reduce the level of nonspecific amplifications due to the hybridization of the primers on sequences without relationship with the sequence of interest. We can also reduce the concentration of KCl until eliminated or increase the concentration of $MgCl_2$ [1, 5]. Indeed, some pairs of primers work better with solutions enriched with magnesium. On the other hand, with high concentrations of dNTP, the concentration of magnesium should be increased because of stoichiometric interactions between magnesium and dNTPs that reduce the amount of free magnesium in the reaction medium. dNTPs (deoxyribonucleoside triphosphates) provide both the energy and the nucleotides needed for DNA synthesis during the chain polymerization. They are incorporated in the reaction medium in excess, that is, about 200 μM final. Depending on the reaction volume chosen, the primer concentration may vary between 10 and 50 pmol per sample. Matrix DNA can come from any organism and even complex biological materials that include DNAs from different organisms. But to ensure the success of a PCR, it is still necessary that the DNA matrix is not too degraded. This criterion is obviously all the more crucial as the size of the sequence of interest is large. It is also important that the DNA extract is not contaminated with inhibitors of the polymerase chain reaction (detergents, EDTA, phenol, proteins, etc.) [6, 7]. The amount of template DNA in the reaction medium initiate that the amplification reaction can be reduced to a single copy. The maximum quantity may in no case exceed 2 μg. In general, the amounts used are in the range of 10–500 ng of template DNA. The amount of Taq polymerase per sample is generally between 1 and 3 units. The choice of the duration of the temperature cycles and the number of cycles depends on the size of the sequence of interest as well as the size and the complementarity of the primers. The durations should be reduced to a minimum not only to save time but also to prevent risk of nonspecific amplification. For denaturation and hybridization of primers, 30 seconds are usually sufficient. For elongation, it takes 1 minute per kilobase of DNA of interest and 2 minutes per kilobase for the final cycle of elongation. The number of cycles, generally between 20 and 40, is inversely proportional to the abundance of DNA matrix [6–8].

4. PCR product detection and analysis

The product of a PCR consists of one or more DNA fragments (the sequence or sequences of interest). The detection and analysis of the products can be very quickly carried out by agarose gel electrophoresis (or acrylamide). The DNA is revealed by ethidium bromide staining [2, 3, 5]. Thus, the products are instantly visible by ultraviolet transillumination (280–320 nm). Very small products are often visible very close to the migration front in the form of more or less diffuse bands. They correspond to primer dimers and sometimes to the primers themselves. Depending on the reaction conditions, nonspecific DNA fragments may be amplified to a greater or lesser extent, forming net bands or "smear" [6–9]. On automated systems, a fragment analyzer is now used. This apparatus uses the principle of capillary electrophoresis. Fragment detection is performed by a laser diode. This is only possible if the PCR is performed with primers coupled to fluorochromes [10].

5. Overview of molecular techniques based on PCR technology

Microsatellites are hypervariable; on a locus, they often show dozens of different alleles from each other in the number of repetitions. They are still the markers of choice for studies on the diversity, paternity analysis and mapping of quantitative effects loci (QTL), although this could change, in the near future, through the elaboration inexpensive SNP assay methods. Minisatellites have the same characteristics as microsatellites, but repetitions range from ten to a few hundred base pairs. Micro- and minisatellites are also known as variable number of tandem repeat (VNTR) polymorphisms. Amplified fragment length polymorphisms.

5.1 Microsatellites

Microsatellites are now the most used markers in genetic characterization studies of farmed animals [11]. The high mutation rate and codominant nature favor the estimation of intra and interracial diversity, and the genetic mixing between races, even if they are very close. Challenges have surrounded the choice of a mutation model—the infinite or progressive allele mutation model [12] for the analysis of microsatellite data. However, simulation studies have indicated that the infinite allele mutation model is generally valid for the evaluation of intraracial diversity [13]. The low number of alleles per population and observed and expected heterozygosity are the most commonly used parameters for assessing intraracial diversity. The simplest parameters for evaluating interracial diversity are genetic differentiation or fixation indices. Several estimators have been proposed (e.g., FST—fixation index and GST—glutathione S transferase), and the most widely used is FST [14], which measures the degree of genetic differentiation of subpopulations by calculation standardized variances of allele frequencies of populations. Statistical significance is calculated for FST values between population pairs to test the null hypothesis of a lack of genetic differentiation between populations and, consequently, the partitioning of genetic diversity [15]. Microsatellite data are also commonly used to assess genetic relationships between populations and subjects through the estimation of genetic distances [16–19]. The measure of genetic distance used most often is the standard genetic distance of Nei [20]. In another case, the modified Cavalli-Sforza distance is recommended [21] for the closest populations, where genetic drift is the main factor of genetic differentiation. The genetic relationship between breeds is often visualized by the reconstruction of a phylogeny, most often using the "neighbor-joining" method [22]. However, the main problem in the reconstruction of the phylogenetic tree is that the evolution of the lines is presumed to be uncrosslinked that is to say that the lines can deviate, but can never come from interbreeding. This assumption is rarely valid for farm animals, as new breeds are often derived from crosses between two or more ancestral breeds. The visualization of breed evolution by phylogenetic reconstruction must therefore be interpreted with great attention.

5.2 SNP

Single nucleotide polymorphisms (SNPs) are used as an alternative to microsatellites in genetic diversity studies. Several technologies are available to detect the type of SNP markers [23]. As biallelic markers, SNPs have relatively low amounts of information, and to reach the information level of a standard panel of 30 microsatellite loci, larger amounts must be used. However, ever-evolving molecular technologies increase automation and reduce the cost of typing SNPs, which will likely allow, in the near future, the parallel analysis of a large number of markers at a reduced cost. In this perspective, large-scale projects are being implemented for several livestock species to identify millions of SNPs [24] and validate several thousands and identify haplotype in the genome. As with sequence information, SNPs allow for direct comparison and joint analysis of different experiments. SNPs are likely to be interesting markers for future use in genetic diversity studies because they can be easily used in the assessment of functional or neutral variation. However, the preliminary phase of SNP discovery or selection of SNPs from databases is critical. SNPs can be generated through various experimental protocols, such as sequencing, single-stranded coformational polymorphism (SSCP) or denaturing high-performance liquid chromatography (DHPLC) or in silico, aligning and comparing multiple sequences from the same region from public databases on genomes and sequential expression tags (ESTs). If the data were obtained randomly, the standard population genetic parameter estimators cannot be applied. A common example is when SNPs initially identified in a small sample (panel) of individuals are then typed into a larger sample of chromosomes. By preferably performing sampling of SNPs at intermediate frequencies, such a protocol will affect the distribution of allele frequencies with respect to the probable values for a random sample. SNPs present a modern tool in the context of genetic analyzes of the population; however, it is necessary to develop statistical methods that will take into account each SNP operating method and their locations [25, 26].

5.3 Amplification of fragment length polymorphism (AFLP)

AFLPs are dominant biallelic markers [27]. Variations on many loci can be arranged simultaneously to detect single nucleotide variations of unknown genomic regions, where a given mutation may often be present in undetermined functional genes. The disadvantage is that they show a dominant mode of inheritance, which reduces their power during genetic analyses of the population on intraracial diversity and consanguinity. However, AFLP profiles are highly informative in the evaluation of race relations [28–32] and related species [33].

5.4 Restriction fragment length polymorphism (RFLP)

Restriction fragment length polymorphisms (RFLPs) are identified using restriction enzymes that cut DNA only at specific “restriction sites” (e.g., EcoRI cuts at the site defined by the palindrome GAATTC sequence). At present, the most common use of RFLPs is downstream PCR (PCR-RFLP) to detect alleles that differ in sequence at a given restriction site. A gene fragment is first amplified using PCR and then exposed to a specific restriction enzyme that cuts only one of the allelic forms. The digested amplicons are usually resolved by electrophoresis. Microsatellites or SSRs (simple sequence repeats) or STRs (short tandem repeats) consist of a few nucleotides—2–6 base pair DNA sequence—epeated several times in tandem (e.g., CACACACACACACACA). They are spread on a eukaryotic genome. Microsatellites are relatively small in size and, therefore, are easily amplified using DNA PCRs extracted from different sources, such as blood, hair, skin, or even feces. Polymorphisms can be visualized on a sequencing gel, and the availability of automated DNA sequencers allows high-throughput analysis of a large number of samples [34, 35].

5.5 Mitochondrial DNA markers

Mitochondrial DNA polymorphisms (mtDNA) have been widely used in analyzes of phylogenetic and genetic diversity. The haploid mtDNA transported by the mitochondria of the cellular cytoplasm has a maternal mode of inheritance (the animals inherit the mtDNA from their mothers and not from their fathers) and a high mutation rate; it does not recombine. These features allow biologists to reconstruct intra and interracial evolutionary relationships by evaluating mtDNA mutation patterns. mtDNA tags can also provide a quick way to detect hybridization between farmed species and subspecies [36]. Polymorphisms in the hypervariable region of the D-loop or the mtDNA control region have largely contributed to the identification of wild ascendants of domestic species and to the establishment of geographical models of genetic diversity.

6. Applications

6.1 Acellular cloning

This is one of the most remarkable applications of PCR. It makes it possible to isolate, that is to say, to purify a gene without resorting to traditional methods of molecular cloning which consist in inserting a DNA library in a plasmid vector which is then used to transform a bacterial strain whose clones after selection are screened. The realization is much faster and much less random using PCR. Acellular cloning is used when using PCR because it is useless to use a cellular system (bacteria, yeast, and animal or plant cell) to amplify the clone. The realization of molecular cloning by PCR depends on two major criteria: the choice of DNA extract (matrix DNA) and primers. It is indeed essential to have more or less reliable data on the sequence of the gene that is to be cloned and/or flanking sequences in order to synthesize the sets of primers necessary for its amplification in whole or in part. On the other hand, is it still necessary to perform the PCR on the appropriate matrix DNA [37, 38]. We can choose the genomic DNA that includes the total sequence of the genome and therefore all the genes of the species. In this case, the genes include both exons and introns and their amplification results in the cloning of the complete gene sequence and even, depending on the primers that have been chosen, regulatory regions. But we can also choose to extract the messenger RNA (mRNA), that is to say the only coding sequences of the gene—the transcripts. Since RNAs are unstable, messenger RNAs are transformed into complementary DNA (cDNA) by RT-PCR (see below), a variant of PCR that uses reverse transcriptase and allows changing the RNA sequences into DNA. It is on this cDNA library that PCR is then performed to clone the gene of interest. In this case, the deal is more complex. The presence of the gene transcript in the extract depends on the cell type, tissue, or organ from which the mRNA extraction was performed. Indeed, transcription is specific to the cell type. More serious, the expression of a gene is often regulated by physiological factors, environmental, in this case the gene of interest is not necessarily transcribed and the cDNA library may not contain it. Finally, it must be said that transcription is itself regulated and is often accompanied by alternative splicing. This phenomenon leads to exon elimination at the time of excision of the introns and leads to the expression of different proteins from the same gene. It follows that depending on the cell type and regulatory profiles, we may not be dealing with the same transcript. It is nevertheless very interesting to clone a transcript since its nucleotide sequence corresponds to the amino acid sequence resulting from the translation. On the other hand, with a cDNA, it is easier to carry out the expression of the gene and thus the functional evaluation of the corresponding protein or proteins in a cellular model of expression. Very frequently, PCR cloning is practiced in parallel on genomic DNA (genomic library) and different cDNA libraries so as to determine the complete sequence of the gene, its expression profile, the modalities of splice regulation [8, 39], etc.

6.2 Reverse transcriptase PCR (RT-PCR)

As discussed in the previous chapter, it may be relevant to extract the mRNAs to then generate cDNA copies. This reaction is catalyzed by retrovirus reverse transcriptase (reverse transcriptase) which synthesizes a DNA chain from an RNA template. At first, the total RNAs are extracted. The mRNAs are isolated from the total RNA by affinity chromatography using oligodT (polyT oligonucleotide) because the messenger RNAs are characterized by a 3′polyA sequence. Then, the mRNAs are subjected to reverse transcriptase which will generate a copy of DNA (cDNA) of each mRNA. After the reverse transcription, the mRNAs are hydrolyzed (alkaline treatment, RNase, or temperature). The following steps are carried out in the enclosure of the thermal cycler. The single-stranded cDNAs are then replicated by the DNA polymerase during a first temperature cycle [40, 41]. Other cycles are repeated to amplify double-stranded cDNAs in large quantities. In a given cell phenotype, an estimated 10–15,000 genes are expressed in humans and most mammals. Some cell transcripts are expressed at a few hundred or even a few thousand copies per cell, but the majority of transcripts represent a low copy number. The expression profiles of transcripts undergo qualitative or quantitative variations that reflect the biological dynamics of the cell. The identification of variations in gene expression in a given physiological or pathological context can therefore provide valuable information concerning the function of genes and the influence of modulation factors on their expression, whether they are physiological or of environmental origin. The analysis of the expression variations of genes involved in a pathology can lead to new therapeutic or diagnostic targets. Finally, from a fundamental point of view, studying the gene expression profile makes it possible to advance in understanding the mechanisms of cellular physiology [40–42].

6.3 Quantitative PCR in real time (quantitative real-time PCR)

Developed in the mid-1980s, quantitative PCR can determine the level of specific DNA or RNA in a biological sample. The method is based on the detection of a fluorescent signal that is produced in proportion to the amplification of the PCR product, cycle after cycle. It requires a thermal cycler coupled to an optical reading system that measures fluorescence emission. A nucleotide probe is synthesized so that it can hybridize selectively to the DNA of interest between the sequences where the primers hybridize. The probe is labeled on the 5′ end with a fluorochrome signal (e.g., 6-carboxyfluorescein), and on the 3′ end with a quencher (e.g., 6-carboxytetramethyl rhodamine). This probe must show temperature hybridization (Tm) greater than that of the primers so that it hybridizes 100% during the elongation phase (critical parameter) [43–45].

As long as the two fluorochromes remain present at the probe, the extinguisher prevents the fluorescence of the signal. In this step, the proximity of the quencher and the signal induces a lack of fluorescence emission. During this phase of elongation, Taq polymerase, which has an intrinsic 5′–3′ nuclease activity, degrades the probe and thus releases the fluorochrome signal. The level of fluorescence then released is proportional to the amount of PCR products generated in each cycle. The thermal cycler is designed so that each sample (the PCR is generally carried out in 96-well plates) is connected to an optical system. This includes a laser transmitter connected to an optical fiber. The laser, via the optical fiber, excites the fluorochrome within the PCR reaction mixture. The fluorescence emitted is retransmitted, always through optical fiber, to a digital camera connected to a computer. A software then analyzes and stores the data. Quantitative PCR is a method of high specificity and sensitivity. It is very timely for countless applications. A conventional PCR only provides qualitative data (presence or absence of the DNA of interest, purification of this DNA). Quantitative PCR, as its name suggests, makes it possible to know more precisely the quantity of the DNA of interest (or RNA, since it is possible to conduct a quantitative RT-PCR with the same apparatus) [45–47]. It is indeed very often used for this purpose, for example, in order to determine the viral load, in particular in cases of hepatitis C or AIDS. One of the most remarkable and useful applications is the analysis of gene expression through the quantitative measurement of transcripts.

6.4 Semi-quantitative or competitive PCR

This is in most cases RT-PCR. In the case of quantitative PCR, the level of RNA or DNA of interest is measured as the absolute amount. In the case of semi-quantitative PCR or competitive PCR, it is a question of measuring relative quantities by means of standards that correspond to RNA or more rarely to DNA. This is in most cases RT-PCR. These standards can be internal or external. External standards may be homologous or heterologous. The standard is an RNA (more rarely a DNA) which is present in the RNA extract (internal standard) or which is added in known quantity in the reaction mixture (external standard). The standard is amplified at the same time as the RNA of interest. There is therefore competition between the amplification of the standard and that of the DNA of interest. The higher the standard quantity, the less the RNA of interest will be amplified and therefore its quantity will be small. Of course, the method of analysis of the PCR sample must make it possible to discriminate the standard with respect to the RNA of interest on the one hand and on the other hand to evaluate the relative amount of DNA of interest by comparison with the amount of standard that is known [48]. The internal standards are endogenous RNA, corresponding to RNA genes whose expression is presumed constant (actin, beta2-microglobulin, etc.) and which are present in the population of RNA matrices during reverse transcription. These standards have a major disadvantage: they require the use of primers different from those used for the RNA of interest. The kinetics of amplification are therefore substantially different, and it is very difficult or impossible to guarantee a constant expression between different samples. The homologous external RNA standards are synthetic RNAs that share the same priming hybridization sites as the RNA of interest and that have the same overall sequence, with a slight mutation, deletion, or insertion that will allow the identification and quantification thereof with respect to the signal rendered by the RNA of interest. These standards make it possible on the one hand to appreciate the variability introduced at the level of the RT and, on the other hand, generally have the same amplification efficiency as the RNA of interest whether it is at the RT level or PCR [48, 49].

The heterologous external RNA standards are exogenous RNAs and their rate can therefore be controlled. However, unlike homologous external standards, they have a different amplification efficiency compared to that of the RNA of interest. In the case of quantitative RT-PCR (semi-quantitative PCR), the standard consists of a titrated solution of DNA of sequence identical to that of the DNA of interest to be quantified. A dilution series is performed, each being used for amplification. It is then a question of defining the ideal number of cycles to be placed in the exponential phase of the reaction while ensuring an effective amplification. Then, each standard DNA dilution as well as the DNA extracted from the sample to be quantified are submitted in parallel to the PCR reaction. A standard curve is established with standard dilutions [signal = f (concentration)]. Knowing the value of the signal measured on the sample to be quantified, the corresponding number of copies can be extrapolated from the curve. In the case of competitive PCR, a series of synthetic external homologous standard RNA dilutions are co-amplified with equivalent amounts of total RNA (and thus an equivalent amount of the native gene) [50, 51]. The standard competes with the RNA of interest for polymerase and primers. As the standard concentration increases, the signal of the gene of interest decreases. Here, the PCR does not need to be performed in the exponential phase and the results show a correct reproducibility. However, the method is cumbersome and does not allow to manage many samples simultaneously [52].

6.5 PCR applied to diagnosis

PCR is a fabulous diagnostic tool. It is already widely used in the detection of genetic diseases. The amplification of all or part of a gene responsible for a genetic disease makes it possible to reveal the deleterious mutations (s), their positions, their sizes, and their natures. It is thus possible to detect deletions, inversions, insertions, and even point mutations, either by direct analysis of PCR products by electrophoresis or by combining PCR with other techniques [53]. But PCR can still be used to detect infectious diseases (viral, bacterial, parasitic, etc.), as is already the case for AIDS, hepatitis C, or chlamydia infections. Although other diagnostic tools are effective at detecting these diseases, PCR has the enormous advantage of producing very reliable and rapid results from minute biological samples in which the presence of the pathogen is not always detectable with other techniques [53, 54].

6.6 Detection of genetic diseases

In the context of genetic diseases, it is a question of detecting a mutation on the sequence of a gene. Several situations arise. The simplest ones concern insertions and deletions. In these cases, the mutation is manifested by the change in the size of the gene or part of the gene. Insofar as the mutation is known and described, it suffices to amplify all or part of the gene. In the case of an insertion, the PCR product from a patient's DNA is longer than that from a healthy person. A deletion presents a contrary result [55]. The analysis of PCR products by electrophoresis, and therefore the evaluation of their size, leads directly to the diagnosis. The detection of inversions and point mutations is more delicate. The difference in size between healthy and diseased DNA is zero in the case of an inversion and almost zero in the case of a point mutation. We cannot therefore retain the size criterion of the PCR products to achieve the result. It is therefore necessary to resort to techniques complementary to PCR. Three approaches can be selected, the southern blot, the restriction fragment length polymorphism (RFLP), or the detection of mismatch. The southern blot consists in hybridizing on the PCR product an oligonucleotide probe marked, thanks to a radioactive isotope or a fluorochrome, whose sequence is complementary and therefore specific to that which corresponds to the mutation. This strategy is well suited to inversion cases [56, 57].

The RFLP can detect inversions such as point mutations. It involves a restriction enzyme capable of hydrolyzing the PCR product at the sequence which sets the mutation. This approach is only possible if a restriction site is indeed present on this sequence, whether it is the mutated allele or the wild-type allele. The restriction enzyme thus hydrolyzes either the PCR product derived from healthy DNA or that which is derived from the diseased DNA. From these PCR products, one or two DNA fragments are thus obtained which are then revealed by electrophoresis. Mismatch detection is, like the RFLP, adapted to inversions and point mutations [57–59]. The PCR product from the patient's DNA (sample DNA) is mixed with the PCR product from the DNA of a healthy person (reference DNA). This mixture is then denatured by the temperature and then rehybridized. Yes the sample DNA is mutated; the pairings between sample DNA and reference DNA will be incomplete at the level of the mutation. The mismatches concern a single base pair in the case of a point mutation and several base pairs in the case of an inversion. These mismatches are then degraded by S1 nuclease, an enzyme that degrades only single-stranded DNAs. Another solution is to cleave the mismatches chemically (osmium tetroxide, then piperidine), but it is more suitable for point mutations. In summary, mutation induces a mismatch at the level of enzymatic or chemical cleavage which leads to the generation of two fragments from a single PCR product. These fragments are analyzed by electrophoresis.

6.7 Detection of infectious diseases

Contamination with viruses or microorganisms (bacteria, parasites, etc.) necessarily results in the presence of their genetic material in all or part of the infected organism. PCR is therefore a tool all the more effective in detecting the presence of a pathogen in a biological sample that its sensitivity and specificity are very large. The performance of the PCR diagnosis is essentially based on a criterion: the choice of primers capable of very selectively amplifying a sequence of the DNA of the virus or microorganism [57–59]. Matrix DNA, on the other hand, must be extracted from a tissue in which the microorganism is present. It is therefore sufficient to amplify a specific sequence of the pathogen from a sample taken on the patient and to analyze the PCR product by electrophoresis. The size of the amplified DNA fragment, which must conform to the expected size, guarantees the reliability of the result and therefore of the diagnosis. In the case of AIDS (HIV) testing, for example, routine testing is based on the ELISA method of detecting HIV antibodies or viral antigens in the patient's serum by an immunoassay technique. This method, quite reliable and inexpensive, nevertheless has some disadvantages. False positives are quite common because of cross-reactivities. Positive samples are therefore tested for control by another routine technique, Western blot. There remains the problem of HIV-positive people who do not carry the virus, such as children whose mothers have AIDS. The blood of these newborns usually contains anti-HIV antibodies of maternal origin and they are therefore seropositive. On the other hand, they do not necessarily carry the virus. In this type of case, the PCR diagnosis is relevant [57–60]. The method involves amplifying a specific sequence of the provirus from a lymphocyte extract. The same principle is used for the detection of toxoplasma in newborns whose mother is a carrier. It is of course possible to diagnose AIDS by RT-PCR by looking for viral RNA in the patient's serum. Quantitative or semi-quantitative methods have been developed which also make it possible to evaluate the viral load.

6.8 PCR applied to identification

PCR is remarkably effective at identifying species, varieties, or individuals by genetic fingerprinting. This application is based on the knowledge acquired on genome structure. It is simply to amplify nucleotide sequences that are specific to species, variety, or individual. In eukaryotes, in particular, these sequences are very numerous and offer a vast palette that allows identification in a very precise and very selective way. Indeed, the genomes of eukaryotic organisms have, unlike prokaryotes, coding sequences and noncoding sequences. The coding sequences correspond to the genes and are therefore translated into proteins. The noncoding sequences, which are therefore not translated, represent a large proportion of eukaryotic genomic DNA (up to 98%). The coding sequences are highly homologous in individuals of the same species. Indeed, the species is characterized by characters and common traits that are guaranteed by its genes. The phenotypic differences between the individuals that compose it are based on the allelic variations and the different alleles of the same gene show sequence differences that are minute (of the order of 1 base pair per 1000) [61, 62]. From one species to another, depending on the phylogenetic distance that separates them, the sequences of the genes that code for the same function have very strong homologies, all the more so that the function of the gene is essential to the embryogenesis or metabolism. As a result, coding sequences are of little relevance in terms of identification. On the other hand, the noncoding sequences are very polymorphous between species as between individuals of the same species. They thus present a large choice of genetic markers that make it possible to establish identification tests which are highly discriminating. Among these markers are minisatellites (or variable number of tandem repeats) and microsatellites (or STR, short tandem repeats) [61–63]. VNTRs and STRs are repetitive polymorphisms composed of sequences that are repeated in tandem. These repeat sequences measure from 10 to 40 base pairs for VNTRs and from 1 to 5 base pairs for STRs. From one individual to another, the repeated sequence of a VNTR or STR is identical but the number of repetitions and therefore the size of the VNTR or the STR can be very variable (we speak of alleles). On the other hand, there is a wide variety of VNTRs and STRs on eukaryotic genomes. Detection of STR or VNTR polymorphism is by PCR using primers that hybridize to nonpolymorphic flanking sequences. The amplification products are then either analyzed by electrophoresis or undergo fragment analysis using a capillary sequencer. It is now possible to simultaneously amplify several STRs or VNTRs by using several pairs of primers. The variety of amplification products obtained leads to footprints that are specific individuals. On the other hand, the power of PCR makes it possible to amplify micro- and minisatellites from very little DNA. DNA fingerprinting has become much more commonplace in recent years in the context of judicial investigations. But these techniques are equally as effective in other species as humans and allow not only identifying individuals but also varieties or species. The type of identification depends simply on the choice of markers. Similarly, for varietal identification purposes, one can commonly proceed according to protocols derived from the PCR [64–66].

Two techniques that are relevant are the random amplification of polymorphic DNA (RAPD) and the amplification of fragment length polymorphism (AFLP). (Random amplification of polymorphic DNA (RAPD) is a PCR for varietal identification that uses pairs of random primers of reduced size (about 10 base pairs). These primers will hybridize randomly, but PCR usually results in an electrophoresis amplification profile which is specific to the variety from which the matrix DNA is derived. Amplification of fragment length polymorphism (AFLP) is a much more efficient method. It first consists hydrolyzing the genomic DNA with one or better two restriction endonucleases. Then, we proceed with the ligation of adapters (defined sequences of DNA of about 15 nucleotides) at the level of the generated cohesive ends by restriction enzymes. Finally, the product of the ligation is amplified by PCR with a pair of primers that hybridizes at the level of the adapters. The

AFLP gives a result comparable to the RAPD. However, the AFLP shows cleaner and more reproducible results. This is the most successful method to date applied to varietal identification.

7. Conclusion

The extension of genotyping approaches to all living organisms has made significant advances in the reconstruction of the history of life. At the population level, the distribution and frequency of known genetic polymorphisms in a species can highlight the evolving forces at play, reveal the effects of natural selection, and infer demographic change. Moreover, the comparison of the sequences of the same genes between different species and that of whole genomes is at the origin of the molecular phylogenies that currently prevail in the classification. They make it possible to trace the relationships between species on the basis of the divergence of their DNA sequences. As such, the PCR is a key stage at two levels. The first concerns the isolation of homologous genes in several species and their characterization. The second is the production of amplified total genomic DNA for genome sequencing and comparative analysis. But PCR is also used to identify the genetic heritage of missing organisms. The DNA breaks down by fragmentation after the death of the body. If we can recover these fragments and amplify them, it becomes possible, in spite of its state, to deduce all or part of the initial genome of the individual. PCR has thus become the primary tool in the field of palaeogenetics, which consists in recovering and analyzing DNA sequences of more or less old organisms, and this as well from the remains preserved in museum collections, from historical site where the skeletal or mummified remains of extinct organisms for hundreds thousands or even hundreds of thousands of years. The uses of the PCR thus quickly stopped being limited to the studies of biology, to gain other disciplines or fields of activities.

Author details

Karim Kadri[1,2]

1 Regional Research Center on Oasis Agriculture, Laboratory of Biotechnology and Genetic Resources, Degache, Tunisia

2 National Institute for Agronomic Research in Tunis, Laboratory of Biotechnology Applied on Agriculture, Ariana, Tunisia

*Address all correspondence to: kadrikarim2001@yahoo.fr

References

[1] Pelt-Verkuil E, Belkum A, John P. A brief comparison between in vivo DNA replication and in vitro PCR amplification. Principles and Technical Aspects of PCR Amplification. Netherlands: Springer; 2008. pp. 9-15

[2] Polymerase Chain Reaction (PCR). National Center for Biotechnology Information [Online]. Available from: http://www.ncbi.nlm.nih.gov/probe/docs/techpcr/

[3] PCR Optimization: Reaction Conditions and Components. Applied Biosystems. 2017. Available from: https://www3.appliedbiosystems.com/cms/groups/mcb_marketing/documents/generaldocuments/cms_042520.pdf

[4] Lawyer FC, Stoffel S, Saiki RK, Myambo K, Drummond R, Gelfand DH. Isolation, characterization, and expression in *Escherichia coli* of the DNA polymerase gene from Thermus aquaticus. Biological Chemistry. 1989;**264**:6427-6437

[5] Primer Design Tips & Tools. Thermo Fisher Scientific, Inc. 2015. Available from: http://www.thermofisher.com/ca/en/home/products-and-services/product-types/primers-oligosnucleotides/invitrogen-custom-dna-oligos/primer-design-tools.html

[6] Mammedov TG, Pienaar E, Whitney SE, TerMaat JR, Carvill G, Goliath R, et al. A fundamental study of the PCR amplification of GC-rich DNA templates. Computational Biology and Chemistry. Dec 2008;**32**(6):452-457

[7] Strien SJ, Mall GJ. Enhancement of PCR amplification of moderate GC-containing and highly GC-rich DNA sequences. Molecular Biotechnology. 2013;**54**

[8] Hubé F, Reverdiau P, Iochmann S, Gruel Y. Improved PCR method for amplification of GC-rich DNA sequences. Molecular Biotechnology. September 2005;**31**(1):81-84

[9] Su XZ, Wu Y, Sifri CD, Wellems TE. Reduced extension temperatures required for PCR amplification of extremely A+T-rich DNA. Nucleic Acids Research. 15 Apr 1996;**24**(8):1574-1575

[10] Pelt V, Belkum EV, Hays AV. Principles and Technical Aspects of PCR Amplification. Switzerland: Springer Science & Business Media; 2008

[11] Korbie DJ, Mattick JS. Touchdown PCR for increased specificity and sensitivity in PCR amplification. Nature Protocols. 2008;**3**(9):1452-1456

[12] Goldstein DB, Linares AR, Cavalli-Sforza LL, Feldman MW. An evaluation of genetic distances for use with microsatellite loci. Genetics. 1995;**139**:463-471

[13] Takezaki N, Nei M. Genetic distances and reconstruction of phylogenetic trees from microsatellite DNA. Genetics. 1996;**144**:389-399

[14] Weir BS, Basten CJ. Sampling strategies for distances between DNA sequences. Biometrics. 1990;**46**:551-582

[15] Mburu DN, Ochieng JW, Kuria SG, Jianlin H, Kaufmann B. Genetic diversity and relationships of indigenous Kenyan camel (*Camelus dromedarius*) populations: Implications for their classification. Animal Genetics. 2003;**34**(1):26-32

[16] Beja-Pereira A, Alexandrino P, Bessa I, Carretero Y, Dunner S, Ferrand N, et al. Genetic characterization of southwestern European bovine breeds: A historical and biogeographical reassessment with a set of 16

microsatellites. Journal of Heredity. 2003;**94**:243-250

[17] Ibeagha-Awemu EM, Jann OC, Weimann C, Erhardt G. Genetic diversity, introgression and relationships among west/central African cattle breeds. Genetics Selection Evolution. 2004;**36**:673-690

[18] Joshi MB, Rout PK, Mandal AK, Tyler-Smith C, Singh L, Thangaraj K. Phylogeography and origin of Indian domestic goats. Molecular Biology and Evolution. 2004;**21**:454-462

[19] Tapio M, Tapio I, Grislis Z, Holm LE, Jeppsson S, Kantanen J, et al. Native breeds demonstrate high contributions to the molecular variation in northern European sheep. Molecular Ecology. 2005;**14**:3951-3963

[20] Nei M. Genetic distance between populations. The American Naturalist. 1972;**106**:283-292

[21] Nei M, Tajima F, Tateno Y. Accuracy of estimated phylogenetic trees from molecular data. II. Gene frequency data. Journal of Molecular Evolution. 1983;**19**:153-170

[22] Saitou N, Nei M. The neighbor-joining method: A new method for reconstructing phylogenetic trees. Molecular Biology and Evolution. 1987;**4**:406-425

[23] Syvänen AC. Accessing genetic variation genotyping single nucleotide polymorphisms. Nature Reviews Genetics. 2001;**2**:930-941

[24] Wong GK, Liu B, Wang J, Zhang Y, Yang X, Zhang Z, et al. A genetic variation map for chicken with 2.8 million singlenucleotide polymorphisms. Nature. 2004;**432**:717-722

[25] Nielsen R, Signorovitch J. Correcting for ascertainment biases when analyzing SNP data: Applications to the estimation of linkage disequilibrium. Theoretical Population Biology. 2003;**63**:245-255

[26] Clark AG, Hubisz MJ, Bustamante CD, Williamson SH, Nielsen R. Ascertainment bias in studies of human genomewide polymorphism. Genome Research. 2005;**15**:1496-1502

[27] Vos P, Hogers R, Bleeker M, Reijans M, van de Lee T, Hornes M, et al. AFLP: A new technique for DNA fingerprinting. Nucleic Acids Research. 1995;**23**:4407-1444

[28] Ajmone-Marsan P, Negrini R, Milanesi E, Bozzi R, Nijman IJ, Buntjer JB, et al. Genetic distances within and across cattle breeds as indicated by biallelic AFLP markers. Animal Genetics. 2002;**33**:280-286

[29] Negrini R, Milanesi E, Bozzi R, Pellecchia M, Ajmone-Marsan P. Tuscany autochthonous cattle breeds: An original genetic resource investigated by AFLP markers. Journal of Animal Breeding and Genetics. 2006;**123**:10-16

[30] De Marchi M, Dalvit C, Targhetta C, Cassandro M. Assessing genetic diversity in indigenous Veneto chicken breeds using AFLP markers. Animal Genetics. 2006;**37**:101-105

[31] SanCristobal M, Chevalet C, Haley CS, Joosten R, Rattink AP, Harlizius B, et al. Genetic diversity within and between European pig breeds using microsatellite markers. Animal Genetics. 2006;**37**:189-198

[32] Paun O, Schönswetter P. Amplified Fragment Length Polymorphism (AFLP) - an invaluable fingerprinting technique for genomic, transcriptomic and epigenetic studies. Methods in Molecular Biology. 2012;**862**:75-87

[33] Buntjer JB, Otsen M, Nijman IJ, Kuiper MT, Lenstra JA. Phylogeny of bovine species based on AFLP fingerprinting. Heredity. 2002;**88**:46-51

[34] Goldstein DB, Schlötterer C. Microsatellites: Evolution and Applications. New York, Etats-Unis d'Amérique: Oxford University Press; 1999

[35] Jarne P, Lagoda PJL. Microsatellites, from molecules to populations and back. Tree. 1996;**11**:424-429

[36] Nijman IJ, Otsen M, Verkaar EL, de Ruijter C, Hanekamp E. Hybridization of banteng *(Bos javanicus)* and zebu *(Bos indicus)* revealed by mitochondrial DNA, satellite DNA, AFLP and microsatellites. Heredity. 2003;**90**:10-16

[37] Marcela AAV, Rafael LG, Lucas ACB, Paulo RE, Alessandra ATC, Sergio C. Principles and applications of polymerase chain reaction in medical diagnostic fields: A review. Brazilian Journal of Microbiology. 2009;**40**:1-11

[38] Lynch JR, Brown JM. The polymerase chain reaction: Current and future clinical applications. Journal of Medical Genetics. 1990;**27**:2-7

[39] Shafique S. Polymerase Chain Reaction. Riga, Latvia: LAP Lambert Academic Publishing; 2012. p. 3659134791

[40] Freeman WM, Walker SJ, Vrana KE. Quantitative RT-PCR: Pitfalls and potential. BioTechniques. 1999;**26**(1):112-122. 124-125

[41] Joyce C. Quantitative RT-PCR. A review of current methodologies. Methods in Molecular Biology. 2002;**193**:83-92

[42] Rajeevan MS, Vernon SD, Taysavang N, Unger ER. Validation of array-based gene expression profiles by real-time (kinetic) RT-PCR. The Journal of Molecular Diagnostics. 2001;**3**(1):26-31

[43] Annapaula G, Lut O, Dirk V, Brigitte D, Roger B, Chantal M. An overview of real-time quantitative PCR: Applications to quantify cytokine gene expression. Methods. 2001;**25**:386-401

[44] Bustin SA, Benes V, Nolan T, Pfaffl MW. Quantitative real-time RT-PCR—A perspective. Journal of Molecular Endocrinology. 2005;**34**:597-601

[45] Bustin SA, Nolan T. Pitfalls of quantitative real-time reverse-transcription polymerase chain reaction. Methods. 2001;**25**:386-401

[46] David G, Ginzinger H. Gene quantification usingreal-time quantitative PCR: An emerging technology hits the mainstream. Experimental Hematology. 2002;**30**:503-512

[47] Jochen W, Alfred P. Real-time polymerase chain reaction. Chembiochem. 2003;**4**:1120-1128

[48] Schmittgen TD, Livak KJ. Analyzing real-time PCR data by the comparative C(T) method. Nature Protocols. 2008;**3**(6):1101-1108

[49] Tse C, Capeau J. Quantification des acides nucléiques par PCR quantitative en temps réel. Annale de Biologie Clinique. 2003;**61**:279-293

[50] Yong-l O, Alexandra I. Quantitative real-time PCR: A critique of method and practical considerations. Hematology. 2002;**7**(1):59-67

[51] Simone M, Carlos RR, Pierluigi P, Donato N, Francesco MM. Quantitative real-time PCR: A powerful ally in cancer research. Trends in Molecular Medicine. 2003;**9**(5):189-195

[52] Chumming D, Charles RC. Quantitative analysis of nucleic acids—The last few years of progress. Biochemistry and Molecular Biology. 2004;**37**(1):1-10

[53] Cavé H, Acquaviva C, Bièche I, Brault D, de Fraipont F, Fina F, et al.

La RT-PCR en diagnostique clinique. Annale de Biologie Clinique. 2003;**61**:635-644

[54] Stephen B, Mueller R. Realtime reverse transcription PCR (qRT-PCR) and its potential use in clinical diagnosis. Clinical Science. 2005;**109**:365-379

[55] Phillip S, Bernard C, Wittwer T. Reamtime PCR technology for cancer diagnostics. Clinical Chemistry. 2002;**48**(8):1178-1185

[56] Lin MH, Chen TC, Kuo TT, Tseng C, Tseng CP. Real-time PCR for quantitative detection of *Toxoplasma gondii*. Journal of Clinical Microbiology. 2000;**38**:4121-4125

[57] Martell M, Gomez J, Esteban JI, Sauleda S, Quer J, Cabot B, et al. High-throughput real-time reverse transcription-PCR quantitation of Hepatitis C virus RNA. Journal of Clinical Microbiology. 1999;**37**:327-332

[58] Chen W, Martinez G, Mulchandani A. Molecular beacons: A real time polymerase chain reaction assay for detecting *Salmonella*. Analytical Biochemistry. 2000;**280**:166-172

[59] Fortin NY, Mulchandani A, Chen W. Use of real time polymerase chain reaction and molecular beacons for the detection of *Escherichia coli* O157:H7. Analytical Biochemistry. 2001;**289**:281-288

[60] Jeyaseelan K, Ma D, Armugam A. Real-time detection of gene promotor activity: Quantification of toxin gene transcription. Nucleic Acids Research. 15 June 2001;**29**(12):e58

[61] Gibson UE, Heid CA, Williams PM. A novel method for real time quantitative RT-PCR. Genome Research. 1996;**6**:995-1001

[62] Giesendorf BA, Tyagi JA, Mensink S, Trijbels EJ, Blom HJ. Molecular beacons: A new approach for semiautomated mutation analysis. Clinical Chemistry. 1998;**44**:482-486

[63] Higuchi R, Dollinger G, Walsh PS, Griffith R. Simultaneous amplification and dectection of specific DNA sequences. Biotechnology. 1992;**10**:413-417

[64] Poddar SK. Detection of adenovirus using PCR and molecular beacon. Journal of Virological Methods. 1999;**82**:19-26

[65] Yong IO, Alexandra I. Quantitative real-time PCR: A critique of method and practical considerations. Hematology. 2002;**7**(1):59-67

[66] Ravasi DF, Peduzzi S, Guidi V, Peduzzi R, Wirth, SB, Gilli A, et al. Development of a real-time PCR method for the detection of fossil 16S rDNA fragments of phototrophics ulfur bacteria in the sediments of Lake Cadagno. Geobiology. 2012;**10**:196-204

Chapter 10

Annealing Temperature of 55°C and Specificity of Primer Binding in PCR Reactions

Marjanca Starčič Erjavec

Abstract

In our study, we used PCR to clone *papA*, *papEF*, *papG* and *F17G* genes of *Escherichia coli* isolated from faecal samples of dogs with diarrhoea. Annealing temperature of 55°C was used in the PCR. Nucleotide sequence analysis of 26 cloned PCR products showed that in PCRs with *papA* primers, six out of eight obtained PCR products were false due to non-specific binding of the forward primer on both DNA strands; in PCRs with the *papEF* primers, all seven obtained PCR products originated from specific binding of the forward primer on the 3′ → 5′ DNA strand and non-specific binding of the forward primed on the 5′ → 3′ DNA strand; and in PCRs with the *F17G* primers, four out of eight obtained PCR products were false due to non-specific binding of forward and reverse primer. The anticipated annealing sites for non-specific primer binding in analysed nucleotide sequences are presented. In the case of PCR products obtained with *papG*-specific primers, all PCR products were amplifications of the *papG* sequence. When the annealing temperature of *papA* PCRs was raised to 60°C, all obtained PCR products were amplifications of the correct DNA sequences.

Keywords: primer binding, annealing temperature, sequence analysis, *Escherichia coli*, adhesin, P-fimbriae, F17-fimbriae

1. Introduction

Since polymerase chain reaction (PCR) was invented in the mid-1980s, it has made its way into all molecular biology, genetic, microbiology or biochemistry laboratories, where it is, due to its simplicity and efficiency, used in a very wide range of (PCR)-based techniques and applications [1, 2]. In just a few hours with a certain amount of cycles consisting of three simple steps—DNA denaturation, annealing of primers and extension [2]—the desired DNA sequence is multiplied about a million fold [3]. The crucial step in PCR is the annealing of primers, where the annealing temperature determines the specificity of primer annealing. The annealing temperature of a standard PCR protocol is either 55°C [2, 3] or 60°C [4]. The chosen temperature depends on the strand-melting temperature of the primers and the desired specificity. For greater stringency higher temperatures are recommended [2].

PCR is very often used to amplify specific DNA fragments that are later cloned as inserts in plasmid vectors and used then in subsequent experiments. Examples of such subsequent experiments are nucleotide sequencing, in order to determine the nucleotide sequence of the insert or in vitro transcription, and translation, in order to obtain a certain protein.

In our experiments, the aim was to determine the nucleotide sequence of several fimbrial genes from different *Escherichia coli* (*E. coli*) strains isolated from faecal samples of dogs with diarrhoea. The genes of interest were *papA*, *papG*, *papEF* of the P-fimbriae and *F17G* of the F17-fimbriae. Therefore, from a collection of 24 clinical haemolytic *E. coli* strains from faecal samples of dogs with diarrhoea [5], genomic DNA was isolated and used as the matrix DNA to amplify these genes of interest with gene-specific primers with PCR. Further, the obtained PCR products were cloned into a TA cloning vector, and the nucleotide sequence was determined.

2. *Escherichia coli*

Escherichia coli is one of the best studied organisms. It belongs to the family of *Enterobacteriaceae*. It is a Gram-negative rod-shaped bacterium, non-sporulating, non-motile or motile by peritrichous flagella, chemoorganotrophic, facultative anaerobic, producing acid from glucose, catalase positive, oxidase negative and mesophilic [6].

It is a well-known commensal bacterium that is part of the gut microbiota of humans and other warm-blooded organisms. However, also pathogenic strains of *E. coli* do exist and can cause a variety of intestinal and extraintestinal infections in humans and many animal hosts. *E. coli* is considered to be one of the most important pathogens; it is the most frequently isolated species in clinical microbiology laboratories [7]. Intestinal pathogenic *E. coli* (IPEC) strains, also called diarrhoeagenic *E. coli* (DEC) strains, are divided into six different well-described categories, i.e. pathotypes: enteropathogenic *E. coli* (EPEC), enterohaemorrhagic *E. coli* (EHEC), enterotoxigenic *E. coli* (ETEC), enteroaggregative *E. coli* (EAEC), enteroinvasive *E. coli* (EIEC) and diffusely adherent *E. coli* (DAEC) [8]. DEC causes diarrhoea syndromes that vary in clinical presentation and pathogenesis depending on the strain's pathotype [7]. *E. coli* strains involved in diarrhoeal diseases are one of the most important among the various etiological agents of diarrhoea [9]. The extraintestinal pathogenic *E. coli* (ExPEC) strain group is comprised of different *E. coli* associated with infections of extraintestinal anatomic sites [10]. Traditionally, the ExPEC isolates are separated into groups determined by disease association, i.e. uropathogenic *E. coli* (UPEC), neonatal meningitis-associated *E. coli* (NMEC) and sepsis-causing *E. coli* (SEPEC), naming the most important ExPEC groups. But ExPEC strains are also implicated in infections originating from abdominal and pelvic sources (e.g. biliary infections, infective peritonitis and pelvic inflammatory disease) and also associated with skin and soft tissue infections and hospital-acquired pneumonia [11]. Due to its genotypic and phenotypic diversity, *E. coli* is known as the paradigm for a versatile bacterial species [12].

The pathogenic strains possess specialised virulence factors such as adhesins, toxins, iron acquisition systems, polysaccharide coats and invasins that are not present in commensal strains [7].

3. Adhesins

Adhesins play a very important role in the host-microbe interactions, as they convey the adherence to the epithelial host's cells, surface structures or molecules.

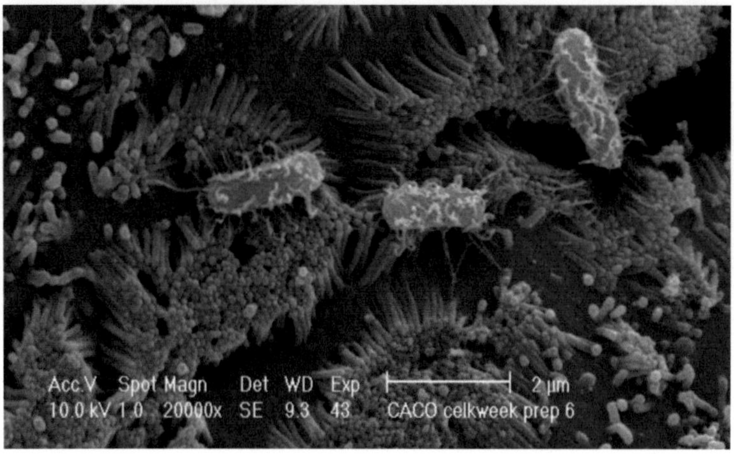

Figure 1.
Scanning electron microscopy of Escherichia coli strain 963 adhering to 19-day-old Caco-2 cells [5]. The fimbrial structures on the bacterial surfaces are promoting the bacterial adherence to receptors on host cells.

Adhesion is the essential first step for most commensal and pathogenic bacteria in order to colonise and persist within the host [13]. While adhesion to abiotic surfaces is usually mediated by non-specific interactions, adhesion to biotic surfaces typically involves specific receptor-ligand interaction [14]. Adhesins are structures on the bacterial surface that help the bacteria to bind to receptors on host's cells (**Figure 1**).

Adhesins are not just involved in adherence but also in bacterial invasion, survival, biofilm formation, serum resistance and cytotoxicity [15]. Moreover, they are also involved in bacterial motility and DNA transfer [13]. They differ in their architecture and receptor specificities. Types of adhesin vary depending on the Gram nature of bacteria [15].

Adhesins are among the most important virulence-associated properties of *E. coli*, as they are the main virulence factors of bacteria needed in bacterial colonisation. There are two types of bacterial adhesins: fimbrial and afimbrial [16].

Fimbrial adhesins, i.e. fimbriae, are rodlike structures with a diameter of 5–7 nm. Each fimbria consists out of several hundred copies of a protein, whose generic name is 'major subunit', and other proteins, present in one or a very few copy number and called 'minor subunits' that are positioned either at the basis or at the top of the fimbriae or intercalated between the 'major subunits' [16]. Fimbriae can be even longer than 1 µm [13]. On the bacterial surface of wild-type *E. coli* strains, there are around 500 fimbriae [17]. P-fimbriae and F-17 fimbriae belong to the fimbrial adhesins.

Non-fimbrial adhesins are monomeric or trimeric structures that decorate the surface of bacteria. These adhesins are anchored to the surface of the outer membrane and due to their small size, the size of non-fimbrial adhesins is approximately 15 nm, allow an intimate contact between the bacterial cell surface and specific substrates. One of the major classes of non-fimbrial adhesins is autotransporter adhesins [13].

3.1 P-fimbriae

P-fimbriae are the most extensively studied adhesins. They are also the first virulence-associated factor found among uropathogenic *E. coli*. These fimbriae bind to Gal(α1–4)Galβ moieties of the membrane glycolipids on human erythrocytes

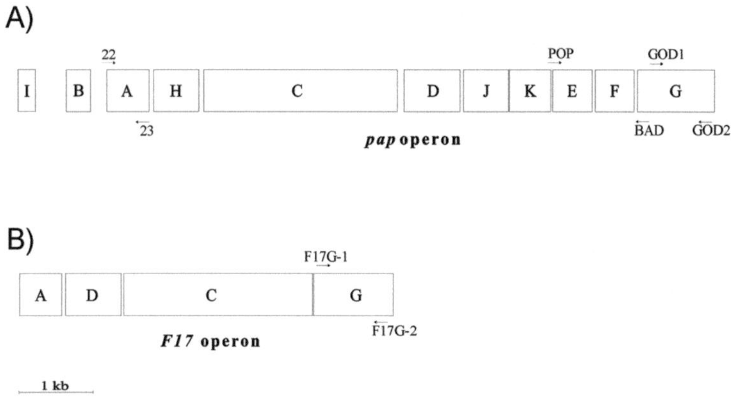

Figure 2.
Scheme of pap and F17 operon and annealing sites of the used primers. Genes in the operon are presented as boxes. The positions of used primers to amplify the studied genes are marked with arrows.
(A) Scheme of pap operon. The scheme of pap operon was drawn based on the GenBank deposited nucleotide sequence X61239.1 [20] and (B) scheme of F17 operon. The scheme of F17 operon was drawn based on the GenBank deposited nucleotide sequence L77091.1 [26].

of the P blood group and on uroepithelial cell fimbriae [18]. Further receptors for P-fimbriae are present on erythrocytes from pigs, pigeon, fowl, goats and dogs but not on those from cows, guinea pigs or horses [19]. These fimbriae are encoded in the *pap* operon, consisting of 11 different genes (see **Figure 2A**): *papA* (558 bp), *papB* (315 bp), *papC* (2511 bp), *papD* (720 bp), *papE* (522 bp), *papF* (504 bp), *papG* (1008 bp), *papH* (588 bp), *papI* (234 bp), *papJ* (582 bp) and *papK* (537 bp) [20].

The product of the *papA* gene is the major subunit protein A (19.5 kDa) [19]. In *papB* a regulatory protein (13 kDa) is encoded. PapB is necessary for the activation of the *papA* expression [21]. PapC (80 kDa) is located in the outer membrane and forms the assembly platform for fimbrial growth. PapD (27.5 kDa) is present in the periplasmic space and is involved in the translocation of fimbrial subunits across the periplasmic space to the outer membrane prior to assembly. PapE (16.5 kDa), PapF (15 kDa) and PapG (35 kDa) are minor fimbrial components. PapG is the adhesin molecule conferring the binding specificity [19]. PapH (20 kDa) terminates fimbrial assembly and helps anchor the fully grown fimbriae to the cell surface [22]. PapI (12 kDa) is another regulatory protein involved in *papA* expression due to activation of *papB* promoter [21]. PapJ (18 kDa) is a periplasmic protein required to maintain the integrity of P-fimbriae [23]. PapK (20 kDa) regulates the length of the tip fibrillum and joins it to the rod [24].

Many variants of P-fimbriae exist. PapA molecules from different P-fimbrial serovariants have a high degree of similarity at the N and C termini, while the central portions of PapA exhibit a great variation in the primary structure. This central part of PapA is hydrophilic and exposed and hence under selective pressure from the host immune system. Substantial heterogeneity is also between different minor fimbrial subunits (PapE, PapF and PapG) [19]. In addition also P-fimbria-related fimbriae, the so-called Prs-fimbriae, exist. Prs-fimbriae are encoded in the *prs* (*pap*-related sequence) operon [18].

3.2 F17-fimbriae

F17-fimbriae are found on pathogenic *E. coli* strains, isolated from infections in domestic animals. They are mainly detected on bovine and ovine *E. coli* associated with diarrhoea or septicaemia but also on *E. coli* from other hosts, including humans. The F17 adhesin binds to N-acetyl-D-glucosamin receptors of bovine intestinal cells;

however, F17 subtypes were also found to bind to N-acetyl-D-glucosamin receptors of human uroepithelial and intestinal cells [25]. The F17-fimbriae are encoded in the *F17* operon, consisting of four genes: *F17A* (546 bp), *F17D* (723 bp), *F17C* (2469 bp) and *F17G* (1035 bp) (see **Figure 2B**) [26].

F17A protein (20 kDa [25]) is the structural component of the F17-fimbriae (major subunit protein). The F17A protein is homologous to PapA protein of the P-fimbriae [27]. F17C protein (90 kDa) probably functions as a base protein on which the fimbrial subunits are polymerised. F17D protein (28 kDa) has a close homology to the PapD protein of the P-fimbriae [28]. It functions as the periplasmic transport protein [29]. F17G protein (36 kDa [25]) is the minor fimbrial component required for the binding of the F17-fimbriae to its receptor on the host cell [30].

Several variants of F17-fimbriae exist. The diversity is based on differences in F17A and F17G genes. The variant of F17-fimbriae found in humans is designated as G-fimbriae, encoded in the *gaf* operon [25].

4. Materials and methods

4.1 Bacterial strains, growth media and conditions

The analysed 24 clinical haemolytic *E. coli* strains [5] originated from dogs with diarrhoea and were isolated at the Veterinary Microbiological Diagnostics Centre of Utrecht University, the Netherlands. Some more details about the strains are given in **Table 1**. As positive control strains, a dog uropathogenic *E. coli* strain (strain 1473) and a cattle mastitis *E. coli* strain (strain E5) from Wim Gaastra's *E. coli* collection were used [31].

All used bacterial strains were stored at −80°C as a suspension in a 1:1 mixture of L-broth and glycerol as published by Garcia et al. [32]. The strains were grown overnight on LB plates and in liquid LB medium at 37°C. When grown in liquid LB medium, the flasks with the bacterial culture were incubated with aeration.

4.2 Isolation of chromosomal DNA

Chromosomal DNA was isolated from all 24 clinical haemolytic *E. coli* strains [5] and strains used for positive controls [31] using a slightly modified protocol based on the protocol of miniprep of bacterial genomic DNA published by Ausubel et al. [33]. To summarise, 2 ml of an overnight bacterial culture was centrifuged for 2 min at 14,000 rpm at room temperature. The obtained bacterial pellet was resuspended in 567 μl of buffer TE and 6 μl of 0.5 M EDTA. The suspension was incubated for 15 min at −80°C. Following the incubation at −80°C, the suspension was thawed, and 10 μl of 25 mg/ml proteinase K solution was added. The suspension was mixed thoroughly, and 30 μl of 10% SDS was added to the suspension and mixed thoroughly again. A 2-hour incubation at 37°C followed, and then 100 μl of 5 M NaCl was added to the suspension and mixed thoroughly. Next 80 μl of CTAB/NaCl was added, mixed thoroughly again and incubated at 65°C for 10 min. After the incubation the suspension was treated with 200 μl of chloroform/isoamyl alcohol and centrifuged for 5 min at 14,000 rpm at room temperature. The aqueous supernatant was transferred to a fresh microcentrifuge tube and treated with 100 μl of phenol/chloroform/isoamyl alcohol and centrifuged for 5 min at 14,000 rpm at room temperature. The aqueous supernatant was transferred to a fresh microcentrifuge tube, and the DNA in the aqueous supernatant was precipitated with addition of 0.6 volume of isopropanol. The precipitated chromosomal DNA was transferred to a fresh microcentrifuge tube containing 100 μl of 70% ethanol. The precipitated

Strain number	Dog's age	Clinical signs	Serotype	MSHA	MRHA
297	Unknown	Unknown	O78K?	E, P, C	C
333	Young dog	Chronic diarrhoea	O6K53	E, P, C, O	P, O
366	Unknown	Unknown	NT	B, E, P, C, O	B, E, P, O
375	Pup	Sepsis	O20K?	None	P
380	Unknown	Unknown	O6K-	B, E, P, C, O	P, C, O
442	Pup	Sepsis diarrhoea	O4K2	B, P, C, O	E, P, C, O
450	Pup	Sepsis diarrhoea	O42K-	E, P, C	None
467	5 months	Chronic diarrhoea	O6K1	E, P, C, O	P, C
479	Pup	Sepsis diarrhoea	O23K1	B, E, P, C	P, C, O
503	Unknown	Unknown	O42K-	C, O	None
555	Pup	Sepsis diarrhoea	O4K53	E, P, C, O	O
567	3 months	Recurrent diarrhoea	O4K?	E, P, C, O	P, C, O
727	3 months	Unknown	O139K?	E, P, C	P
734	18 months	Chronic diarrhoea	O4K?	E, P, C, O	E, P, C, O
740	4 years	Chronic diarrhoea	O25K13	E, P, C, O	P, C, O
759	12 months	Chronic diarrhoea	O4K?	P, O	P, O
857	9 months	Chronic diarrhoea	NT	P, C, O	P, O
897	Unknown	Chronic diarrhoea	O6K53	B, E, P, C, O	B, E, P, C, O
912	Old dog	Chronic diarrhoea	O4K-	E, P, C, O	E, P, C, O
958	Pup	Sepsis diarrhoea	NT	B, C, O	None
963	Unknown	Chronic diarrhoea	O4K?	B, E, P, C	B, E, P, C
996	4 months	Unknown	O4K?	E, P, C, O	O
1205	Unknown	Chronic diarrhoea	O4K-	E, P, C, O	E, P, C, O
1237	3 months	Bloody diarrhoea	O2K1	B, E, P, C, O	B, E, P, C, O

MSHA is an abbreviation of mannose-sensitive haemagglutination, and MRHA is an abbreviation of mannose-resistant haemagglutination. The erythrocytes are abbreviated as follows: B, bovine erythrocytes; E, equine erythrocytes; C, canine; O, ovine; P, porcine. NT, non-typable.

Table 1.
Characteristics of the 24 studied E. coli strains [5, 31].

DNA in 70% ethanol was pelleted with centrifugation (10 min at 14,000 rpm at room temperature). The 70% ethanol was then removed and the chromosomal DNA pellet air-dried at 37°C. Finally the chromosomal DNA pellet was dissolved in 100 μl of sterile distilled water.

4.3 PCR mixtures for PCR amplification of P- and F17-fimbrial genes

One μl of the isolated chromosomal DNA was used in 50 μl PCR mixtures consisting of 20 pmol of each primer, 0.2 mM dNTP mixture and 0.625 U of *Taq*-polymerase in PCR buffer [5]. In PCRs for P-fimbrial genes for positive control samples, the isolated chromosomal DNA of the dog uropathogenic *E. coli* strain (strain 1473) was used. In PCRs for F17-fimbrial gene for positive control samples, the isolated chromosomal DNA of the cattle mastitis *E. coli* strain (strain E5) was used. In all PCRs for the negative control, sterile distilled water was used [31].

4.4 Primers and PCRs used to amplify P- and F17-fimbrial genes

Primers used in the PCRs to amplify the studied genes are listed in **Table 2**.

PCR for gene(s)	Primers (name, sequence of the primer 5′ → 3′)	Tm (°C) of primers
papA	22	84.1
	ATGATGAATTCGGTTATTGCCGGTGCGG	
	23	68.3
	CTGAGAATTCAGGTTGAAATTCGC	
papEF	POP	63.8
	CCACGTTTGAATTGACATATCG	
	BAD	72.9
	CCGTAGCAATGCCCGGGC	
papG	GOD1	65.5
	ATGGTACCCAGCTTTGTTATTTTCC	
	GOD2	62.4
	TGGCAATATCATGAGAAGCTTT	
F17G	F17G-1	72.4
	CAGGCGGCAGTTTCATTTATTGGC	
	F17G-2	76.4
	CCGGACTGAGGGTGACGTTTCCGT	

Table 2.
Primers and their melting temperatures (Tm) used to amplify the studied genes.

Predicted primer annealing sites of the used primers on the target operons are shown in **Figure 2**.

The PCR amplification in all the reactions for all studied genes was carried out in the following steps: heating at 94°C for 4 min, followed by 35 cycles of denaturation at 94°C for 1 min, annealing at 55°C for 1 min, extension at 72°C for 1 min and the final extension for 10 min at 72°C.

The expected sizes of PCR products were determined with the 'Primer-BLAST' online tool (data set nr organism *Escherichia coli*) on the Internet page of the National Center for Biotechnology Information, US National Library of Medicine (http://www.ncbi.nlm.nih.gov) as follows: *papA*—552 bp (GenBank deposited nucleotide sequence LR134092.1), 555 bp (GenBank deposited nucleotide sequence CP025703.1), 534 bp (GenBank deposited nucleotide sequence CP018957.1), 564 bp (GenBank deposited nucleotide sequence CP029579.1) and 561 bp (GenBank deposited nucleotide sequence CP024886.1); *papEF*—1372 bp (GenBank deposited nucleotide sequence CP027701.1), 1373 bp (GenBank deposited nucleotide sequence CP028304.1), 1367 bp (GenBank deposited nucleotide sequence CP026853.1) and 1371 bp (GenBank deposited nucleotide sequence LR134238.1); *papG*—1000 bp (GenBank deposited nucleotide sequence CP026853.1) and 1003 bp (GenBank deposited nucleotide sequence M20181.1); and *F17G*—888 bp (GenBank deposited nucleotide sequence AF055313.1) and 885 bp (GenBank deposited nucleotide sequence CP001162.1).

4.5 Agarose gel electrophoresis

Samples of isolated chromosomal DNA (5 μl of isolated chromosomal DNA and 1 μl of 6 × loading dye) were subjected to analysis with agarose gel electrophoresis using

1% of agarose gels with 0.5 μg/ml ethidium bromide, run in 0.5 × TBE electrophoresis buffer. Samples of obtained PCR products (25 μl of PCR products, 5 μl of 6 × loading dye) were subjected to analysis with agarose gel electrophoresis using 1% of agarose gels with 0.5 μg/ml ethidium bromide, run in 1 × TAE electrophoresis buffer. Used protocols for agarose gel electrophoresis were based on Sambrook et al. [34]. For DNA ladder the lambda bacteriophage DNA digested with the restriction endonuclease *Pst*I was used.

4.6 Cloning of PCR products and DNA sequencing of cloned PCR products amplified in PCRs for P- and F17-fimbrial genes

Cloning of PCR products and DNA sequencing of cloned PCR products obtained in the PCRs for P- and F17-fimbrial genes was done as described by Starčič et al. [5]. In short, obtained PCR products were cut out of the agarose gel, cleaned with the GeneClean II Kit, inserted into the TA cloning vector pMOSBlue and then transformed to electrocompetent *E. coli* pMOSBlue cells. Subsequently, the plasmid DNA was isolated from pMOSBlue cells using the FlexiPrep Kit, and the nucleotide sequence was determined with the dideoxynucleotide chain termination method using an automated laser fluorescence sequencer. All procedures were performed according to the manufacturers' protocols.

4.7 Analysis of cloned nucleotide sequences of the PCR products amplified in PCRs for P- and F17-fimbrial genes

Sequence analysis of the cloned fragments, originated from PCR products obtained in PCRs for P- and F17-fimbrial genes, was performed with the computer program BLAST on the Internet page of the National Center for Biotechnology Information, US National Library of Medicine (http://www.ncbi.nlm.nih.gov) searching for homology in the GenBank nr database.

5. Results

5.1 Analysis of cloned nucleotide sequences from PCRs with primers specific for *papA*

An annealing temperature of 55°C was used in the PCRs for the amplification of the *papA* gene with primers 22 and 23. The obtained PCR products were all of the expected size (around 600 bp). However, the nucleotide sequence analysis of the eight obtained cloned PCR products revealed that six clones harboured false, non-*papA* inserts. Four of these false clones derived from amplification of part of methylisocitrate lyase gene, and two clones derived from amplification of part of the RNA-binding protein Hfq gene and part of the GTPase HflX gene, as revealed by BLAST analysis. In both cases even though both primers, forward primer 22 and reverse primer 23, were added to the PCR mixture, the primer 22 was used as the forward but also the reverse primer. Further nucleotide analysis revealed that in the case of the amplification of part of the methylisocitrate lyase gene, the forward primer annealed downstream from the c348059 position of the $3' \rightarrow 5'$ strand and reverse primer upstream of the 348539 position on the $5' \rightarrow 3'$ DNA strand of the *E. coli* K-12 MG1655 sequence as deposited in the CP025268.1 nucleotide sequence [35]. The anticipated annealing sites for non-specific *papA*-primer binding in this case are presented in **Figure 3**.

In the case of the amplification of part of the RNA-binding protein Hfq gene and part of the GTPase HflX gene, the forward primer annealed downstream from

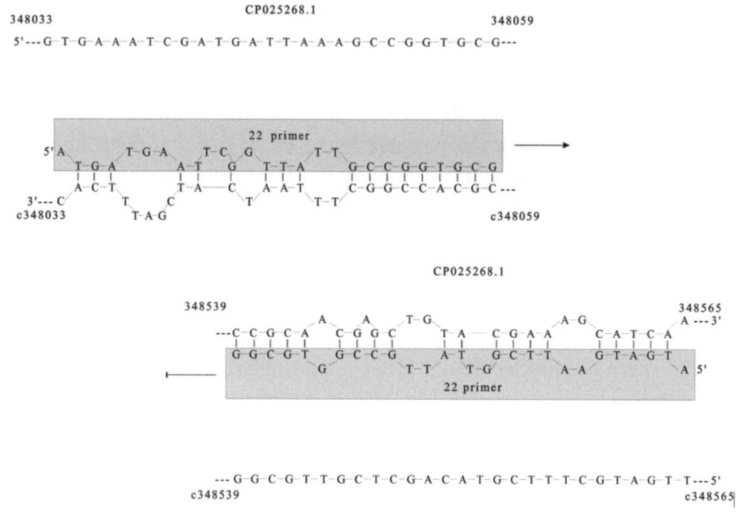

Figure 3.
Anticipated annealing sites for non-specific papA-primer binding in the methylisocitrate lyase gene. The shown sequences are enumerated according to the CP025268.1 GenBank deposited sequence [35]. The sequence and the complement chromosomal sequence are given. For the forward primer annealing site, the sequence from 348033 to 348059 nt is shown, and for the reverse primer annealing site, the sequence from 348539 to 348565 nt is shown. The primer sequence is in the grey box. The arrows mark the direction of DNA elongation in the PCR. The methylisocitrate lyase gene is positioned in the deposited sequence from 347733 to 348623 nt.

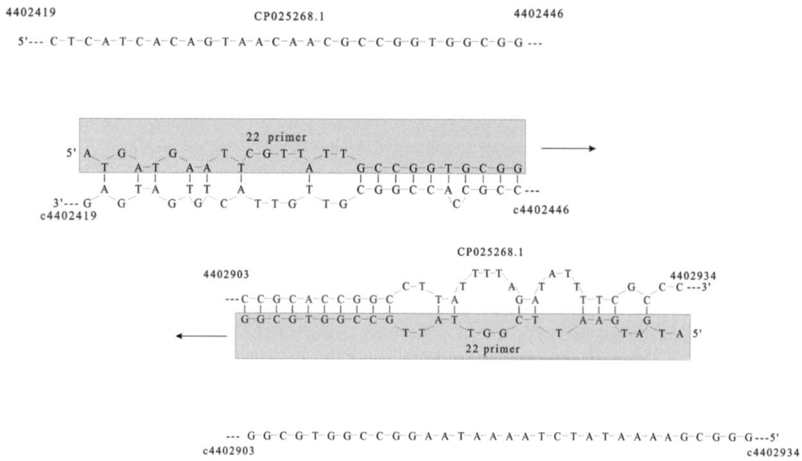

Figure 4.
Anticipated annealing sites for non-specific papA-primer binding in the RNA-binding protein Hfq gene (forward primer) and GTPase HflX gene (reverse primer). The shown sequences are enumerated according the CP025268.1 GenBank deposited sequence [35]. The sequence and the complement chromosomal sequence are given. For the forward primer annealing site, the sequence from 4402419 to 4402446 nt is shown, and for the reverse primer annealing site, the sequence from 4402903 to 4402934 nt is shown. The primer sequence is in the grey box. The arrows mark the direction of DNA elongation in the PCR. The RNA-binding protein Hfq gene is positioned in the deposited sequence from 4402214 to 4402522 nt, and the GTPase HflX gene is positioned from 4402598 to 4403878 nt.

the c4402446 position on the 3′ → 5′ DNA strand, and the reverse primer annealed upstream from the 4402903 position on the 5′ → 3′ DNA strand of the *E. coli* K-12 MG1655 sequence as deposited in the CP025268.1 nucleotide sequence [35]. The anticipated annealing sites for non-specific *papA*-primer binding in this case are presented in **Figure 4**.

5.2 Analysis of cloned nucleotide sequences from PCRs with primers specific for *papEF*

In the PCRs for the *papEF* amplification, also the annealing temperature of 55°C was used. Seven PCR products, all of the expected size, of around 1400 bp, were cloned, and the obtained insert sequences were analysed. All seven clones harboured the amplified *papEF*-related sequence, the *prsEF* sequence of the Prs-fimbriae (GenBank X61238.1 [36]); however, in all seven cases, only the forward POP primer annealed to the correct complementary sequence from c27 to c48 nt on the 3′ → 5′ DNA strand of the X61238.1, while the reverse primer was not as expected the BAD primer but again the POP primer, which annealed at another partially complementary sequence of the *prsEF* gene from 1357 upstream on the 5′ → 3′ DNA strand. Further BLAST analysis showed that the BAD primer has only a partial complementary region of nine nucleotides at the position 3229 to 3237 in the 5′ → 3′ DNA strand and at the position c3238 to c3230 in the 3′ → 5′ strand of the X61238.1 sequence. The anticipated annealing sites of POP primer on the analysed X61238.1 nucleotide sequences are presented in **Figure 5**.

5.3 Analysis of cloned nucleotide sequences from PCRs with primers specific for *papG*

In the PCRs for the *papG* amplification, also the annealing temperature of 55°C was used. Three PCR products, all of the expected size, of around 1000 bp, were obtained and cloned, and the obtained insert sequences were analysed. All three clones harboured the expected *papG* sequence. In all three PCR amplifications, both primers, the forward GOD1 and reverse GOD2 primer, annealed at the expected positions. The anticipated annealing sites for specific *papG*-primer binding

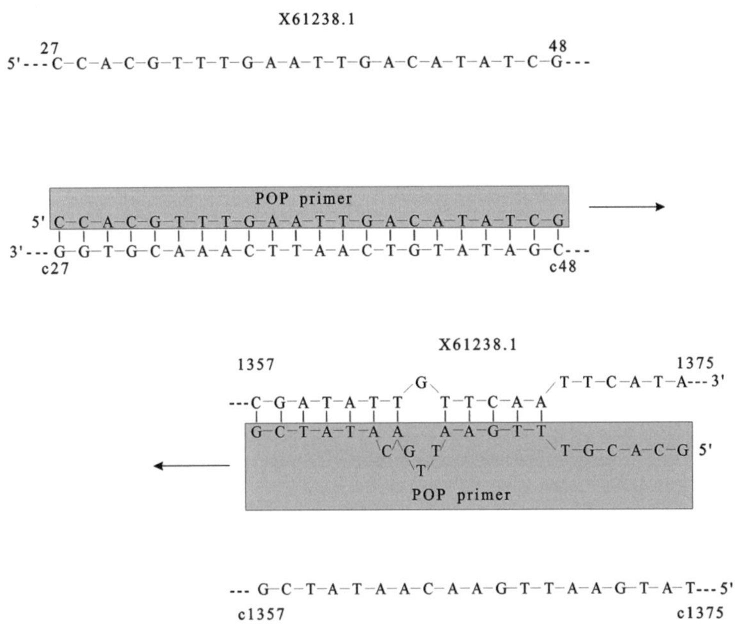

Figure 5.
Anticipated annealing sites of primer POP in the prsEF sequence. The shown sequences are enumerated according the X61238.1 GenBank deposited sequence [36]. The sequence and the complement chromosomal sequence are given. For the forward primer annealing site, the sequence from 27 to 48 nt is shown, and for the reverse primer annealing site, the sequence from 1357 to 1375 nt is shown. The primer sequence is in the grey box. The arrows mark the direction of DNA elongation in the PCR. The prsE gene is positioned in the deposited sequence from 79 to 600 nt, and the prsF gene is positioned from 676 to 1179 nt.

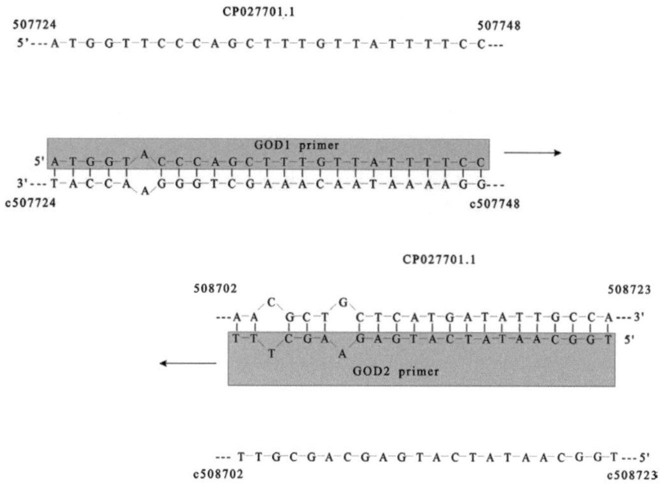

Figure 6.
Anticipated annealing sites of primer GOD1 and primer GOD2 in the papG sequence. The shown sequences are enumerated according the CP027701.1 GenBank deposited sequence [37]. The sequence and the complement chromosomal sequence are given. For the forward primer annealing site, the sequence from 507724 to 507748 nt is shown, and for the reverse primer annealing site, the sequence from 508702 to 508723 nt is shown. The primer sequence is in the grey box. The arrows mark the direction of DNA elongation in the PCR. The papG gene is positioned in the deposited sequence from 507716 to 508726 nt.

of GOD1 and GOD2 as revealed by analysis of the nucleotide *E. coli* sequence CP027701.1 [37] are presented in **Figure 6**.

5.1 Analysis of cloned nucleotide sequences from PCRs with primers specific for *F17G*

At the annealing temperature of 55°C with primers specific for the *F17G* gene, eight PCR products, again all of the expected size of approximately 900 bp, were obtained and cloned. Nucleotide sequence analysis of all eight clones showed that

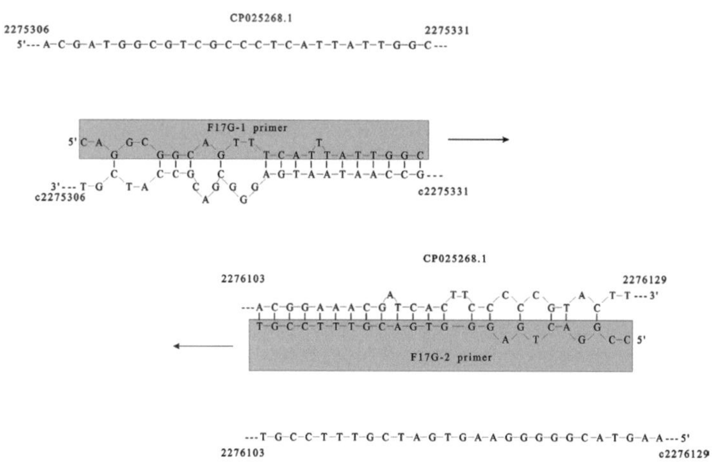

Figure 7.
Anticipated annealing sites for non-specific F17G-primer binding in the rtn gene. The shown sequences are enumerated according the CP025268.1 GenBank deposited sequence [35]. The sequence and the complement chromosomal sequence are given. For the forward primer, F17G-1, annealing site, the sequence from 2275306 to 2275331 nt is shown, and for the reverse primer, F17G-2, annealing site, the sequence from 2276103 to 2276129 nt is shown. The primer sequence is in the grey box. The arrows mark the direction of DNA elongation in the PCR. The rtn gene is positioned in the deposited sequence from 2274762 to 2276318 nt.

four harboured correct and four harboured false inserts. All four false inserts were, as BLAST revealed, sequences of the protein *rtn* gene of the *E. coli* K-12 MG1655 chromosome, as deposited in the CP025268.1 nucleotide sequence [35]. Further nucleotide analysis revealed that in the case of the *rtn* gene amplification, the forward primer F17G-1 annealed downstream from the c2275331 position on the 3′ → 5′ DNA strand and reverse primer F17G-2 upstream of the 2276103 position on the 5′ → 3′ DNA strand of the *E. coli* K-12 MG1655 CP025268.1 nucleotide sequence. The anticipated annealing sites for non-specific *F17G*-primer binding in analysed nucleotide sequences are presented in **Figure** 7.

6. Discussion

The main aim of our research was to determine the sequences of chosen P- and F17-fimbriae genes among *E. coli* isolated from faecal samples of diarrhoeic dogs. As we assumed that the fimbriae of such *E. coli* strains, due to already known variations of P- and F17-fimbriae, might have nucleotide differences, the annealing temperature of 55°C in the PCRs was used. To our surprise, even though only PCR products of expected sizes were cloned, many of the obtained PCR clones, in the case of PCR products obtained with *papA* primers 75% and in the case of PCR product obtained with *F17G* primers 50%, carried false inserts. Nucleotide sequence analysis revealed that also in the case of *papEF* clones, even though the cloned inserts were as hoped for fimbrial inserts, even if they were Prs-fimbrial genes, the binding site of the reverse primer was not the expected one. The high percentages of false PCR products were obtained when PCR primers with a high melting temperature (Tm) were used at the annealing temperature of 55°C—primer 22 has the Tm of 84.1°C, and 75% of false PCR products were obtained with this primer; primers F17G-1 and F17G-2 have the Tm of 72.4°C and 76.4°C, respectively, and 50% of false PCR products were obtained with them. In the consecutive PCR amplifications with the primers 22 and 23, the annealing temperature was raised to 60°C, and from these PCRs more PCR products were obtained, namely, 16. All 16 were cloned and analysed, and all clones were with correct inserts (data not shown).

7. Conclusion

To conclude, we all know that with PCR, we can obtain false unspecific products, and we believe that such PCR products will be distinguished from right PCR products, because the false PCR products will not be of the correct expected size; however, our results showed that also PCR products of the expected size can be false PCR products. In order to avoid false positive PCR results, it is therefore essential to use the right annealing temperature that should not be too different from the primer's melting temperature.

Acknowledgements

The author is very thankful to Wim Gaastra for the primer nucleotide sequences. This analysis was supported by the Slovenian Research Agency (P1-0198).

Conflict of interest

The author has no conflict of interest.

Author details

Marjanca Starčič Erjavec
Biotechnical Faculty, University of Ljubljana, Ljubljana, Slovenia

*Address all correspondence to: marjanca.starcic.erjavec@bf.uni-lj.si

References

[1] Watson JD, Gilman M, Witkowski J, Zoller M, Recombinant DNA. 2nd ed. New York: Scientific American Books; 1994

[2] White BA. PCR Protocols. Current Methods and Applications. 1st ed. Totowa: Humana Press Inc.; 1993

[3] Erlich HA. PCR Technology. Principles and Applications for DNA Amplification. 1st ed. New York: M Stockton Press; 1989

[4] McPherson MJ, Hames BD. PCR2: A Practical Approach. 1st ed. Oxford: IRL Press at Oxford University Press, Inc; 1995

[5] Starčič M, Johnson JR, Stell AL, van der Goot J, Hendriks HG, van Vorstenbosch C, et al. Haemolytic *Escherichia coli* isolated from dogs with diarrhea have characteristics of both uropathogenic and necrotoxigenic strains. Veterinary Microbiology. 2002;**85**:361-377

[6] Madigan MT, Martinko JM, Bender KS, Buckley DH, Stahl DA. Brock Biology of Microorganisms. 14th ed. London: Pearson Education, Inc; 2015

[7] Vila J, Sáez-López E, Johnson JR, Römling U, Dobrindt U, Cantón R, et al. *Escherichia coli*: An old friend with new tidings. FEMS Microbiology Reviews. 2016;**40**:437-463. DOI: 10.1093/femsre/fuw005

[8] Kaper JB, Nataro JP, Mobley HL. Pathogenic *Escherichia coli*. Nature Reviews. Microbiology. 2004;**2**:123-140

[9] Gomes TA, Elias WP, Scaletsky IC, Guth BE, Rodrigues JF, Piazza RM, et al. Diarrheagenic *Escherichia coli*. Brazilian Journal of Microbiology. 2016;**47**(Suppl 1): 3-30. DOI: 10.1016/j.bjm.2016.10.015

[10] Russo TA, Johnson JR. Proposal for a new inclusive designation for extraintestinal pathogenic isolates of *Escherichia coli*: ExPEC. The Journal of Infectious Diseases. 2000;**181**:1753-1754

[11] Dale AP, Woodford N. Extra-intestinal pathogenic *Escherichia coli* (ExPEC): Disease, carriage and clones. Journal of Infection. 2015;**71**:615-626. DOI: 10.1016/j.jinf.2015.09.009

[12] Leimbach A, Hacker J, Dobrindt U. *E. coli* as an all-rounder: The thin line between commensalism and pathogenicity. Current Topics in Microbiology and Immunology. 2013;**358**:3-32. DOI: 10.1007/82_2012_303

[13] Vo JL, Martínez Ortiz GC, Subedi P, Keerthikumar S, Mathivanan S, Paxman JJ, et al. Autotransporter adhesins in *Escherichia coli* pathogenesis. Proteomics. 2017;**17**:1600431. DOI: 10.1002/pmic.201600431

[14] Berne C, Ducret A, Hardy G, Brun YV. Adhesins involved in attachment to abiotic surfaces by Gram-negative bacteria. Microbiology Spectrum. 2015;**3**(4). DOI: 10.1128/microbiolspec.MB-0018-2015

[15] Patel S, Mathivanan N, Goyal A. Bacterial adhesins, the pathogenic weapons to trick host defense arsenal. Biomedicine & Pharmacotherapy. 2017;**93**:763-771. DOI: 10.1016/j.biopha.2017.06.102

[16] Mainil J. *Escherichia coli* virulence factors. Veterinary Immunology and Immunopathology. 2013;**152**:2-12. DOI: 10.1016/j.vetimm.2012.09.032

[17] Hacker J. Role of fimbrial adhesins in the pathogenesis of *Escherichia coli* infections. Canadian Journal of Microbiology. 1992;**38**:720-727

[18] Lane MC, Mobley HL. Role of P-fimbrial-mediated adherence in

pyelonephritis and persistence of uropathogenic *Escherichia coli* (UPEC) in the mammalian kidney. Kidney International. 2007;**72**:19-25

[19] Johnson JR. Virulence factors in *Escherichia coli* urinary tract infection. Clinical Microbiology Reviews. 1991;**4**:80-128

[20] GenBank X61239.1 [Internet]. 2005. Available from: http://www.ncbi.nlm.nih.gov/nuccore/x61239.1 [Accessed: 2019-25-01]

[21] Båga M, Göransson M, Normark S, Uhlin BE. Transcriptional activation of a Pap pilus virulence operon from uropathogenic *Escherichia coli*. EMBO Journal. 1985;**4**:3887-3893

[22] Båga M, Norgren M, Normark S. Biogenesis of *E. coli* Pap pili: papH, a minor pilin subunit involved in cell anchoring and length modulation. Cell. 1987;**49**:241-251

[23] Tennent JM, Lindberg F, Normark S. Integrity of *Escherichia coli* P pili during biogenesis: Properties and role of PapJ. Molecular Microbiology. 1990;**4**:747-758

[24] Jacob-Dubuisson F, Heuser J, Dodson K, Normark S, Hultgren S. Initiation of assembly and association of the structural elements of a bacterial pilus depend on two specialized tip proteins. EMBO Journal. 1993;**12**:837-847

[25] Le Bouguénec C, Bertin Y. AFA and F17 adhesins produced by pathogenic *Escherichia coli* strains in domestic animals. Veterinary Research. 1999;**30**:317-342

[26] GenBank L77091.1 [Internet]. 1996. Available from: http://www.ncbi.nlm.nih.gov/nuccore/L77091.1 [Accessed: 2019-25-01]

[27] Lintermans P, Pohl P, Deboeck F, Bertels A, Schlicker C, Vandekerckhove J, et al. Isolation and nucleotide sequence of the F17-A gene encoding the structural protein of the F17 fimbriae in bovine enterotoxigenic *Escherichia coli*. Infection and Immunity. 1988;**56**:1475-1484

[28] Lintermans P, Bertels A, Van Driessche E, De Greve D. Identification of the F17 gene cluster and development of adhesion blockers and vaccine components. In: Pusztai A, Bardocz S, editors. Lectins: Biomedical Perspectives. e-Library ed. London: Taylor & Francis Ltd.; 2005. pp. 246-261

[29] Bertels A, De Greve H, Lintermans P. Function and genetics of fimbrial and nonfimbrial lectins from *Escherichia coli*. In: Kilpatrick DC, Van Driessche E, B0g-Hansen TS, editors. Lectin Reviews 1. 1st ed. St. Louis: Sigma Chemical Co; 1991. pp. 53-67

[30] Lintermans PF, Bertels A, Schlicker C, Deboeck F, Charlier G, Pohl P, et al. Identification, characterization, and nucleotide sequence of the F17-G gene, which determines receptor binding of *Escherichia coli* F17 fimbriae. Journal of Bacteriology. 1991;**173**:3366-3373

[31] Starčič M, Virulenčni dejavniki sevov bakterije *Escherichia coli*, izoliranih iz psov z drisko [Virulence determinants of *Escherichia coli* strains isolated with diarrheic dogs]. Magistrska naloga [Master of Science Thesis]. Ljubljana: Univerza v Ljubljani, Medicinska fakulteta; 1997 [Ljubljana: University of Ljubljana, Medical Faculty; 1997]

[32] Garcia E, Bergmans HE, van den Bosch JF, Orskov I, van der Zeijst BA, Gaastra W. Isolation and characterisation of dog uropathogenic *Escherichia coli* strains and their fimbriae. Antonie Van Leeuwenhoek. 1988;**54**:149-163

[33] Ausubel FM, Brent R, Kingston RE, Moore DD, Seidman JG, Smith JA, et al.,

editors. Short Protocols in Molecular Biology. 2nd ed. New York: Green Publishing Associates and John Wiley & Sons; 1992

[34] Sambrook J, Fritsch EF, Maniatis T. Molecular Cloning: A Laboratory Manual. 2nd ed. New York: Cold Spring Harbor Laboratory Press; 1989

[35] GenBank CP025268.1 [Internet]. 2017. Available from: http://www.ncbi.nlm.nih.gov/nuccore/CP025268.1 [Accessed: 2019-25-01]

[36] GenBank X61238.1 [Internet]. 2005. Available from: http://www.ncbi.nlm.nih.gov/nuccore/X61238.1 [Accessed: 2019-25-01]

[37] GenBank CP027701.1 [Internet]. 2018. Available from: http://www.ncbi.nlm.nih.gov/nuccore/CP027701.1 [Accessed: 2019-25-01]

Chapter 11

Real-Time Quantitative PCR as a Tool for Monitoring Microbiological Quality of Food

Amanda Teixeira Sampaio Lopes
and Bianca Mendes Maciel

Abstract

Microbiological parameters of food provide quality information regarding the processing, storage, and distribution conditions, shelf life, as well as whether the food poses a health risk to the population. In this context, the concern with food safety is a competitive advantage, as the pressure of consumers, who are increasingly interested and concerned about what they are consuming, directs the trade to reach the quality of products and services offered. With regard to microbiological analyses, researchers have been developing sensitive techniques to produce rapid results, since traditional methods of microbiological culture are time-consuming and very laborious. Thus, the real-time quantitative PCR technique (qPCR) offers the possibility of quantifying the total bacterial DNA in a food sample without the need of the microbial growth step. That is, the result can be expressed on the same day, and it is possible to perform a simultaneous quantification of more than one pathogen in a single assay. Therefore, it can be a useful tool for monitoring microbiological quality in food industries. In this chapter, we will present the advantages and disadvantages of this methodology for food microbiology emphasizing the challenge of differentiating viable cells from nonviable cells.

Keywords: pathogen quantification, food microbiology, food safety, quantitative microbial risk assessment, propidium monoazide qPCR, ethidium monoazide qPCR

1. Introduction

The quality term has undergone variations over time. In the last century, the food quality was expressed only by the intrinsic and extrinsic characteristics of different individual units of a product which would determine its acceptability [1]. Currently, the term quality has already a broader aspect: it is related to the ability to plan and develop continuous actions during all stages of processing, aiming at maintaining the product characteristics and performance to reach the requirements that satisfy the needs and expectations of the consumer [2]. Thus, food companies seek to achieve more and more the quality standard of their products that will be delivered to the final consumer. In turn, the perception of quality by consumers is closely linked to the attributes they most value: nutrition and food safety.

IntechOpen

Food safety practices aim to ensure the appropriate physical, chemical, and microbiological conditions for product quality. For food industries, the safety aspect is always a determining factor about quality, since any problem can compromise the consumer health, culminating in serious financial losses and diminishing the reliability of their products. Thus, the industry advocates the application of food safety management system in the entire food production chain, as a preventative approach toward identifying, preventing, and reducing foodborne hazards, to ensure the food is safe for consumption and with nutritional value. Only then, the total quality of food can be reached [3–5].

One of the main parameters that determine the food quality is its microbiological characteristic, since microbial contamination is responsible for most foodborne disease (FBD) outbreaks in worldwide, affecting individuals of all ages, particularly children under 5 years of age and persons living in low-income regions of the world [6]. The microbiological evaluation is performed with the objective of establishing the absence of pathogens or their toxins and to enumerate total or indicator microorganisms that provide information about the conditions of processing, storage, distribution, shelf life, and the health risk of the population [7]. As such examples, we can cite the increased numbers of *Staphylococcus aureus* when detected in a food processing step might imply in contamination by handling, the increased numbers of *Escherichia coli* might suggest fecal contamination, and the detection of *Salmonella* spp. might indicate that the processing has not been able to eliminate pathogenic microorganisms [8].

The microbiological quality should be effectively focused on traceability, with emphasis on the "farm-to-fork" approach, reaching the entire food chain. For this, rapid diagnostic methods are highly recommended so that early interventions of control strategies can be applied, ensuring the consumer's health and reducing the financial losses of the industry, as well as the costs with public health in cases of FBD outbreaks. In addition, these methods are essential for assessment of food safety objectives (maximum levels of hazards at the point of consumption) in food safety management, which require results in a shorter time than those obtained by culture cultivation [9]. Among rapid methods, real-time quantitative polymerase chain reaction (qPCR) has been shown to be a good tool for monitoring microbiological quality of food, since this technique is evolving to improve the sensitivity and specificity in detection and quantification of pathogens. According to "MIQE guidelines" [10], we chose to use the abbreviation qPCR for real-time quantitative PCR in entire chapter, avoiding confusion with other abbreviations that designate reverse transcription-qPCR (RT-qPCR).

2. Advantages and disadvantages of real-time quantitative PCR for microbiological assessment of food quality

For more than a century, the identification and isolation of pathogens in food and clinical samples were performed exclusively by microbiological culture techniques. The analyses use a wide variety of selective, nonselective, and differential media. The suspect microbial colonies in these media are selected and isolated and need to go through yet another confirmation step, the biochemical tests. If a pathogen is detected, serological typing and more detailed biochemical tests are performed, and the data from these tests facilitate epidemiological analyses. However, even though these conventional methods are valuable, there is a great need of time (around 1 week) and material, making this technique inadequate in the event of a food outbreak. One of the main criticisms of conventional methods is that the results are available relatively late in clinical disease, limiting the overall value of the test. Treatment decisions are usually based on the clinical severity of the disease prior to receipt of confirmation of isolation of the microbial culture. This long period to diagnose foodborne diseases by traditional microbiological methods may have an impact on the clinical pathway for each patient. However, for isolation and identification of bacterial pathogens transmitted by food, these classical methods are still considered as the "gold standard," especially by regulatory agencies, since they are harmonized methods in worldwide [7, 11, 12].

In the last decades, several alternative methods have been developed with the purpose of producing fast microbiological results to ensure food safety and allowing manipulation of multiple samples in the same analysis [12]. These methods are based on chromogenic culture media, immunoassays for antigen detection, bacteriophage analysis, biosensors, or molecular methods that detect nucleic acids [11–15]. Among the molecular methods, polymerase chain reaction (PCR) is the most versatile and widely used amplification technique [12].

2.1 Principle of real-time quantitative PCR techniques

The real-time quantitative PCR technique (qPCR) is a variant of conventional PCR and offers the possibility of quantifying the pathogen DNA in a sample in real time, without the need of microbial growth steps. That is, the result can be expressed on the same day. In addition, it is possible to perform multiplex analyses, allowing simultaneous quantification of more than one pathogen in the same assay [16]. For absolute quantification of pathogens, it is necessary to design a standard curve through serial dilutions of a known amount of target DNA [17]. In this curve, the lowest DNA amount detectable by the technique may be included (< 10 copies of a target gene) to attest its sensitivity. The high sensitivity, specificity, and speed of results have allowed qPCR to be widely used for specific pathogen quantification in which microbial amount is low.

The use of qPCR, by reducing the time associated with generating quantitative data, offers the potential to increase the robustness of the quantitative microbial risk assessment, thus allowing a subsequent early intervention of control strategies. The quantification of a pathogen in a food product and the prevalence of contamination are important parts of the quantitative microbial risk assessment modeling process, because it needs to determine the probability of exposure as well as the amount of exposure to a pathogen [18].

The quantification through qPCR is based on the exponential increase of the initial DNA amount during PCR amplification cycles. After amplifying a specific sequence, the amplification progress is monitored in real time using fluorescence technology. As soon as the fluorescent signal reaches a threshold level, correlation with the amount of original target sequence occurs, thus allowing DNA quantification in a sample. In addition, the final product may further be characterized by gradual raising temperature during a melt curve to determine the "melt temperature." This point is reached when half of the DNA strand is on single strand and the other half on double strands. It depends on the length and composition of nucleotide sequence of the target gene, which increases the specificity of technique [19].

Among fluorescent reagents, the DNA intercalating agents (such as SYBR Green) and hydrolysis probes (also known as TaqMan™ probes) are the most popularly used. SYBR Green dye is a nonspecific detection system that promotes intercalation, followed by surface binding to double strands of newly amplified DNA [20]. As the DNA is amplified, the fluorescent signal is emitted by the reagent and detected by the equipment. As any DNA amplification can be detected and quantified, to help ensure the reaction specificity, the melt curve of the amplified product can be analyzed to determine the melt temperature (Tm). If there are two or Tm peaks, it is suggested that more than one sequence was amplified, and one may not be the specific DNA target [19] or even primer dimer.

The principle of detection system using the hydrolysis probes is based on Förster resonance energy transfer, when a non-radiative energy is transferred from a fluorescent donor (the fluorophore) to a lower energy acceptor (the quencher) via long-range dipole-dipole interactions [21, 22]. It occurs because the hydrolysis probes are small dual-labeled oligonucleotide sequences: in one side, it is labeled by a specific fluorophore, and the other side by the quencher. As the fluorophore and quencher are in close proximity, the quencher adsorbs the reporter fluorophore signal. When the DNA amplification occurs during qPCR reaction, the probe is hydrolyzed by the Taq DNA polymerase, due to its 5′-nuclease activity, and the fluorophore and quencher are separated, emitting fluorescence that corresponds to specific amplification of the target DNA [19]. The great advantage of qPCR using hydrolysis probes is that when the probes are labeled with fluorophores that emit fluorescence at different wavelengths, there is the possibility of performing a multiplex qPCR reaction in which more than two targets are detected and quantified simultaneously in a specific way [23]; therefore, it is a good alternative for use as a rapid test in large number of samples, providing real-time results, and to diminish the cost of analyses.

2.2 qPCR *versus* traditional culture method in food microbiology

Some studies comparing qPCR and microbial culture observed that qPCR for the detection of a single pathogen (singleplex assay) demonstrated to be statistically more sensitive than the conventional technique. Real-time PCR assay specific for detection of *Salmonella enterica* serotype enteritidis analyzed 422 naturally contaminated environmental samples from integrated poultry houses, being the same samples also evaluated by traditional microbiology. The diagnostic sensitivity of the qPCR assay for these samples was significantly higher than those using the culture method. In addition, the result of real-time PCR was obtained in 2 days, while the traditional method took 4–8 days [24]. Another study comparing standard culture methods, conventional PCR, and real-time PCR for the detection of *Listeria monocytogenes* in milk, cheese, fresh vegetables, and raw meat showed that the real-time PCR assay was statistically more sensitive, reducing the time of analysis and laborious work [25]. The targeted gene coding for a protein of the ribosome large subunit was used in qPCR for quantifying Enterobacteriaceae in 51 food products naturally contaminated. The results showed high specificity to differentiate Enterobacteriaceae of non-Enterobacteriaceae based on the cycle threshold (Ct) values; by comparing qPCR and culture methods, only a < 1log difference between methods was obtained in 81.8% of these samples [26]. In seafood products and sediments, conventional PCR, real-time PCR, and culture methods were used to detect pathogenic *Vibrio* spp. (*V. parahaemolyticus*, *V. cholerae*, and *V. alginolyticus*) in 113 fish, 83 clams, 30 seawater samples, and 21 sediment samples. Of the 247 samples analyzed, 41.3% were positive for traditional microbiological method, while 51% were positive for the molecular methods, without prior isolation of pathogens [27].

However, by using multiplex qPCR assay for detection/quantification of more than one pathogen, the sensitivity of the technique may decrease compared to the traditional culture technique (or even compared with singleplex assay), probably due to the competitive nature of the process [8]. In our lab, we compared multiplex qPCR assay for quantification of *Escherichia coli, Staphylococcus aureus,* and *Salmonella* spp. with singleplex assays (by hydrolysis probes and by SYBR Green) in 28 naturally contaminated oyster samples containing pools of 40 oysters collected from natural estuarine environment (1120 in total). The multiplex assay presented lower sensitivity and higher specificity than both singleplex assays (data not published). This can be caused by the competition of the primers by the reagents available in the reaction mix or by the non-varying concentrations of the reaction components (which are used in the same way in the singleplex and multiplex reactions). In addition, the amplification of one target DNA present in the reaction can be overcome by more efficient amplification of other targets (including nonspecific products), thereby reducing the efficiency of the multiplex reaction and consequently decreasing its sensitivity [28]. The same methodology was applied in different food matrices (ground beef, milk, and oyster samples) artificially contaminated by *E coli, S. aureus*, and *Salmonella enteritidis*. Differences <1log in *E. coli* and *S. aureus* quantities were observed comparing multiplex qPCR and traditional culture method in milk and ground beef, with no statistic difference. However, in oyster samples, the multiplex qPCR demonstrated to be more sensitive than culture methods for *E. coli* quantification [8]. Thus, we can affirm that the food matrix can interfere in the sensitivity of the results due to the intrinsic nature of PCR inhibitors present in such food.

	Singleplex qPCR	Multiplex qPCR	Traditional culture
Advantages			
Shorter analysis time	++	+++	0
Specificity	+++	++	+
Sensitivity	+++	+	++
Reproducibility	+++	+++	++
Monitoring the results in real time	+++	+++	0
Simultaneous quantification of different pathogens	0	+++	0
Distinguishing of living cells from dead cells	0	0	+++
Detection of "viable but non-culturable" (VBNC) microorganisms	+++	++	0
Colony isolation for further genotyping/phenotyping analysis	0	0	+++
Potential of automation	+++	+++	0
Standardized method in worldwide	+	0	+++
"Gold standard" for regulatory agencies	0	0	+++
Fast screening of large number of samples	+++	++	0
Useful for microbiological quality control	+++	+++	+
Useful for the quantitative microbial risk assessment	+++	++	+
Disadvantages			
Cost of material, equipment, and infrastructure	---	---	---
Competitive amplification (decrease of the efficiency)	0	---	0
Interference of food sample	---	---	0
Labor-intensive analysis	---	---	---
Need for qualified personnel	---	---	---

**Based on Refs. [8, 12].*
(+) advantage score; (−) disadvantage score; (0) no score for such characteristic.

Table 1.
Advantage and disadvantage scores of real-time quantitative PCR (singleplex/multiplex qPCR) and traditional culture methods for microbiological analysis of food.*

To increase sensitivity, a pre-enrichment step may be applied prior to qPCR reaction. However, this stage favors microbial growth making it impossible to quantify the pathogens in the original sample; only their detection is possible [29]. Therefore, for simultaneous quantification of pathogens in food, multiplex qPCR can be a potential tool for rapid screening of large number of samples in food industries, leading to faster product release for sale [8].

The high cost of equipment investment and its maintenance can be an obstacle to qPCR implementation in routine food analysis laboratories. We must not forget the training of skilled labor. This is because, despite the potential of automation of the technique, the interpretation of the results must be done in a thorough way, so that the "noises" produced by the technique are not interpreted as real signals. However, what really limits the use of this technique in microbiological analysis of foods is the impossibility of distinguishing living cells from dead cells [30]. That is, this technique is able of amplifying any target DNA present in the sample, even being from nonviable cells, which can generate false-positive results by overestimating the number of pathogens present in the food. The **Table 1** summarizes some advantages and disadvantages of qPCR (singleplex and multiplex) and traditional culture methods for microbiological analysis of food.

3. Potential of qPCR for the monitoring microbiological quality of foods: the challenge of differentiating viable cells from nonviable cells

The changes in consumption, diversity, and food mobility, due to globalization, world population growth, and increasing purchasing power, have increased the need of analyzing food qualitatively and quantitatively, especially from the perspective of standardization, authentication, and certification. In this sense, real-time PCR is undergoing continuous improvement and becoming a method present in food analysis both to detect and quantify pathogens, allergens, and plant species or animals that are present in food, with high sensitivity and specificity. Many fluorescent probes are available, and nowadays, nanoparticles are opening up new diagnostic opportunities using this methodology due to it high sensitivity and providing results in a short time [31].

As already mentioned, the inability of qPCR to differentiate viable cells from nonviable (dead) cells is one of its main limitations in microbiological food analysis [30]. As DNA persists in samples even after the cell have lost its viability, the DNA-based detection methods cannot differentiate whether positive signals originate from living or dead bacterial targets. Thus, in order to detect only viable microorganisms in foods, DNA intercalating dyes, such as propidium monoazide (PMA) or ethidium monoazide (EMA), have been used in a step prior to PCR methods (**Table 2**). These agents selectively penetrate in damaged cell membranes and cross-link to DNA, thereby reducing the amplification capacity of the DNA template [32]. Both EMA and PMA are being used for detection of viable cells from different human pathogens, including those that assume the physiological status of "viable but non-culturable" (VBNC), such as *Campylobacter jejuni, Escherichia coli, Helicobacter pylori, Klebsiella pneumoniae, Listeria monocytogenes, Pseudomonas aeruginosa, Salmonella typhimurium*, *Shigella dysenteriae*, and *Vibrio cholerae*, which may be viable, but cannot grow outside their natural habitat [33].

PMA has been reported to be more effective than EMA in eliminating qPCR signals from dead cells [32]. Studies comparing EMA and PMA have shown that EMA can also penetrate in living cells of some bacterial species, such as *Anoxybacillus flavithermus* [34], *Staphylococcus aureus, Listeria monocytogenes, Micrococcus luteus, Mycobacterium avium, Streptococcus sobrinus*, and *Escherichia coli* O157: H7 [32],

Food matrix	Microorganisms	Cell viability dye-PCR method	References
Meat			
Chicken breasts and legs	*Campylobacter jejuni*	EMA-qPCR	[37]
Chicken rinses and egg broth	*Salmonella* spp.	EMA-qPCR	[38]
Poultry	*Campylobacter jejuni*; *Campylobacter coli*	EMA/PMA-qPCR	[39]
Chicken carcasses	*Campylobacter* spp.	PMA-qPCR	[40]
Ground beef	*E. coli* O157:H7	EMA-qPCR	[41]
		PMA-qPCR	[42]
	Salmonella spp.	PMA-qPCR	[43]
Broiler carcass rinses	*Campylobacter jejuni; Campylobacter coli*	PMA-qPCR	[44]
Meat products	*Staphylococcus aureus*	PMA-qPCR	[45]
Meat exudates	*Listeria monocytogenes*	PMA-qPCR	[46]
Frozen and chilled broiler carcasses	*Campylobacter* spp.	PMA-qPCR	[47]
Ground beef meatballs	*E. coli* O157:H7*	PMA-qPCR	[48]
Dairy products			
Gouda cheese	*Listeria monocytogenes*	EMA-qPCR	[49]
Infant formula	*Cronobacter sakazakii*	EMA-qPCR	[50]
Pasteurized milk	Coliform bacteria; Enterobacteriaceae	EMA/PMA-qPCR	[51]
UHT milk	*Bacillus sporothermodurans*	PMA-semi-nested PCR	[52]
	Bacillus cereus group	PMA-qPCR	[53]
Milk powder	*Staphylococcus aureus*	PMA-qPCR	[45]
Ice cream	*Salmonella typhimurium*	PMA-qPCR	[54]
Milk and milk products	*Cronobacter sakazakii; Bacillus cereus*; *Salmonella* spp.	PMA-multiplex qPCR	[55]
Milk	*E. coli* O157: H7; *Salmonella* spp.	PMA-multiplex qPCR	[56]
Probiotic yogurt	*Bifidobacterium*	EMA-qPCR	[57]
	Lactobacillus paracasei	PMA-qPCR	[58]
Seafood			
Fish fillets	16S rDNA	EMA-qPCR	[59, 60]
		PMA-qPCR	[61]
Raw seafood (oyster, scallop, shrimp, and crab)	*Vibrio parahaemolyticus*	PMA-qPCR	[62]
Raw shrimp	*Vibrio parahaemolyticus; Listeria monocytogenes*	PMA-multiplex qPCR	[63]
Shrimp, pomfret fish, and scallop	*Vibrio parahaemolyticus**	PMA-qPCR	[64]
Smoked salmon juice	*Listeria monocytogenes*	PMA-qPCR	[46]

Food matrix	Microorganisms	Cell viability dye-PCR method	References
Water and vegetables			
Water	*Campylobacter jejuni; Campylobacter coli*	EMA-qPCR	[65]
Lettuce	*Salmonella typhimurium*	PMA-qPCR	[66]
Lettuce and soya sprouts	*E. coli* O157:H7	PMA-qPCR	[67]
Fresh spinach	*Salmonella* spp.	PMA-qPCR	[43]

**Bacterial culture in physiological status of "viable but nonculturable" (VBNC).*

Table 2.
Summary of the studies using PMA or EMA prior to PCR methods for microbiological analysis applied in different food matrices.

causing loss of genomic DNA during extraction [35] and reducing the efficiency of PCR. However, PMA has been shown to be highly selective in penetrating only bacterial cells with compromised membrane integrity, but not in cells with intact cell membranes. After the DNA intercalation of nonviable cells, the azide group, present in the dye molecule, forms a covalent grid and when exposed to halogen light makes the DNA insoluble, which results in its loss during the extraction process of the genomic DNA. Thus, exposing a bacterial population composed of living and dead cells to PMA treatment results in the selective removal of DNA from dead cells [32]. Nevertheless, the dose of PMA must be carefully adjusted because this reagent becomes increasingly toxic to cells at higher concentrations. It is important to note that the cost of method may become prohibitive in the case of increasing concentration of PMA for its use in different food matrix, or its use in large scale [36].

4. Conclusion

The qPCR came with the intention of reducing the time of analysis and laborious work of the microbiological culture method. The analysis of a food sample performed by qPCR allows the monitoring of amplification while it runs; therefore, it does not need to perform any postreaction processing, such as the electrophoresis gel, allowing results available in around 2 h. Nevertheless, the difficulty of distinguishing living cells from dead cells is the great obstacle when using this methodology as routine food analysis laboratories. In this way, the pretreatment of food samples using PMA (or EMA) aims at eliminating false-positive results, as it only allows the quantification of viable cells. Thus, the PMA/EMA-qPCR promises to be a valuable tool in food safety management and microbiological quality control, especially as a method for quantitative microbial risk assessment. It is critical, therefore, that assays are comparatively evaluated in different food matrices for the detection and quantification of different pathogens and their reproducibility must be validated with intralaboratory experiments to ensure their effectiveness in the intended testing situation prior to implementation.

Acknowledgements

The authors thank Universidade Estadual de Santa Cruz for the financial support. This study was financed in part by the Coordenação de Aperfeiçoamento de Pessoal de Nível Superior, Brasil (CAPES), Finance Code 001, for the scholarship granted to Amanda Teixeira Sampaio Lopes.

Conflict of interest

The authors declare no conflict of interest.

Author details

Amanda Teixeira Sampaio Lopes[1] and Bianca Mendes Maciel[1,2]*

1 Graduation Program in Animal Science, Santa Cruz State University, Ilhéus, BA, Brazil

2 Department of Biological Sciences, Santa Cruz State University, Ilhéus, BA, Brazil

*Address all correspondence to: bmmaciel@uesc.br

References

[1] Kramer A, Twigg BA, editors. Fundamentals of Quality Control for the Food Industry. 2nd ed. Westport, Connectcut: AVI Publishing Company; 1970. 190 p

[2] Peri C. The universe of food quality. Food Quality and Preference. 2006;**17**:3-8. DOI: 10.1016/j.foodqual.2005.03.002

[3] Talamini E, Pedrozo EA, Silva AL. Gestão da cadeia de suprimentos e a segurança do alimento: Uma pesquisa exploratória na cadeia exportadora de carne suína. Gestão & Produção. 2005;**12**:107-120. DOI: 10.1590/S0104-530X2005000100010

[4] Figueiredo VF, Neto PLOC. Implantação do HACCP na indústria de alimentos. Gestão & Produção. 2001;**8**:100-111. DOI: 10.1590/S0104-530X2001000100008

[5] Barendz AW. Food safety and total quality management. Food Control. 1998;**9**:163-170. DOI: 10.1016/S0956-7135(97)00074-1

[6] WHO. WHO estimates of the global burden of foodborne diseases: Foodborne disease burden epidemiology reference group (2007-2015). In WHO Library Cataloguingin- Publication Data [Internet]. 2016. Available from: http://apps.who.int/iris/bitstream/10665/199350/1/9789241565165 eng.pdf?ua=1 [Accessed: 10 January 2019]

[7] Hoorfar J. Rapid detection, characterization and enumeration of foodborne pathogens. Acta Pathologica, Microbiologica et Immunologica Sacandinavica. 2011;**19**:1-24. DOI: 10.1111/j.1600-0463.2011.02767.x

[8] Lopes ATS, Albuquerque GR, Maciel BM. Multiplex real-time polymerase chain reaction for simultaneous quantification of *Salmonella* spp., *Escherichia coli*, and *Staphylococcus aureus* in different food matrices: Advantages and disadvantages. BioMed Research International. 2018;**2018**:1-12. DOI: 10.1155/2018/6104015

[9] Santana AS, Franco BDG. Microbial quantitative risk assessment of foods: Concepts, systematics and applications. Brazilian Journal of Food Technology. 2009;**12**:266-276. DOI: 10.4260/BJFT2009800900021

[10] Stephen A, Bustin SA, Benes V, Garson JA, Hellemans J, Huggett J, et al. The MIQE guidelines: Minimum information for publication of quantitative real-time PCR experiments. Clinical Chemistry. 2009;**55**:611-622. DOI: DOI 10.1373/clinchem.2008.112797

[11] Mandal PK, Biswas AK, Choi K, Pal UK. Methods for rapid detection of foodborne pathogens: An overview. American Journal of Food Technology. 2011;**6**:87-102. DOI: 10.3923/ajft.2011.87.102

[12] Jasson V, Jacxsens L, Luning P, Rajkovic A, Uyttendale M. Alternative microbial methods: An overview and selection criteria. Food Microbiology. 2010;**27**:710-730. DOI: 10.1016/j.fm.2010.04.008

[13] Tang Y, Procop GW, Persing DH. Molecular diagnostic of infectious diseases. Clinical Chemistry. 1997;**43**:2021-2038. PMID: 9365385

[14] Abubakar I, Irvinr L, Aldus CF, Wyatt GM, Fordham R, Schelenz S, et al. A systematic review of the clinical, public health and cost-effectiveness of rapid diagnostic tests for the detection and identification of bacterial intestinal pathogens in faeces and food. Health Technology Assessment. 2007;**11**:1-230. DOI: 10.3310/hta11360

[15] Wain J, Hosoglu S. The laboratory diagnosis of enteric fever. The Journal

of Infection in Developing Countries. 2008;**2**:421-425. DOI: 10.3855/jidc.155

[16] Kurkela S, Brown DWG. Molecular diagnostic techniques. Medicine. 2009;**37**:535-540. DOI: 10.1016/j.mpmed.2009.07.012

[17] Mackay IM. Real-time PCR in the microbiology laboratory. Clinical Microbiology and Infection. 2004;**10**:190-212. DOI: 10.1111/j.1198-743X.2004.00722.x

[18] Malorny B, Löfström C, Wagner M, Krämer N, Hoofar J. Enumeration of *Salmonella* bacteria in food and feed samples by real-time PCR for quantitative microbial risk assessment. Applied and Environmental Microbiology. 2008;**74**:1299-1304. DOI: 10.1128/AEM.02489-07

[19] Valasek MA, Repa JJ. The power of real-time PCR. Advances in Physiology Education. 2005;**29**:151-159. DOI: 10.1152/advan.00019.2005

[20] Zipper H, Brunner H, Bernhangen J, Vitzthum F. Investigations on DNA intercalation and surface binding by SYBR Green I, its structure determination and methodological implications. Nucleic Acids Research. 2004;**32**:e103. DOI: 10.1093/nar/gnh101

[21] Förster T. Zwischenmolekulare energiewanderung und fluoreszenz. Ann. Phys. 1948;**437**:55-75. DOI: 10.1002/andp.19484370105

[22] Chou KF, Dennis A. Förster resonance energy transfer between quantum dot donors and quantum dot acceptors. Sensors (Basel). 2015;**15**:13288-13325. DOI: 10.3390/s150613288

[23] Klein D. Quantification using real-time PCR technology: Applications and limitations. Molecular Medicine. 2002;**8**:257-260. DOI: 10.1016/S1471-4914(02)02355-9

[24] Lungu B, Waltman WD, Berghaus RD, Hofacre CL. Comparison of a real-time PCR method with a culture method for the detection of *Salmonella enterica* serotype enteritidis in naturally contaminated environmental samples from integrated poultry houses. Journal of Food Protection. 2012;**75**:743-747. DOI: 10.4315/0362-028X.JFP-11-297

[25] Kim DH, Chon JW, Kim H, Kim HS, Choi D, Kim YJ, et al. Comparison of culture, conventional and real-time PCR methods for *Listeria monocytogenes* in foods. Korean Journal for Food Science of Animal Resources. 2014;**34**:665-673. DOI: 10.5851/kosfa.2014.34.5.665

[26] Takahashi H, Saito R, Miya S, Tanaka Y, Miyamura N, Kuda T, et al. Development of quantitative real-time PCR for detection and enumeration of Enterobacteriaceae. International Journal of Food Microbiology. 2017;**246**:92-97. DOI: 10.1016/j.ijfoodmicro.2016.12.015

[27] Gdoura M, Sellami H, Nasfi H, Trabelsi R, Mansour S, Attia T, et al. Molecular detection of the three major pathogenic *Vibrio* species from seafood products and sediments in Tunisia using real-time PCR. Journal of Food Protection. 2016;**79**:2086-2094. DOI: 10.4315/0362-028X.JFP-16-205

[28] Elnifro EM, Ashshi AM, Cooper RJ, Klapper PE. Multiplex PCR: Optimization and application in diagnostic virology. Clinical Microbiology Reviews. 2000;**13**:559-570. DOI: 10.1128/CMR.13.4.559

[29] Maciel BM, Dias JCT, Romano CC, Sriranganathan N, Brendel M, Rezende RP. Detection of *Salmonella* enteritidis in asymptomatic carrier animals: Comparison of quantitative real-time PCR and bacteriological culture methods. Genetics and Molecular Research. 2011;**10**:2578-2588. DOI: 10.4238/2011.October.24.1

[30] Wang S, Levin RE. Discrimination of viable *Vibrio vulnificus* cells from dead cells in real-time PCR. Journal of Microbiological Methods. 2006;**64**:1-8. DOI: 10.1016/j.mimet.2005.04.023

[31] Salihah NT, Hossain MM, Lubis H, Ahmed MU. Trends and advances in food analysis by real-time polymerase chain reaction. Journal of Food Science and Technology. 2016;**53**:2196-2209. DOI: 10.1007/s13197-016-2205-0

[32] Nocker A, Cheung CY, Camper AK. Comparison of propidium monoazide with ethidium monoazide for differentiation of live vs. dead bacteria by selective removal of DNA from dead cells. Journal of Microbiological Methods. 2006;**67**:310-320. DOI: 10.1016/j.mimet.2006.04.015

[33] Zeng D, Chen Z, Jiang Y, Xue F, Li B. Advances and challenges in viability detection of foodborne pathogens. Frontiers in Microbiology. 2016;**7**: 1829-1833. DOI: 10.3389/fmicb.2016.01833

[34] Rueckert A, Ronimus RS, Morgan HW. Rapid differentiation and enumeration of the total, viable vegetative cell and spore content of thermophilic bacilli in milk powders with reference to *Anoxybacillus flavithermus*. Journal of Applied Microbiology. 2005;**99**:1246-1255. DOI: 10.1111/j.1365-2672.2005.02728.x

[35] Nocker A, Camper AK. Selective removal of DNA from dead cells of mixed bacterial communities by use of ethidium monoazide. Applied and Environmental Microbiology. 2006;**72**:1997-2004. DOI: 10.1128/AEM.72.3.1997-2004.2006

[36] Taylor MJ, Bentham RH, Ross K. Limitations of using propidium monoazide with qPCR to discriminate between live and dead *Legionella* in biofilm samples. Microbiology Insights. 2014;**7**:15-24. DOI: 10.4137/MBI.S17723

[37] Rudi K, Moen B, Drømtorp SM, Holck AL. Use of monoazide and PCR in combination for quantification of viable and dead cells in complex samples. Applied and Environmental Microbiology. 2005;**71**:1018-1024. DOI: 10.1128/AEM.71.2.1018-1024.2005

[38] Wang L, Mustapha A. EMA-real-time PCR as a reliable method for detection of viable *Salmonella* in chicken and eggs. Journal of Food Science. 2010;**75**:134-139. DOI: 10.1111/j.1750-3841.2010.01525.x

[39] Seinige D, Krischek C, Klein G, Kehrenberg C. Comparative analysis and limitations of ethidium monoazide and propidium monoazide treatments for the differentiation of viable and nonviable *Campylobacter* cells. Applied and Environmental Microbiology. 2014;**80**:2186-2192. DOI: 10.1128/AEM.03962-13

[40] Josefsen MH, Löfström C, Hansen TB, Christensen LS, Olsen JE, Hoorfar J. Rapid quantification of viable *Campylobacter* bacteria on chicken carcasses, using real-time PCR and propidium monoazide treatment, as a tool for quantitative risk assessment. Applied and Environmental Microbiology. 2010;**76**:5097-5104. DOI: 10.1128/AEM.00411-10

[41] Wang L, Li Y, Mustapha A. Detection of viable *Escherichia coli* O157:H7 by ethidium monoazide real-time PCR. Journal of Applied Microbiology. 2009;**107**:1719-1728. DOI: 10.1111/j.1365-2672.2009.04358.x

[42] Liu Y, Mustapha A. Detection of viable *Escherichia coli* O157:H7 in ground beef by propidium monoazide real-time PCR. International Journal of Food Microbiology. 2014;**170**:48-54. DOI: 10.1016/j.ijfoodmicro.2013.10.026

[43] Li B, Chen JQ. Development of a sensitive and specific qPCR assay in conjunction with propidium

monoazide for enhanced detection of live *Salmonella* spp. in food. BioMed Center Microbiology. 2013;**13**:273. DOI: 10.1186/1471-2180-13-273

[44] Duarte A, Botteldoorn N, Coucke W, Denayer S, Dierick K, Uyttendaele M. Effect of exposure to stress conditions on propidium monoazide (PMA)-qPCR based *Campylobacter* enumeration in broiler carcass rinses. Food Microbiology. 2015;**48**:182-190. DOI: 10.1016/j.fm.2014.12.011

[45] Zhang Z, Liu W, Xu H, Aguilar ZP, Shah NP, Wei H. Propidium monoazide combined with real-time PCR for selective detection of viable *Staphylococcus aureus* in milk powder and meat products. Journal of Dairy Science. 2015;**98**:1625-1633. DOI: 10.3168/jds.2014-8938

[46] Overney A, Jacques-André-Coquin J, Ng P, Carpentier B, Guillier L, Firmesse O. Impact of environmental factors on the culturability and viability of *Listeria monocytogenes* under conditions encountered in food processing plants. International Journal of Food Microbiology. 2017;**244**:74-81. DOI: 10.1016/j.ijfoodmicro.2016.12.012

[47] Castro AGSA, Dorneles EMS, Santos ELS, Alves TM, Silva GR, Figueiredo TC, et al. Viability of *Campylobacter* spp. in frozen and chilled broiler carcasses according to real-time PCR with propidium monoazide pre treatment. Poultry Science. 2018;**97**:1706-1711. DOI: 10.3382/ps/pey020

[48] Zhong J, Zhao X. Detection of viable but non-culturable *Escherichia coli* O157:H7 by PCR in combination with propidium monoazide. 3 Biotech. 2018;**8**:28. DOI: 10.1007/s13205-017-1052-7

[49] Rudi K, Naterstad K, Drømtorp SM, Holo H. Detection of viable and dead *Listeria monocytogenes* on gouda-like cheeses by real-time PCR. Letters in Applied Microbiology. 2005;**40**:301-306. DOI: 10.1111/j.1472-765X.2005.01672.x

[50] Minami J, Soejima T, Yaeshima T, Iwatsuki K. Direct real-time PCR with ethidium monoazide: A method for the rapid detection of viable *Cronobacter sakazakii* in powdered infant formula. Journal of Food Protection. 2012;**75**:1572-1579. DOI: 10.4315/0362-028X

[51] Soejima T, Minami J, Yaeshima T, Iwatsuki K. An advanced PCR method for the specific detection of viable total coliform bacteria in pasteurized milk. Applied Microbiology and Biotechnology. 2012;**95**:485-497. DOI: 10.1007/s00253-012-4086-0

[52] Cattani F, Ferreira CA, Oliveira SD. The detection of viable vegetative cells of *Bacillus sporothermodurans* using propidium monoazide with semi-nested PCR. Food Microbiology. 2013;**34**:196-201. DOI: 10.1016/j.fm.2012.12.007

[53] Cattani F, Barth VC Jr, Nasário JSR, Ferreira CAS, Oliveira SD. Detection and quantification of viable *Bacillus cereus* group species in milk by propidium monoazide quantitative real-time PCR. Journal of Dairy Science. 2016;**99**:2617-2624. DOI: 10.3168/jds.2015-10019

[54] Wang Y, Yang M, Liu S, Chen W, Suo B. Detection of viable *Salmonella* in ice cream by TaqMan real-time polymerase chain reaction assay combining propidium monoazide. Journal of Food and Drug Analysis. 2015;**23**:480-485. DOI: 10.1016/j.jfda.2015.03.002

[55] Yu S, Yan L, Wu X, Li F, Wang D, Xu H. Multiplex PCR coupled with propidium monoazide for the detection of viable *Cronobacter sakazakii*, *Bacillus cereus*, and *Salmonella* spp. in milk and milk products. Journal of Dairy Science. 2017;**100**:7874-7882. DOI: 10.3168/jds.2017-13110

[56] Zhou B, Liang T, Zhan Z, Liu R, Li F, Xu H. Rapid and simultaneous quantification of viable *Escherichia coli* O157:H7 and *Salmonella* spp. in milk through multiplex real-time PCR. Journal of Dairy Science. 2017;**100**:8804-8813. DOI: 10.3168/jds.2017-13362

[57] Meng XC, Pang R, Wang C, Wang LQ. Rapid and direct quantitative detection of viable bifidobacteria in probiotic yogurt by combination of ethidium monoazide and real-time PCR using a molecular beacon approach. The Journal of Dairy Research. 2010;**77**:498-504. DOI: 10.1017/S0022029910000658

[58] Scariot MC, Venturelli GL, Prudêncio ES, Arisi ACM. Quantification of *Lactobacillus paracasei* viable cells in probiotic yogurt by propidium monoazide combined with quantitative PCR. International Journal of Food Microbiology. 2018;**264**:1-7. DOI: 10.1016/j.ijfoodmicro.2017

[59] Lee JL, Levin RE. Use of ethidium bromide monoazide for quantification of viable and dead mixed bacterial flora from fish fillets by polymerase chain reaction. Journal of Microbiological Methods. 2006;**67**:456-462. DOI: 10.1016/j.mimet.2006.04.019

[60] Lee JL, Levin RE. Quantification of total viable bacteria on fish fillets by using ethidium bromide monoazide real-time polymerase chain reaction. International Journal of Food Microbiology. 2007;**118**:312-317. DOI: 10.1016/j.ijfoodmicro.2007.07.048

[61] Lee JL, Levin RE. A comparative study of the ability of EMA and PMA to distinguish viable from heat killed mixed bacterial flora from fish fillets. Journal of Microbiological Methods. 2009;**76**:93-96. DOI: 10.1016/j.mimet.2008.08.008

[62] Zhu RG, Li TP, Jia YF, Song LF. Quantitative study of viable *Vibrio parahaemolyticus* cells in raw seafood using propidium monoazide in combination with quantitative PCR. Journal of Microbiological Methods. 2012;**90**:262-266. DOI: 10.1016/j.mimet.2012.05.019

[63] Zhang Z, Liu H, Lou Y, Xiao L, Liao C, Malakar PK, et al. Quantifying viable *Vibrio parahaemolyticus* and *Listeria monocytogenes* simultaneously in raw shrimp. Applied Microbiology and Biotechnology. 2015;**99**:6451-6462. DOI: 10.1007/s00253-015-6715-x

[64] Yufei L, Qingping Z, Juan W, Shuwen L. Enumeration of *Vibrio parahaemolyticus* in VBNC state by PMA-combined real-time quantitative PCR coupled with confirmation of respiratory activity. Food Control. 2018;**91**:85-91. DOI: 10.1016/j.foodcont.2018.03.037

[65] Seinige D, von Köckritz-Blickwede M, Krischek C, Klein G, Kehrenberg C. Influencing factors and applicability of the viability EMA-qPCR for a detection and quantification of *Campylobacter cells* from water samples. PLoS One. 2014;**20**(9):1-17. DOI: 10.1371/journal.pone.0113812

[66] Liang N, Dong J, Luo L, Li Y. Detection of viable *Salmonella* in lettuce by propidium monoazide real-time PCR. Journal of Food Science. 2011;**76**:234-237. DOI: 10.1111/j.1750-3841.2011.02123.x

[67] Elizaquível P, Sánchez G, Aznar R. Application of propidium monoazide quantitative PCR for selective detection of live *Escherichia coli* O157:H7 in vegetables after inactivation by essential oils. International Journal of Food Microbiology. 2012;**159**:115-121. DOI: 10.1016/j.ijfoodmicro.2012.08.006